SELECTED METHODS IN CELLULAR IMMUNOLOGY

SELECTED METHODS
IN CELLULAR IMMUNOLOGY

Edited by

Barbara B. Mishell and Stanley M. Shiigi

University of California, Berkeley

Editorial Consultants

Claudia Henry and Robert I. Mishell

University of California, Berkeley

W. H. FREEMAN AND COMPANY
San Francisco

Sponsoring Editor: Arthur C. Bartlett
Project Editor: Nancy Flight
Manuscript Editor: Ruth C. Veres
Designer: Marie Carluccio
Production Coordinator: Linda Jupiter
Illustration Coordinator: Cheryl Nufer
Cover Designer: Marjorie Spiegelman
Artists: Evan Gillespie and Judith Tulenko Morley
Compositor: Bi-Comp, Inc.
Printer and Binder: The Maple-Vail Book Manufacturing Group

NOTE: In the United Kingdom, Denmark, and France, a special license is required if it is judged by the instructor that the experiments present a risk of discomfort to the animals or interfere with their ordinary state of well-being.

Cover illustration based on photograph by Gregory L. Finch, Laboratory for Energy-Related Health Research, University of California, Davis.

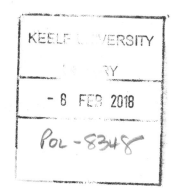

Library of Congress Cataloging in Publication Data

Main entry under title:

Selected methods in cellular immunology.

    Includes bibliographies and index.
    1. Cellular immunity—Technique. 2. Cell separation. I. Mishell, Barbara B., 1936–
II. Shiigi, Stanley M., 1944–   [DNLM: 1. Immunity, Cellular. QW568 S464]
QR185.5.S44   574.2'9   79-19990
ISBN 0-7167-1106-0

Printed in the United States of America

2 3 4 5 6 7 8 9

To our children,
Jacob Mishell,
David Shiigi,
and
Cassis Henry

Contents

2   Generation of Humoral Responses

3   Hemolytic Plaque Assays

IV

ADDITIONAL METHODS   305

APPENDIXES   441

A Preparation and Testing of Reagents

B Washing and Sterilization of Laboratory Glassware

C Sterilization of Liquid Reagents

Preface

This book originated as a manual for teaching students and research personnel in our laboratory and for use in a graduate course in cellular immunology offered by our department. Because a number of individuals outside our department found the manual useful both in their research programs and in laboratory courses, we decided to prepare a manuscript for publication. In doing so, we reorganized the original manual and, to broaden its scope, added many contributions from investigators at other institutions. The text now contains most of the principal methods used by cellular immunologists working with murine cells. In addition to its usefulness to cellular immunologists, we anticipate that this book will be helpful to other biologists who wish to apply cellular immunological methods to their work.

The aim of this book is to help the reader use these methods successfully. Towards this end, we have emphasized the details of procedures and minimized general theoretical discussion. Because seemingly trivial differences in technique often have profound effects on experimental results, we have tried to impart to the written descriptions the degree and kind of detail that is ordinarily communicated only by personal instruction at the laboratory bench. We hope that the methods as described will sufficiently convey the technical experiences of the authors to enable beginning graduate students and research personnel to perform the procedures with ease and reliability.

As an aid to the readers, we frequently list suppliers of reagents or equipment found to be satisfactory. In many instances, similar products are available through alternative sources. Since comparative evaluations have been done for only a few products, we do not wish to imply through omission that other products are any less reliable than those cited.

We have tried to alert our readers to many potential hazards that might not be self-evident. Obviously, a reagent now considered safe may in the future be found to have hazardous properties. We therefore recommend that reasonable precautions be taken, especially with organic chemical reagents and biological materials.

Because we have modified or reorganized many of the contributions of others to fit the general format of the book, we bear responsibility for any inaccuracies that may have been introduced inadvertently. While we sincerely hope that all errors or ambiguities have been eliminated from the published text, we request readers to notify us should any be found so that corrections can be made in later printings or editions.

July 1979   *Barbara B. Mishell*
                                                             Stanley M. Shiigi

Acknowledgments

We deeply appreciate the work done by the many individuals who have contributed to this book. They have participated in many ways: writing detailed descriptions of methods, reading portions of the manuscript, testing the effectiveness of written procedures at the bench, checking references and supply sources, and proofreading. The collaborative effort was such that recognition of specific contributions to some sections of this book is difficult.

The knowledge and experience of Claudia Henry and Robert Mishell are reflected throughout the book. In addition to contributing a large number of procedures, each has critically reviewed the manuscript at every stage of its development. We are grateful both for the time they spent on this endeavor and for the quality of their contributions. Anne Good wrote descriptions of many of the immunochemical procedures and reviewed much of the manuscript and galley proofs. Her extensive experience in developing and directing the graduate laboratory courses offered by our department proved invaluable, and we are grateful for her efforts.

Many other members of our department made important contributions and provided an incalculable amount of help in reviewing and preparing the final text. We deeply appreciate their efforts. Leon Wofsy enabled us to include several procedures developed by him and his associates. John North made significant contributions to several sections of the book, and Linda Bradley, Kenneth Grabstein, and Elizabeth Mather each assumed responsibility for entire chapters. Eva Chan, Yu-hua Una Chen, John Kimura, Elaine Kwan, Kathleen Miller, Yvonne McHugh, Maxwell Slomich, and Mary Rodrick contributed to the written descriptions. Kathryn Crossland, Michael Gold, Geri Hecker, George Lamson, Alexander Lucas, Ellen Wallace, and Mayumi Yagi helped with the galley proofs.

A number of the procedures included in this book were contributed by investigators at other institutions. We are especially pleased that John Marbrook participated in this project, contributing two methods developed by him, the diffusion culture system and the acrylamide raft technique, as well as other methods. We are indebted to several contributors who provided detailed descriptions of techniques that have only recently been introduced to cellular immunological research and that seem destined to have wide application in the near future. Vernon Oi and Leonard Herzenberg described methods for the production of antibody-secreting hybridomas. Theta Tsu and Leonore Herzenberg contributed a description of solid-phase radioimmunoassays and Patricia Jones provided a description of one- and two-dimensional gel electrophoretic methods for the analysis of cell membrane components.

We also thank Luciano Adorini, Jessica Clarke, Geraldine Dettman, Erich Eipert, Ruth Gallily, Roberta Kamin, Dale Kipp, Kwok-Choy Lee, George Lewis, Alexander Miller, David Parks, Donald Raidt, Susan Swain, Harley Tse, Douglas Vann, James Watson, and Stanley Wilbur, who provided us with carefully prepared, detailed descriptions of methods they have used and, in some cases, developed. We are grateful to Jirayr Roubinian for the descriptions of surgical procedures he has employed in conducting immunological studies with mice. We also wish to express our appreciation to Dankward Kodlin and Carla Wofsy for their constructive comments on the chapter on dilution analysis, to Robert Stout for reviewing the original draft of this book and offering useful suggestions and criticism, and to Richard Dutton, James Goding, and Nathan Sharon for critically reviewing portions of the final draft of the manuscript.

Several other individuals deserve acknowledgment for their efforts on behalf of this project. Much of the success we have had in using the methods we have described has depended on the quality of the mice from which the cells were obtained. We appreciate very much the excellent management of our mouse colony by Zollie A. Griffin. We also want to thank Barbara White, who typed the manuscript, portions of it many times, with cheer and good humor; Sandra Pruitt, who helped locate sources of reagents and equipment; and Boyd Sleeth, who read portions of the manuscript for consistency. We are especially indebted to James

Lecce, who reviewed the final manuscript and helped us to clarify ambiguous portions. We have relied on both the laboratory and the artistic skills of June Shiigi. In addition to contributing methodological material, she helped us with the accuracy and clarity of many portions of the book, prepared some of the art work for the manuscript, spent long hours putting the manuscript in final form, and proofread the book at every stage of production.

Finally, we wish to thank Ruth C. Veres for her excellent professional editorial assistance with the manuscript, and the staff at W. H. Freeman and Company, especially Nancy Flight, who shepherded the book through editing and production, and Arthur C. Bartlett, who helped to guide the project from its inception.

Contributors

Luciano Adorini
    Department of Microbiology
    University of California
    Los Angeles, California 90024

Linda M. Bradley
    Department of Microbiology and
      Immunology
    University of California
    Berkeley, California 94720

Eva Lee Chan
    Department of Microbiology and
      Immunology
    University of California
    Berkeley, California 94720

Yu-hua Una Chen
    Department of Microbiology and
      Immunology
    University of California
    Berkeley, California 94720

Jessica Clarke
    Department of Microbiology
    University of California
    Los Angeles, California 90024

Geraldine L. Dettman
    Department of Radiological
      Sciences
    College of Medicine
    University of California
    Irvine, California 92717

Erich F. Eipert
    National Marine Fishery Service
    2725 Montlake Boulevard, East
    Seattle, Washington 98112

Ruth Gallily
    Department of Immunology
    The Hebrew University
    Jerusalem, Israel

Anne H. Good
    Department of Microbiology and
        Immunology
    University of California
    Berkeley, California 94720

Kenneth Grabstein
    Department of Microbiology and
        Immunology
    University of California
    Berkeley, California 94720

Claudia Henry
    Department of Micobiology and
        Immunology
    University of California
    Berkeley, California 94720

Leonard A. Herzenberg
    Department of Genetics
    Stanford University
    Stanford, California 94305

Leonore A. Herzenberg
    Department of Genetics
    Stanford University
    Stanford, California 94305

Patricia P. Jones
    Department of Biological Sciences
    Stanford University
    Stanford, California 94305

Roberta Kamin
    Cancer Research Institute
    University of California
    San Francisco, California 94143

John Kimura
    Department of Microbiology and
        Immunology
    University of California
    Berkeley, California 94720

Dale Kipp
    Department of Microbiology
    University of California
    Los Angeles, California 90024

Dankward Kodlin
    Department of Biometry
    Medical Center
    Louisiana State University
    New Orleans, Louisiana 70113

Elaine Kwan
    Department of Microbiology and
        Immunology
    University of California
    Berkeley, California 94720

Kwok-Choy Lee
    Department of Immunology
    University of Alberta
    Edmonton, Alberta, Canada

George K. Lewis
    Department of Microbiology
    University of California
    San Francisco, California 94143

John Marbrook
    Department of Cell Biology
    University of Auckland
    Auckland, New Zealand

Elizabeth L. Mather
    Department of Microbiology and
        Immunology
    University of California
    Berkeley, California 94720

Yvonne E. McHugh
    Department of Microbiology and
        Immunology
    University of California
    Berkeley, California 94720

Alexander Miller
Department of Microbiology
University of California
Los Angeles, California 90024

Kathleen Miller
Division of Parasitology
National Institute for Medical
Research
The Ridgeway
Mill Hill, London, NW 7, IAA
England

Barbara B. Mishell
Department of Microbiology and
Immunology
University of California
Berkeley, California 94720

Robert I. Mishell
Department of Microbiology and
Immunology
University of California
Berkeley, California 94720

John North
Department of Pathology
University of Bristol Medical
School
Bristol, B58 ITD England

Vernon T. Oi
Department of Genetics
Stanford University
Stanford, California 94305

David Parks
Department of Genetics
Stanford University
Stanford, California 94305

Donald J. Raidt
Department of Pediatrics
School of Medicine
University of California, San Diego
La Jolla, California 92093

Mary L. Rodrick
Laboratory for Surgical Research
Peter Bent Brigham Hospital at the
Harvard Medical School
25 Shattuck Street
Boston, Massachusetts 02115

Jirayr Roubinian
Department of Medicine
University of California
San Francisco, California 94121

June M. Shiigi
Department of Microbiology and
Immunology
University of California
Berkeley, California 94720

Stanley M. Shiigi
Department of Microbiology and
Immunology
University of California
Berkeley, California 94720

Maxwell Slomich
Department of Microbiology and
Immunology
University of California
Berkeley, California 94720

Robert Stout
Rosenstiel Basic Medical Sciences
Research Center
Brandeis University
Waltham, Massachusetts 02154

Susan L. Swain
   Department of Biology
   University of California
   San Diego, California 92037

Harley Y. Tse
   Laboratory of Immunology
   National Institute of Allergy and
      Infectious Diseases
   National Institutes of Health
   Bethesda, Maryland 20014

Theta T. Tsu
   Department of Genetics
   Stanford University
   Stanford, California 94305

Douglas C. Vann
   Department of Genetics
   John A. Burns School of Medicine
   University of Hawaii at Manoa
   Honolulu, Hawaii 96822

James Watson
   Department of Medical
      Microbiology
   California College of Medicine
   University of California
   Irvine, California 92717

Stanley M. Wilbur
   Department of Microbiology and
      Immunology
   School of Medicine
   University of California
   Los Angeles, California 90024

Carla Wofsy
   Department of Mathematics and
      Statistics
   University of New Mexico
   Albuquerque, New Mexico 87131

Leon Wofsy
   Department of Microbiology and
      Immunology
   University of California
   Berkeley, California 94720

Abbreviations

Ab	antibody
Ag	antigen
AO	acridine orange
AO/EB	acridine orange-ethidium bromide
Ars	azophenyl arsonate or arsanilic acid
Ars-HB	azophenyl arsonate coupled to methyl-*p*-hydroxybenzimidate
Ars-HGG	human gamma globulin modified with azophenyl arsonate
Ars-KLH	keyhole limpet hemocyanin modified with azophenyl arsonate
Ars-MB	*Mycobacterium* modified with azophenyl arsonate
BBS	borate-buffered saline
BDB	bis-diazotized benzidine
BDF_1	C57BL/6 $\times$ DBA/2 hybrid mice
BGG	bovine gamma globulin
BSA	bovine serum albumin
BSS	balanced salt solution
BSS-FCS	balanced salt solution containing fetal calf serum

BUdR	5-bromo-2-deoxyuridine
°C	degree Celsius
CFA	complete Freund's adjuvant
Ci	curie
CM	carboxymethyl
CMC	cell-mediated cytotoxicity
Con A	concanavalin A
cpm	counts per minute
CR	complement receptor
DEAE	diethylaminoethyl
DMSO	dimethyl sulfoxide
DNP	dinitrophenyl
DNP-BGG	bovine gamma globulin modified with dinitrophenyl hapten
2-D PAGE	two-dimensional polyacrylamide gel electrophoresis
DTT	dithiothreitol
ϵ	extinction coefficient
E	erythrocytes
EA	erythrocytes coated with antibodies
EAC	erythrocytes coated with non-hemolytic IgM antibodies and reacted with mouse complement
EB	ethidium bromide
ECDI	1-ethyl-3-(3-dimethylaminopropyl)-carbodiimide hydrochloride
EDTA	ethylenediamine tetraacetic acid
FCS	fetal calf serum
FITC	fluorescein isothiocyanate
g	gram
g	acceleration of gravity
GAMB	goat anti–mouse brain
Glu	azophenyl glucoside
Glu-KLH	keyhole limpet hemocyanin modified with azophenyl glucoside
Glut	azobenzoyl glutamate
Glut-HB	azobenzoyl glutamate coupled to methyl-*p*-hydroxybenzimidate
Gly	azobenzoyl glycine
G-PBS	glucose-phosphate-buffered saline
GRBC	goat red blood cells
HAT	hypoxanthine-aminopterin-thymidine
HB	methyl-*p*-hydroxybenzimidate hydrochloride
HBSS	Hanks' balanced salt solution

HEPES	4-2(hydroxyethyl)-1-piperazineethanesulfonic acid
HGG	human gamma globulin
HPBS	high-phosphate-buffered saline
HPBS-FCS	high-phosphate-buffered saline solution containing fetal calf serum
HRBC	horse red blood cells
HT	hypoxanthine-thymidine
HuRBC	human red blood cells
Ia	I region associated (antigen)
IEF	isoelectric focusing
Ig	immunoglobulin
KLH	keyhole limpet hemocyanin
Lac	azophenyl lactoside
Lac-BGG	bovine gamma globulin modified with azophenyl lactoside
Lac-KLH	keyhole limpet hemocyanin modified with azophenyl lactoside
Lac-KLH-Ars	keyhole limpet hemocyanin modified with both azophenyl lactoside and azophenyl arsonate
LPS	lipopolysaccharide
M	molar (moles/liter)
mA	milliampere
mCi	millicurie
2-ME	2-mercaptoethanol
MEM	Eagle's minimum essential medium
mg	milligram
min	minute
ml	milliliter
MLR	mixed lymphocyte response
mmol	millimole
mol	mole
mOsm	milliOsmole
M_r	molecular weight
mS	milliSiemen
μCi	microcurie
μl	microliter
μm	micrometer
NCS	newborn calf serum
NEPHGE	nonequilibrium pH gradient electrophoresis
NIP	nitro-iodophenyl
nm	nanometer

NP40	Nonidet P40
NS-1	P3-NS 1-1 myeloma cell line
OD	optical density
PAGE	polyacrylamide gel electrophoresis
PBS	phosphate-buffered saline
PEG	polyethylene glycol
PFC	plaque-forming cells
PHA	phytohemagglutinin
PMSF	phenylmethyl sulfonyl fluoride
PNA	peanut agglutinin
POPOP	p-bis-[2-(5-phenyloxazolyl)] benzene
PPC	plaque-forming cells per culture
PPM	plaque-forming cells per million cells recovered
PPO	2,5-diphenyloxazole
PVP	polyvinylpyrrolidone
R	roentgen
RAMB	rabbit anti–mouse brain (serum)
RBC	red blood cells
RIA	radioimmunoassay or radioimmune assay
rpm	revolutions per minute
RPMI 1640	Roswell Park Memorial Institute medium number 1640
RPMI-FCS	RPMI 1640 containing fetal calf serum
RPMI-NCS	RPMI 1640 containing newborn calf serum
S	siemens
SaC	*Staphylococcus aureus* Cowans strain adsorbent
SAS	saturated ammonium sulfate
SBA	soybean agglutinin
SDS	sodium dodecyl sulfate
SRBC	sheep red blood cells
Sulf	azophenyl sulfonate
TCA	trichloroacetic acid
TEMED	N,N,N',N'-tetramethyl-1,2-diaminoethane
TNBS	2,4,6-trinitrobenzene sulfonic acid
TNP	trinitrophenyl
TNP-KLH	keyhole limpet hemocyanin modified with trinitrophenyl hapten
TNP-SRBC	sheep red blood cells modified with trinitrophenyl hapten
Tris	tris(hydroxymethyl)aminomethane
TRITC	tetramethylrhodamine isothiocyanate
UV	ultraviolet
V	volt

v/v   volume/volume; concentration of a solution based on:

$$\frac{\text{number of milliliters of solute}}{\text{100 milliliters of solution}} \times 100\%$$

w/v   weight/volume; concentration of a solution based on:

$$\frac{\text{number of grams of solute}}{\text{100 milliliters of solution}} \times 100\%$$

SELECTED METHODS IN CELLULAR IMMUNOLOGY

I

IN VITRO
IMMUNE RESPONSES

The principal methods for generating immune reactions *in vitro* with murine cells and for assaying immune responses at the cellular level are described in Part I. Included are methods for generating humoral and cell-mediated immunity utilizing both suspension and diffusion culture systems. Hemolytic plaque assays for detecting antibody-forming cells, chromium release assays for measuring cytotoxicity, and thymidine incorporation methods for assessing cell proliferation are also described. The methods originally developed in the 1960s have been modified frequently to facilitate the use of many different kinds of antigens, to permit the independent analysis of carrier-specific and hapten-specific immune reactions, and to permit the quantitative assessment of antigen-reactive precursor cells. The major modifications of these procedures that are generally used by cellular immunologists working with murine cells are included in this portion of the book.

In vitro methods have been widely employed by cellular immunologists investigating the roles of various cell subpopulations in the generation and regulation of specific immunity. These methods are valuable because they permit efficient multiple measurements, allow a uniform suspension of cells to be used for experimental and control observations, and enable the investigator to use an intrinsically simpler system for analysis than is true when intact animals are employed. *In vitro* methods have been particularly useful in studying macrophages and in investigating the occurrence and functions of cell-free mediators.

Data from *in vitro* studies should be interpreted with caution because the systems used inherently impose arbitrary constraints and because cultured cells are not subject to many of the mechanisms they would encounter under physiological conditions. Finally, immunologically reactive cells are very sensitive to substances in the culture environment; it is therefore important to avoid the inadvertent contamination of reagents with microorganisms or potentially toxic chemicals.

1

Preparation of
Mouse Cell Suspensions

The material for this chapter was provided by Barbara B. Mishell,
Stanley M. Shiigi, Claudia Henry, Eva Lee Chan, John North,
Ruth Gallily, Maxwell Slomich, Kathleen Miller, John Marbrook,
David Parks, and Anne H. Good.

1.1 INTRODUCTION

Murine cells for use *in vitro* can be obtained from several organ sites. In this chapter, techniques are described for obtaining cells from the spleen, lymph node, peritoneal cavity, thymus, and bone marrow of donor mice. Also described is the preparation of thioglycollate-activated peritoneal cells and cortisone-resistant thymocytes. Because of the nature of *in vitro* systems, it is especially important that care be taken to minimize trauma during the preparation of cell suspensions. While any technique that disrupts an organ will inevitably kill or damage some cells, the techniques described yield cell suspensions that contain a high percentage of viable cells.

Five methods commonly used to determine cell viability are described. Three of these methods are based on dye exclusion and can be evaluated with the light microscope. The dyes used are trypan blue, eosin Y, and nigrosin. Live cells exclude the dyes, whereas dead cells take up the dyes and appear blue, red, or brown-black, respectively. Fluorescein diacetate and acridine orange-ethidium bromide can be used to determine cell viability with the fluorescence microscope. Fluorescein diacetate is taken in by all cells but is only hydrolyzed inside live cells to reveal green fluorescence. Acridine orange is taken up by live cells, whereas ethidium bromide is taken up by dead cells; under ultraviolet (UV) light live cells appear green, while dead cells appear orange-red. Because cell viability is determined with hemacytometer counting chambers, a description of the use of the hemacytometer is included.

Although it is not generally necessary to remove either dead cells or red blood cells from a cell suspension prior to culture, removal of one or both may be desirable in certain situations. Several methods for removing these cells are described. The superiority of one method for all experimental purposes has not been established. However, none of the procedures outlined appear to have any deleterious effects on immunization *in vitro*, fluorescence staining, or the preparation of cells for electron microscopy.

Cell debris remaining after the lysis of lymphocytes or red blood cells can be removed by filtering the cell suspension through a glass wool column or by centrifuging the suspension through fetal calf serum. Both procedures are described below.

1.2 SPLEEN CELLS

MATERIALS AND REAGENTS

Balanced salt solution (BSS; Appendix A.3)
150-ml beaker containing 50–75 ml of 95% ethanol
Alcohol lamp containing 95% ethanol
Squeeze bottle containing 70% ethanol
Curved scissors (Codman, #54-1076)
Tapered mouse tooth forceps (Codman, #30-4150)
Flat forceps (Codman, #30-6585)
Plastic tissue culture dishes (Petri dishes), 60 × 15 mm; 1 for every 6 spleens (Falcon, #3002 or similar)
Centrifuge tubes, graduated 12 ml (Bellco Glass, #3041-00012) with stainless steel closures (Bellco Glass, #2005-00016)
Pasteur pipettes and rubber bulbs
Paper towels
Beaker or plastic bag large enough to hold the mice, containing 70% ethanol

PROCEDURE

1. Kill mice by cervical dislocation or CO_2 inhalation and place in the beaker or plastic bag containing 70% ethanol to wet them

completely. This reduces the possibility of hair and dander becoming airborne.

2. Place the mice on paper towels soaked with 70% ethanol. Arrange the mice so that left sides face up.

3. In each mouse, make a cut through the loose skin in the inguinal region, and, with fingers on either side of the cut, pull toward the head and tail of the mouse until the peritoneal wall is widely exposed. Flood the peritoneal wall with 70% ethanol to remove any loose hair.

4. Dip the scissors and mouse tooth forceps into the beaker of 95% ethanol and quickly pass them through the flame from the alcohol lamp (flame only long enough to ignite the alcohol on the instruments). When the flame on the instruments has gone out, lift the peritoneal wall over the spleen with the forceps and make a large U-shaped cut around the spleen. Fold back the peritoneum; lift the spleen with the forceps and separate it from the vessels and connecting tissue with the scissors. Place up to 6 spleens in a Petri dish containing 8–10 ml of BSS.

5. Gently tease the spleens with the forceps. Avoid breaking the spleens into small fragments since this makes the procedure more tedious.

6. Once the spleens have been teased, transfer the cell suspension from the dish to a graduated conical tube with a Pasteur pipette and allow the clumps of cells to settle for 5 or 6 minutes. Transfer the cell suspension to another tube and pellet the cells at $200 \times g$ for 10 minutes.

COMMENTS

1. For most experimental work, it is best to hold pelleted cells on ice; in some situations, however, it is preferable to avoid chilling the cells—for example, prior to T cell depletion.

2. The nucleated cell yield per normal spleen is 5×10^7 to 2×10^8, depending on the mouse strain; 0.1 ml of packed spleen cells contains approximately 2×10^8 nucleated cells.

3. As an alternative to flaming, the instruments can be stored in 70% ethanol and then placed in a loosely covered sterile Petri dish where the ethanol is allowed to evaporate prior to use.

4. Alternative methods of obtaining cell suspensions are used by other investigators: pressing spleens through a stainless steel grid, using a glass tissue homogenizer, or pressing spleen segments between the frosted ends of two microscope slides.

1.3 NORMAL PERITONEAL CELLS

MATERIALS AND REAGENTS

As described in Section 1.2 with the following additions:

Disposable syringes, 6 ml, one per mouse
Needles, 18 gauge
Plastic culture dishes, 100 × 15 mm (Lux Scientific, #5211)

PROCEDURE

1. Assemble syringes and needles. Fill syringes with 5 ml of BSS. (It is convenient to fill syringes from Petri dishes containing BSS.)
2. Kill mice by CO_2 inhalation or cervical dislocation and wet completely with 70% ethanol. Place mice, abdomens up, on paper towels soaked in 70% ethanol (or pin to a dissecting board). Make a transverse cut in the inguinal area and pull back skin to completely expose the peritoneal wall. Flood the peritoneal wall with 70% ethanol.
3. Lift the peritoneal wall with forceps and carefully inject about 4.5 ml of BSS into the peritoneal cavity. (Leave about 0.5 ml of BSS in the syringe to dislodge fat from the needle if necessary.) With the needle in place (tip up), massage the peritoneum and then carefully draw fluid back into the syringe. Approximately 4 ml of fluid can be recovered.
4. Pool cells, centrifuge (200 × g, 10 min), and wash once with BSS. Approximately $1–3 × 10^6$ peritoneal cells are obtained per mouse.

COMMENTS

1. Female mice, approximately 2 months of age, are the easiest to use. Male mice, especially older ones, have so much fat in the peritoneum that the needle gets clogged in the process of withdrawing the fluid.
2. Care must be taken to avoid puncturing the gut during the removal of cells, since this would contaminate the cell preparation.

1.4 THIOGLYCOLLATE-STIMULATED PERITONEAL CELLS

The method described (Gallily and Feldman 1967) is a modification of Bang's method (Gallily et al. 1964). Stimulation with thioglycollate increases the yield of peritoneal cells to $3–4.5 × 10^7$ cells per mouse.

MATERIALS AND REAGENTS

Preparation of Thioglycollate Medium (3%)

Thioglycollate medium, dehydrated (Difco Laboratories)
Autoclavable bottles 50–100 ml
Bunsen burner, tripod

Thioglycollate Stimulation

Aged thioglycollate medium (see below)
Syringes, 3–6 ml
Needles, 23 or 24 gauge

Harvesting of Peritoneal Cells

Phosphate-buffered saline (PBS; Appendix A.8) or Hanks' balanced
  salt solution (Hanks' BSS) containing penicillin (100 units/ml),
  streptomycin (50 μg/ml), and heparin (5 USP units/ml)
70% ethanol
Needles, 20 and 24 gauge
Glass syringes, 5 ml, Luer-lock
Centrifuge tubes
Scissors and forceps
Pasteur pipettes and rubber bulb

PROCEDURE

Preparation of Thioglycollate Medium (3%)

1. Suspend 30 g of dehydrated thioglycollate medium in 1000 ml of
   cold distilled water and heat to a boil to dissolve the medium
   completely (very important).
2. Aliquot medium into 50–100-ml bottles and autoclave (15 lb/in^2,
   121°C, for 15 min with slow exhaust).
3. After cooling, store the medium in a dark place at room temperature for at least a month. Two- to four-month-old thioglycollate is
   more effective in increasing the yield of peritoneal macrophages.

Thioglycollate Stimulation

1. For mice 2 months and older, inject 2–3 ml thioglycollate intraperitoneally. For mice younger than 2 months, inject 1–1.5 ml
   thioglycollate.

Harvesting of Peritoneal Cells

Four days after the thioglycollate stimulation, the peritoneal cells can
be harvested by one of the following methods:

1. Swab the abdomen of the mouse with 70% ethanol. Inject 5 ml of
   the PBS solution or Hanks' BSS into the peritoneal cavity, using

the 24-gauge needle. After gently massaging the abdominal area of the mouse, withdraw the fluid into a 5-ml glass syringe with 20–21-gauge needle. About 4–4.8 ml can be harvested per mouse. Centrifuge cells (200 × g, 10 min) and wash once or twice with Hanks' BSS. The mice can withstand at least three injection cycles. This is economical for some experimental purposes (e.g., collecting cells for the preparation of anti-macrophage sera). Rest mice 3 weeks after each peritoneal tap.

2. Kill mice by cervical dislocation and pin them to a dissecting board with the extremities fully extended. Wet abdomens with 70% ethanol. Inject 5 ml of PBS or Hanks' BSS intraperitoneally into each mouse and gently massage abdominal area. Make a small cut in the lower abdominal skin and lift skin with forceps. Push the tip of a Pasteur pipette into the peritoneal cavity and aspirate fluid into a centrifuge tube. Wash the cells as previously described.

REFERENCES

Gallily, R., and M. Feldman. 1967. The role of macrophages in the induction of antibody in x-irradiated animals. *Immunology* **12**:197.

Gallily, R., A. Warwick, and F. B. Bang. 1964. Effect of cortisone on genetic resistance to mouse hepatitis virus *in vivo* and *in vitro*. *Proc. Natl. Acad. Sci.* (USA) **51**:1158.

1.5 THYMOCYTES

MATERIALS AND REAGENTS

Mice, 3–6 weeks of age

Saline: 0.85% NaCl (w/v), or balanced salt solution (BSS; Appendix A.3)

Pelikan ink (Accurate Chemicals & Scientific, #C11/1431A)

Plastic tissue culture dishes, 60 × 15 mm (Falcon, #3002 or similar)

Tissue homogenizer (optional)

Forceps, scissors

Centrifuge tubes

PROCEDURE

1. Both lymph node and blood cells should be excluded from the thymocyte preparations. To exclude lymph node cells, inject each donor mouse intraperitoneally with 0.1 ml of black ink (diluted 1:5

in saline) 20–30 minutes before removing the thymus. The parathymic nodes become black and are easily recognized and excluded, especially if a dissecting microscope is used during removal of the thymus. To exclude blood cells, bleed the mice heavily from the tail veins or the retro-orbital plexus. (If the mice do not die from the bleeding, kill the mice by CO_2 inhalation. Do not use cervical dislocation as it causes bleeding in the thymic area.)

2. Remove the thymuses (see Section 15.3 for a description of thymectomy) and place them in a Petri dish containing sterile BSS or saline. Clean each thymus, removing nodes and blood vessels, and transfer them to another Petri dish containing sterile BSS or saline. After removing all blood vessels and nodes, either tease the thymuses with forceps or dissociate them by using a sterile tissue homogenizer. (We use a homogenizer only when the cells are to be used for injections or absorptions.)

3. Transfer the dissociated cells to a tube and allow clumps to settle for 5 to 6 minutes. Avoiding the clumps, transfer the cells to another tube and pellet the cells at $200 \times g$ for 10 minutes. If the cells are to be injected intravenously, resuspend the cells and allow any clumps to settle once again. If the cell suspension contains aggregates, the recipient mice are likely to die when injected.

COMMENTS

1. The size of the thymus decreases with age. The thymuses of mice 3–6 weeks of age contain approximately 2×10^8 cells, whereas those of mice 6–16 weeks of age contain approximately 1×10^8 cells. Mice older than 4 months may have as few as 5×10^7 cells per thymus.

2. The number of thymocytes contained in 0.1 ml packed volume is approximately 3.5×10^8.

1.6 EDUCATED THYMOCYTES

Educated thymocytes can be obtained by injecting irradiated mice simultaneously with syngeneic thymocytes and antigen. The spleens of these animals can later be used to restore the *in vitro* response of T-cell-depleted spleen cell suspensions. (This population of primed T cells also contains numerous activated accessory cells.)

MATERIALS AND REAGENTS

As described in Section 1.5, with the following changes:

Mice, an equal number of syngeneic donors and recipients:
   Donors: 3 to 6 weeks of age
   Recipients: 12 weeks of age or older, x-irradiated with 900 R
      prior to injection (see Chapter 10.4 and Appendix A.17)
Sheep red blood cells (SRBC), washed twice in sterile BSS or in
   saline and resuspended to 10% (v/v) in either diluent; 0.2 ml per
   recipient is required.
Syringes, tuberculin, and 27-gauge needles

PROCEDURE

Sterile conditions and reagents are required since irradiated mice are
given an intravenous injection. Follow steps 1 through 3 of the procedures described in Section 1.5. Continue with step 4 below.

4. Resuspend the thymocytes to 5×10^8 cells/ml in either BSS or
   saline. Note that the cell suspension *must* be free of all aggregates.

5. Mix equal volumes of the thymus cell suspension and 10% SRBC.
   Slowly inject each recipient intravenously with 0.4 ml of the cell
   mixture (rapid injection may kill mice). Each mouse receives 1×10^8 thymocytes and approximately 4×10^8 SRBC.

6. Use the spleens 6 to 8 days later. The spleens will contain approximately $1-2 \times 10^7$ nucleated cells/spleen.

1.7 CORTISONE-RESISTANT THYMOCYTES

Cortisone-resistant thymocytes can be used as a source of T cell help.
Inject each mouse intraperitoneally or subcutaneously with 2.5 mg of
cortisone acetate and remove thymuses 2 days later. Approximately 2.5%
of the thymocytes will survive the treatment. Alternatively, peanut
agglutinin can be used to separate the immunologically immature cortical
thymocytes, which do not provide T helper activity, from the functionally
mature medullary thymocytes, which do. See Section 9.6 for the details of
this procedure.

1.8 BONE MARROW CELLS

Although bone marrow cells can be obtained from any of the long bones, the femur and tibia are usually used since they give the best yields.

MATERIALS AND REAGENTS

As described in Section 1.2, with the following additions:

5 tissue culture dishes for every 3 mice, 60 × 15 mm (Corning Glass Works, #25010, or similar)
Syringes, 3 or 5 ml
Needles, 20 and 25 gauge

PROCEDURE

1. Kill mice by cervical dislocation or CO_2 inhalation and dip them in 70% ethanol.
2. Place mice on their backs and make a long transverse incision through the skin in the middle of the abdominal area of each mouse. Reflect skin completely from the hindquarters, including the hind legs.
3. Flood the hind legs with 70% ethanol.
4. While grasping the hind legs with the mouse tooth forceps, cut away as much muscle as possible with the scissors.
5. Separate legs from the body at the hip joint and remove the feet, taking care not to damage the epiphyses of the long bones during separation of the joints. Place the legs in a culture dish containing BSS. One culture dish can be used for 3 pairs of legs.
6. Begin the removal of adherent muscle tissue from the femur and tibia by grasping the bones with the mouse tooth forceps and scraping them with the flat forceps. Transfer the partially cleaned bones to another culture dish containing BSS.
7. Repeat step 6 until muscle tissue is completely removed from the bones and then transfer the bones to a fresh culture dish containing BSS. (When the bones are fairly clean, separate the tibia and femur with the scissors.)
8. Remove the epiphyses with the scissors and puncture the bone ends with a 20-gauge needle.
9. Using a syringe with a 25-gauge needle attached, expel the marrow by pushing BSS through the center of the bones. Draw the marrow in and out of the needle and syringe to obtain a single-cell suspension.

COMMENT

Yields of 2–6×10^7 cells per mouse can be expected; 0.1 ml packed bone marrow cells contains approximately 2×10^8 cells.

1.9 LYMPH NODE CELLS

Because removal of all lymph nodes is a tedious process, a standard set of lymph nodes is usually selected (Figure 1.1). In mice the cervical, axillary, brachial, inguinal, and popliteal nodes are easily found, and all are bilateral. The mesenteric lymph node is frequently removed because it is comparatively large (2–3×10^7 cells in adult BDF_1 mice). Lymph nodes can be located in a preliminary experiment by performing a dissection upon a mouse that has been injected in the footpads with complete Freund's adjuvant several weeks in advance. The lymph nodes in such mice are greatly enlarged and can easily be located by beginners.

MATERIALS AND REAGENTS

As described in Section 1.2, with the addition of a corkboard and pins.

PROCEDURE

1. Kill mice by CO_2 inhalation or cervical dislocation and pin them to the corkboard with limbs extended.
2. With scissors and forceps, reflect the skin from the body and pin the skin to the board as shown in Figure 1.1.
3. Use forceps to search for the lymph nodes, which are usually buried in connective tissue and fat. The lymph nodes will appear as firm translucent bumps in contrast to the soft fat and connective tissue.
4. To remove the visceral lymph nodes, open the peritoneal cavity. Lift the gut to expose the mesenteric lymph node (usually single and elongated) found in the mesentery of the ascending colon.
5. To remove the popliteal lymph nodes, place mice on their abdomens with the heads facing away from the operator. Make a long transverse incision in the lower back of each mouse and reflect the skin from the hindquarters and rear legs, exposing the popliteal fossa at the rear of the knee joint. The popliteal nodes are hidden by the muscle tissue at the upper end of the popliteal fossa.

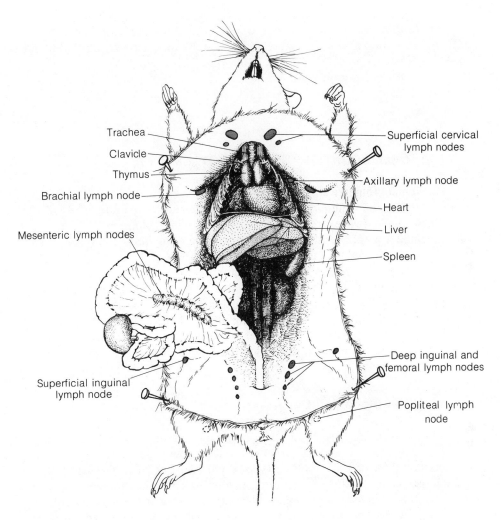

Trachea
Clavicle
Thymus
Brachial lymph node
Mesenteric lymph nodes
Superficial inguinal
lymph node

Superficial cervical
lymph nodes
Axillary lymph node
Heart
Liver
Spleen
Deep inguinal and
femoral lymph nodes
Popliteal lymph
node

FIGURE 1.1
Location of lymph nodes in the mouse. The periaortic lymph nodes, which lie along the course of the aorta, are not shown.

Cut through the outer layer of muscle to expose the nodes. (After footpad injections of complete Freund's adjuvant, the popliteal nodes become very large and are easily detected and removed.)

6. Place the nodes in a tissue culture dish containing BSS. Thoroughly remove all fat and debris. Transfer nodes to a fresh dish containing BSS, and tease as described in Section 1.2.

7. Place dissociated cells into a centrifuge tube and allow clumps to settle for 5–6 minutes. Transfer cells into a centrifuge tube and pellet the cells at $200 \times g$ for 10 minutes. Wash the cells several times to remove all fat.

1.10 CELL COUNTS WITH A HEMACYTOMETER

The hemacytometer chamber (Figure 1.2) is used to count both white and red blood cells. The large square areas indicated by the numbers 1, 2, 3, and 4 in the figure are used for counting white blood cells. The area indicated by the number 5 is used for counting red blood cells. The volume contained by each of these separate areas under a coverslip is 10^{-4} ml (in hemacytometers that are 0.1 mm deep).

Errors can be introduced in a number of ways: dilution errors, loss of cells during pipetting, uneven suspension of cells, overfilling or underfilling of the chamber, and the counting of cells before they settle. Random distribution of cells in the chamber is another source of error but can be compensated for by counting a large number of cells.

A. White Blood Cell Counts

When determining the total white blood cell count, it is advantageous to first remove red blood cells by lysis in dilute acid, to prevent the erroneous counting of red blood cells as small lymphocytes. The addition of gentian violet to the acid solution facilitates counting since it stains the white blood cells. Cell populations that are grown in continuous culture, and thus do not contain red cells, are easily counted in any isotonic diluent.

MATERIALS AND REAGENTS

Cell suspension
Hemacytometer and coverslip (Scientific Products, #B3180-2)
Microscope
Pasteur pipettes and rubber bulb
Hand counters
Counting solution: 3% acetic acid in water (v/v) or 0.01% gentian violet in 3% acetic acid (Turk's solution)

PROCEDURE

1. Make appropriate dilutions of the cell suspension just prior to counting. The optimal concentration of cells for counting is 5–10 $\times$ 10^5 cells/ml (50–100 cells per large square) after dilution in the counting solution.

2. Using a Pasteur pipette with finger control, let the cell suspension flow under the coverslip until the grid area is *just* full and not overflowing into the overflow well. If the chamber is loaded too

Grid

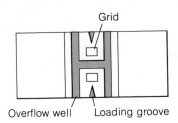

Overflow well   Loading groove

Grid system

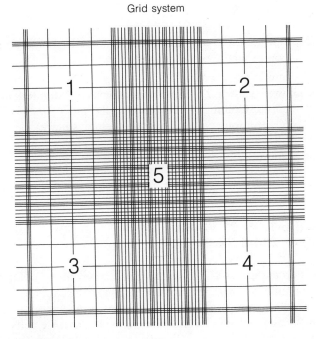

FIGURE 1.2
Hemacytometer.

heavily, clean it and begin again; do not attempt to remove excess liquid. Allow cells to settle.

3. Count all of the cells contained in each of the 4 large squares (1–4 in Figure 1.2). Some cells will be touching the outside borders. Count only those cells touching two of the outside borders (for example, the upper and left). A minimum of 200 cells should be counted. Determine the average number of cells per large square. This is the number of cells per 10^{-4} ml. Thus:

$$\text{cells/ml} = (\text{average number per large square}) \times 10^4/\text{ml} \times \frac{1}{\text{dilution}}.$$

B. Red Blood Cell Counts

MATERIALS AND REAGENTS

Similar to those for white blood cell counts except that the counting solution is a physiological medium such as BSS (Appendix A.3) or PBS (Appendix A.8).

PROCEDURE

1. Make appropriate dilutions of the red blood cells. For example, a 1 : 200 dilution of whole blood is adequate.

2. Count the number of red blood cells, using the large center square (square 5 in Figure 1.2). This large square is divided into 25 smaller squares. Count the red blood cells in 5 of these smaller squares (e.g., the four corners and the center square):

$$\text{cells/ml} = (\text{number in 5 squares}) \times 5 \times 10^4/\text{ml} \times \frac{1}{\text{dilution}}.$$

1.11 DETERMINATION OF VIABILITY BY TRYPAN BLUE EXCLUSION

The number or percentage of viable white blood cells can be determined by staining cell populations with trypan blue. Viable cells exclude the dye, while nonviable cells take up the dye, thereby fostering a visual distinction between unstained viable cells and blue-stained nonviable cells. After being stained with trypan blue, the cells must be counted within 3 minutes; after that time viable cells begin to take up the dye. Also, since trypan blue has a great affinity for proteins (Kruse et al. 1973), elimination of serum from the cell diluent will allow a more accurate determination of cell viability.

MATERIALS AND REAGENTS

Cell suspension at $2–5 \times 10^6$ cells/ml
Trypan blue, 0.2% (w/v) in water
$5\times$ saline: 4.25% NaCl (w/v)

PROCEDURE

1. On the day of use, mix 4 parts of 0.2% trypan blue with 1 part of $5\times$ saline.
2. To 1 part of the trypan blue saline solution, add 1 part of the cell suspension (1 : 2 dilution).
3. Load cells into a hemacytometer (Section 1.10) and count the number of unstained (viable) white blood cells and stained (dead) cells separately. For greater accuracy, count more than a combined total of 200 cells:

viable cells/ml=

$$(\text{average number of viable cells in large square}) \times 10^4/\text{ml} \times \frac{1}{\text{dilution}} \,;$$

$$\% \text{ viable cells} = \frac{\text{number of viable cells}}{\text{number of viable cells} + \text{number of dead cells}} \times 100\%.$$

REFERENCE

Kruse, P. F., Jr., and M. K. Patterson, Jr., Eds. 1973. *Tissue Culture: Methods and Applications*. Academic Press, New York.

1.12 DETERMINATION OF VIABILITY
BY EOSIN Y EXCLUSION

The advantage of using eosin Y as a vital stain is that the time elapsed before examining the cells is less critical than for trypan blue exclusion; The percentage of viable cells remains constant from 1–10 minutes after staining with eosin Y. However, some find red-(eosin Y)-stained cells more difficult to recognize than blue-(trypan blue)-stained cells.

MATERIALS AND REAGENTS

Cell suspension adjusted to 2×10^6 cells/ml

Saline: 0.85% NaCl (w/v)

Eosin Y, 0.2% (w/v) in saline. This solution is stable at room temperature. If precipitate forms, pass the solution through Whatman #1 filter paper.

PROCEDURE

1. To 1 part of cell suspension, add 1 part of 0.2% eosin Y.

2. Determine the number of viable cells/ml and the percent of viable cells by the procedure described in Section 1.11 (Procedure, step 3).

COMMENT

Eosin Y may bind to proteins; therefore, elimination of serum from the cell diluent promotes a more accurate determination of cell viability.

1.13 DETERMINATION OF VIABILITY BY NIGROSIN EXCLUSION

This procedure is especially advantageous in tests where stained cells must remain stained for hours without disintegration and where live cells are not killed by prolonged exposure to the dye. Nigrosin is therefore the dye of choice in microcytotoxicity tests (Section 11.7). Nigrosin exclusion may also be the more accurate measure of macrophage viability since viable macrophages on occasion take up trypan blue and eosin Y. For routine determination of cell viability, nigrosin has disadvantages: The uptake of nigrosin is slower than that of either trypan blue or eosin Y, and inexperienced workers often confuse dead (brown-black) cells and live cells that are not in focus.

MATERIALS AND REAGENTS

Cell suspension adjusted to $2-20 \times 10^6$ cells/ml

Nigrosin, 1% (w/v) in water; filter stock solution through Whatman #1 paper.

Balanced salt solution (BSS; Appendix A.3) or saline (0.85% NaCl, w/v) containing 2.5–5% fetal calf serum

PROCEDURE

1. Dilute the 1% nigrosin stock 1 : 10 in medium containing 2–5% fetal calf serum, just prior to use.
2. Mix the cell suspension with 0.1% nigrosin solution such that the cell suspension : nigrosin solution ratio is between 1 : 2 and 1 : 10.
3. Wait 5–10 minutes; then determine the number of viable cells/ml and the percent of viable cells as described in Section 1.11 (Procedure, step 3).

1.14 DETERMINATION OF VIABILITY WITH FLUORESCEIN DIACETATE

Fluorescein diacetate is taken in by all cells but is only hydrolyzed inside live cells to reveal green fluorescence.

A. Use of Fluorescein Diacetate to Determine Cell Viability

MATERIALS AND REAGENTS

Cell suspension at approximately 10^6 cells/ml in BSS-5% FCS
Fluorescein diacetate, 5 mg/ml in acetone, stored in a tightly capped container at $-20°C$
Phosphate-buffered saline (PBS; Appendix A.8)
Fetal calf serum (FCS)
Balanced salt solution (Appendix A.3) containing 5% fetal calf serum (BSS-5% FCS)
Fluorescence microscope

PROCEDURE

1. Dilute fluorescein diacetate solution (1 : 50) in PBS at room temperature (a fine suspension forms). Immediately, add one volume of the fluorescein diacetate suspension to 9 volumes of the cell suspension.
2. Allow the mixture to stand at room temperature for 15 minutes. Examine cells with a fluorescence microscope as described in Section 13.4. Viable cells will appear bright green.
3. Determine the percent of viable cells as described in Section 1.11 (Procedure, step 3).

B. Use of Fluorescein Diacetate with Rhodamine-Conjugated Anti–Cell Surface Antibodies

The following procedure is used to determine whether cells possessing a particular cell surface marker are viable. The example given is for immunoglobulin-bearing cells.

MATERIALS AND REAGENTS

As described in Section 1.14A, with the following additions:

Rhodamine-conjugated rabbit anti–mouse Ig antibodies (Sections 11.5 and 13.3): Pretitrate the reagent for a maximum of specific fluorescence staining.

Sodium azide solution, 0.2% (w/v) in BSS–5% FCS (optional). Caution: Sodium azide is extremely toxic and should be handled with great care.

PROCEDURE

1. To 5×10^6 cells in a volume of 50 μl BSS–5% FCS, add the appropriate predetermined volume of rhodamine-conjugated antibody (see Section 13.3).

2. Prepare a 1:50 dilution of fluorescein diacetate in BSS-5% FCS as described in Section 1.14A and immediately add a $\frac{1}{10}$ volume of this solution to the cell suspension. Add a $\frac{1}{10}$ volume of sodium azide solution if desired to prevent capping (see Section 13.4).

3. Incubate the mixture for 20 minutes on ice. Then layer the mixture over 100% FCS and centrifuge at $300 \times g$ for 10 minutes (Section 1.22). Wash the cells two times with BSS–5% FCS.

4. Resuspend the cells to the appropriate concentration in 100% FCS and examine the cells with a fluorescence microscope as described in Section 13.4.

COMMENTS

1. First observe for rhodamine stained Ig-bearing cells; then determine whether these cells are stained internally with fluorescein.

2. It may be necessary to decrease the concentration of fluorescein diacetate if nonspecific fluorescein staining of either dead cells or red blood cells is detected, or if fluorescein is visible (as red fluorescence) when the microscope is adjusted to observe rhodamine.

REFERENCE

Rotman, B., and B. W. Papermaster. 1966. The membrane properties of living mammalian cells as studied by enzymatic hydrolysis of fluorogenic esters. *Proc. Nat. Acad. Sci.* (USA) **55**:134.

1.15 DETERMINATION OF VIABILITY WITH ACRIDINE ORANGE-ETHIDIUM BROMIDE

A one-part-per-million solution of acridine orange and ethidium bromide can be used to stain viable and nonviable cells differentially (Parks et al. 1979). Live cells take up acridine orange, whereas nonviable cells take up ethidium bromide. When viewed through a fluorescence microscope, viable cells appear green while nonviable cells appear orange.

MATERIALS AND REAGENTS

Cell suspension at approximately 10^6 cells/ml

Acridine orange (AO; Sigma Chemical or Aldrich Chemical). Caution: AO is hazardous; see 1 under Comments.

Ethidium bromide (EB; Sigma Chemical or Aldrich Chemical). Caution: EB is hazardous; see 1 under Comments.

Phosphate-buffered saline (PBS; Appendix A.8)

Hemacytometer and coverslip (Scientific Products, #B3180-2)

Fluorescence microscope; a tungsten–halogen illuminator is adequate and preferable to a mercury lamp.

Solution of one part per million AO/EB: Dissolve 0.1 mg of both AO and EB in 100 ml of PBS; divide into aliquots and freeze. Once thawed, store in the dark at 4°C.

PROCEDURE

1. Mix one part cell suspension with one part AO/EB solution.

2. Place cells in a hemacytometer (Section 1.10) and determine the number of green (viable) and orange (nonviable) cells, using both UV and visible illumination at the same time. (The fluorescence of the cells is so strong that it is not necessary to turn off the visible illumination while observing the cells.)

COMMENTS

1. Acridine orange and ethidium bromide have been found by the Ames test to be highly mutagenic and thus should be handled with care (McCann et al. 1975).

2. Acridine orange is somewhat unstable at room temperature.

REFERENCES

Lee, S.-K., J. Singh, and R. B. Taylor. 1975. Subclasses of T cells with different sensitivities to cytotoxic antibody in the presence of anesthetics. *Eur. J. Immunol.* **5**:259.

McCann, J., E. Choi, E. Yamasaki, and B. N. Ames. 1975. Detection of carcinogens as mutagens in Salmonella/microsome test: Assay of 300 chemicals. *Proc. Natl. Acad. Sci.* (USA) **72**:5135.

Parks, D. R., V. M. Bryan, V. T. Oi, and L. A. Herzenberg. 1979. Antigen specific identification and cloning of hybridomas with a fluorescence-activated cell sorter (FACS). *Proc. Natl. Acad. Sci.* (USA) **76**:1962.

1.16 LYSIS OF RED BLOOD CELLS BY HYPOTONIC SHOCK

MATERIALS AND REAGENTS

$2\times$ balanced salt solution (BSS; Appendix A.3) or $2\times$ Eagle's minimum essential medium (MEM)

$1\times$ BSS or $1\times$ MEM

$\frac{1}{10}\times$ BSS or $\frac{1}{10}\times$ MEM; readjust to pH 7.2 if necessary.

PROCEDURE

1. To 0.1 ml packed cells, add 0.1 ml $1\times$ diluent (BSS or MEM) and resuspend pellet.

2. Measuring the volume, add 1–2 ml of $\frac{1}{10}\times$ diluent and quickly mix the cells using the same pipette.

3. After exposing cells to 15 seconds of hypotonic shock, quickly add a volume of $2\times$ diluent equal to that used in step 2 and mix thoroughly. Dilute further with $1\times$ diluent. Centrifuge at $200 \times g$ for 10 minutes. Wash once with $1\times$ BSS or $1\times$ MEM.

COMMENT

Clumping can occur when treating double or triple the number of cells described above.

1.17 LYSIS OF RED BLOOD CELLS WITH TRIS-BUFFERED AMMONIUM CHLORIDE

MATERIALS AND REAGENTS

Fetal calf serum (FCS)
NH_4Cl, $M_r = 53.5$
Tris base, $M_r = 121.5$
HCl
Stock solutions
    0.16 M NH_4Cl: 8.3 g/liter
    0.17 M Tris, pH 7.65: Dissolve 20.6 g Tris base in 900 ml water; adjust to pH 7.65 with HCl. Make up to 1000 ml.
Working solution: mix 90 ml of 0.16 M NH_4Cl and 10 ml of 0.17 M Tris, pH 7.65; adjust to pH 7.2 with HCl.

PROCEDURE

1. Pellet the cells and resuspend in Tris-NH_4Cl working solution (0.1 ml packed cells/ml Tris-NH_4Cl). Hold at room temperature for 2 minutes.
2. Underlay the cells with FCS and centrifuge at $300 \times g$ for 10 minutes. Repeat the process if red blood cells are evident in the pellet.
3. Wash cells twice before using.

1.18 LYSIS OF RED BLOOD CELLS WITH HEMOLYTIC GEY'S SOLUTION

MATERIALS AND REAGENTS

Cell suspension
Fetal calf serum (FCS)
Balanced salt solution (Appendix A.3) containing 5% fetal calf serum (BSS-5% FCS)

Stock A:

NH_4Cl	35.0	g
KCl	1.85	g
$Na_2HPO_4 \cdot 12H_2O$	1.5	g
KH_2PO_4	0.12	g
Glucose	5.0	g
Phenol red	50.0	mg

Bring to 1000 ml and autoclave solution.

Stock B:

$MgCl_2 \cdot 6H_2O$	0.42 g
$MgSO_4 \cdot 7H_2O$	0.14 g
$CaCl_2$	0.34 g

Bring to 100 ml and autoclave solution.

Stock C:

$NaHCO_3$	2.25 g

Bring to 100 ml and autoclave solution.

1× Gey's solution:

20 parts Stock A
5 parts Stock B
5 parts Stock C
70 parts distilled water (sterile)

PROCEDURE

1. Resuspend approximately 10^8 pelleted spleen cells in 1 ml of BSS-5% FCS.
2. Add 5 ml of 1× Gey's solution and hold the cells on ice for 3–6 minutes.
3. Underlay the cells with 100% fetal calf serum and centrifuge at 300 × g for 10 minutes. Wash once or twice in BSS-5%FCS prior to use.

1.19 CENTRIFUGATION THROUGH FICOLL-HYPAQUE

This procedure removes both red blood cells and dead cells in a single step with high efficiency.

MATERIALS AND REAGENTS

Cell suspension at 5×10^6–2×10^7 cells/ml
Ficoll-Hypaque solution, $\rho = 1.09$ (see Section 8.7 for the preparation of Ficoll-Hypaque)
Balanced salt solution (Appendix A.3) containing 5% fetal calf serum (BSS-5% FCS)
Polycarbonate tube, 16 × 105 mm (Nalge Co., #3113)
20°C water bath

Centrifuge, 20°C, with rapid acceleration (centrifuge should attain 2000 × g within 20 seconds)

PROCEDURE

1. Prewarm cell suspension and Ficoll-Hypaque to 20°C in a water bath. Prewarm centrifuge to 20°C.
2. Add 4 ml of Ficoll-Hypaque to the polycarbonate tube and gently layer 2 to 6 ml of the cell suspension onto the Ficoll-Hypaque (add the suspension down the wall of the tube).
3. Centrifuge at 2000 × g for 20 minutes. Rapid acceleration is essential for clean separation.
4. To recover the viable white blood cells, collect all of the fluid (which contains the viable cells) above the pellet, add 10 ml of medium or BSS-5% FCS, and centrifuge at 300–350 × g for 15 minutes. Wash twice (250 × g, 10 min) before using cells for further studies.

REFERENCE

Parish, C. R., S. M. Kirov, N. Bowern, N. Blanden, and R. V. Blanden. 1974. A one-step procedure for separating mouse T and B lymphocytes. *Eur. J. Immunol.* **4**:808.

1.20   DEAD CELL AGGLUTINATION

This procedure is rapid and will remove most of the dead cells normally found after the preparation of a spleen cell suspension. It is also effective in removing the majority of dead cells found after carrying out mass cytotoxic procedures (Section 9.2). It is not as reliable for the removal of dead cells from cultured cells. Although dead cells agglutinate most markedly in the high phosphate medium described below, agglutination occurs to some extent in other media.

MATERIALS AND REAGENTS

Cell suspension
Fetal calf serum (FCS)
KH_2PO_4, $M_r = 136.1$
Na_2HPO_4, $M_r = 142.0$
NaCl, $M_r = 58.4$
High phosphate buffered saline (HPBS): Dissolve 4.0 g KH_2PO_4, 17.13 g Na_2HPO_4, and 9.0 g NaCl in 1800 ml of water. Adjust to pH 7.4. Bring volume to 2000 ml.

PROCEDURE

1. Prepare HPBS containing 2–5% FCS (HPBS-FCS). Bring to room temperature.

2. Disperse cell suspension in HPBS-FCS. The initial preparation of lymphoid cell suspensions from whole organs may be made in this medium, or cells may be resuspended in it.

3. Centrifuge at $200 \times g$ for 10 minutes.

4. Remove supernatant.

5. Resuspend pellet in 2–3 ml of HPBS-FCS. Aggregates of debris and dead cells will not disperse readily. Vigorous mixing (avoiding bubbles) with a Pasteur pipette will separate live cells from aggregates. Fill tube with HPBS-FCS and mix.

6. Centrifuge gently at $50 \times g$ for 10–12 seconds to pellet the aggregates but leave viable cells in suspension.

7. Decant supernatant and centrifuge supernatant at $200 \times g$ for 10 minutes to pellet viable cells.

8. Resuspend in desired medium or repeat steps 5–7 if insufficient numbers of dead cells have been removed.

COMMENTS

1. Insufficiently vigorous mixing in step 5 may reduce the yield of viable cells.

2. Excessive centrifugation in step 6 will pellet viable cells and 'thereby reduce the yield.

REFERENCE

North, J. R., J. T. Kemshead, and B. A. Askonas. 1977. Non-specific factor replaces T cells in an IgG response to soluble antigens. *Immunology* 33:321.

1.21 REMOVAL OF DEAD CELLS AND CELL DEBRIS BY FILTRATION THROUGH A GLASS WOOL COLUMN

MATERIALS AND REAGENTS

Balanced salt solution (Appendix A.3) containing 5% fetal calf serum (BSS-5% FCS)

Glass wool (Corning, #3950)

Pasteur pipette
Applicator stick

PROCEDURE

1. Prepare the glass wool column by loosely packing a small amount of glass wool into a Pasteur pipette with an applicator stick. The glass wool should be lightly packed in the large portion of the pipette. The columns may be autoclaved if desired.

2. Rinse columns thoroughly with BSS-5% FCS. Fluid should flow through the columns rapidly. Pass the cell suspension through the column and rinse once with BSS-5% FCS. Pellet cells at $200 \times g$ for 10 minutes.

1.22   CENTRIFUGATION THROUGH FETAL CALF SERUM

MATERIALS AND REAGENTS

Dense cell suspension of $1–2 \times 10^8$ cells/ml in balanced salt solution (BSS; Appendix A.3)
Fetal calf serum (FCS)
Conical centrifuge tubes, 12 ml

PROCEDURE

1. Layer 1–2 ml of the cell suspension over 3 ml FCS in a 12-ml centrifuge tube. Centrifuge at $300 \times g$ for 10 minutes. Carefully remove the supernate and discard. Resuspend the pelleted cells in an appropriate medium or buffer.

2. Alternatively, carefully layer FCS *under* the cell suspension, which will rise as FCS is added. Centrifuge at $300 \times g$ for 10 minutes. This procedure is especially useful both for washing cells after fluorescent staining as an alternative to the method described in Section 13.4 and for avoiding the loss of cells incurred with tube transfers and additional pipetting. With small volumes, use a finely drawn Pasteur pipette for underlayering.

2

Generation of
Humoral Responses

2.1 INTRODUCTION
Robert I. Mishell

Culture methods that enable mouse spleen cells to generate strong primary immune responses have been developed using suspension cultures (Mishell and Dutton 1966, 1967) and diffusion cultures (Marbrook 1967). These systems differ from previously established methods of cell culture, principally in employing low concentrations of oxygen and high cell densities. For each system, special techniques were developed to maintain the pH and supply nutrients to the metabolically active cells. Suspension cultures require daily supplementation of the media with nutrients and base; diffusion cultures utilize a large reservoir of medium in contact with the culture suspension across a dialysis membrane. Both types of systems favor cell interactions and the maintenance of secreted macromolecular mediators at high concentrations, two conditions that may be important in inducing immune responses. Initially developed using heterologous erythrocyte antigens, these culture systems are also useful for generating primary and secondary immunizations to a variety of different antigens (see references at the end of this section for a partial list).

The ability to generate immune responses *in vitro* has provided cellular immunologists with new ways of investigating the generation and regulation of immune responses. Many of the principal phenomena observed with intact animals and with *in vivo* adoptive transfer systems have been reproduced *in vitro*. Culture systems have been particularly useful for comparing the effects of mediators and other immunoregulatory substances, because both the control and the experimental cells are derived from a single uniform cell suspension. Culture methods are also especially well suited for studying how macrophages function, because these cells cannot be removed from the irradiated hosts employed in adoptive transfer techniques. The effects of their removal or manipulation can, however, be examined *in vitro*. The recent development of methods for reducing the volume and the number of cells cultured has improved the usefulness of *in vitro* techniques for limiting dilution analyses and has made possible the study of the biological properties of subpopulations of cells that are obtainable only in small numbers.

It is important to proceed with caution in making use of the various culture techniques. Systematic comparisons of responses obtained with the different methods described in this chapter have been done infrequently and it is not fully known which kinds of experiments would yield similar data with the different techniques. Moreover, since culture methods are frequently modified to suit particular needs, comparisons of data from different laboratories should be interpreted conservatively. The fact that mice are maintained differently in each institution further compounds the problem of making strict comparisons. As greater knowledge of cellular immunology is gained, the ability to recognize and control significant variables will increase. This progress should promote greater uniformity of data and make valid comparisons easier.

REFERENCES

Bullock, W. W., and M. Rittenberg. 1970. Kinetics of *in vitro* initiated secondary antihapten responses: Induction of plaque forming cells by soluble and particulate antigen. *Immunochemistry* 7:310.

Diener, E., and W. D. Armstrong. 1967. Induction of antibody formation and tolerance *in vitro* to a purified protein antigen. *Lancet* ii:1281.

Dutton, R. W., and R. I. Mishell. 1967. Cell populations and cell proliferation in the *in vitro* response of normal mouse spleen to heterologous erythrocytes. Analysis by the hot pulse technique. *J. Exp. Med.* 126:443.

Feldman, M. 1971. Induction of immunity and tolerance to the dinitrophenyl determinant *in vitro*. *Nature* (New Biol.) 231:21.

Henry, C. 1975. *In vitro* anti-hapten response to a lactoside-conjugated protein. *Cell. Immunol.* 19:117.

Hodes, R. J., and A. Singer. 1977. Cellular and genetic control of antibody responses *in vitro*. I. Cellular requirements for the generation of genetically controlled primary IgM responses to soluble antigens. *Eur. J. Immunol.* **7**:892.

Jacobs, D. M., and D. C. Morrison. 1975. Stimulation of a T-independant primary anti-hapten response *in vitro* by TNP-lipopolysaccharide (TNP-LPS). *J. Immunol.* **114**:360.

Kapp, J. A., C. W. Pierce, and B. Benacerraf. 1973. Genetic control of immune responses *in vitro*. I. Development of primary and secondary plaque-forming responses to the random terpolymer L-glutamic acid[60]-L-alanine[30]-L-tyrosine[10] (GAT) by mouse spleen cells *in vitro*. *J. Exp. Med.* **138**:1107.

Kettman, J., and R. W. Dutton. 1970. An *in vitro* primary immune response to 2,4,6-trinitrophenyl substituted erythrocytes: Response against carrier and hapten. *J. Immunol.* **104**:1558.

Marbrook, J. 1967. Primary immune response in cultures of spleen cells. *Lancet* **ii**:1279.

Mishell, R. I., and R. W. Dutton. 1966. Immunization of normal mouse spleen cell suspensions *in vitro*. *Science* **153**:1004.

Mishell, R. I., and R. W. Dutton. 1967. Immunization of dissociated spleen cell cultures from normal mice. *J. Exp. Med.* **126**:423.

Mosier, D. E., B. M. Johnson, W. E. Paul, and P. R. B. McMaster. 1974. Cellular requirements for the primary *in vitro* antibody response to DNP-Ficoll. *J. Exp. Med.* **139**:1354.

North, J. R., and B. A. Askonas. 1976. IgG responses *in vitro*. I. The requirement for an intermediate responsive cell type. *Eur. J. Immunol.* **6**:8.

2.2 PRIMARY IMMUNIZATION IN SUSPENSION CULTURES

Barbara B. Mishell and Robert I. Mishell

The following description of the primary immunization of mouse spleen cell suspensions to heterologous red blood cells (Mishell and Dutton 1966, 1967) is given in great detail because seemingly trivial differences in technique can significantly affect responses. Some of this information is laboratory lore and is perhaps used more because of positive past experience than of strict necessity. We stress the desirability of standardizing all aspects of the procedure since *in vitro* primary responses may be affected by slight nuances in preparative technique.* In our experience, the mag-

---

* Because the requisite conditions for obtaining secondary responses to heterologous red cell antigens *in vitro* are considerably less stringent than those required for primary immunization, some laboratories just beginning to use these procedures have found it beneficial to start by studying secondary responses. Unless there are major problems with the mice, reagents, or techniques, IgM responses with cultured spleen cells from mice immunized within 2 weeks of use should be readily obtainable.

nitude of the response often depends on cell density, on the use of particular lots of fetal calf serum (Mishell and Dutton 1967; Shiigi and Mishell 1975) and sheep red blood cells (Mishell and Dutton 1967; McCarthy and Dutton 1975a, 1975b), and on the inclusion of 2-mercaptoethanol (2-ME) in the medium (Click et al. 1972a, 1972b).

We also stress the desirability of standardizing the care and housing of experimental mice. The conditions of the mice used as spleen cell donors for *in vitro* immunization can critically affect results. On several occasions spleen cells from mice obtained from different suppliers responded poorly in culture, even though the mice appeared healthy; in mixing experiments, these spleen cells often suppressed the responses of cells from genetically similar control animals. We believe that chronic stress, virus infections, high bacterial loads in the diet, water and bedding, and general maintenance procedures are contributing factors. An example of the last point was reported by Silverman and La Via (1976), who traced a decrease in the magnitude of *in vitro* humoral responses to the use of a particular disinfectant in the animal colony.

We maintain mice under controlled conditions designed to reduce stress and exposure to microorganisms. Spleen cells obtained from such mice are less likely to contain nonspecific suppressor cells. However, these spleen cells tend to be hypoactive,* show delayed kinetics, and have a greater dependence on particular lots of fetal calf serum when cultured in the absence of 2-ME. In the presence of 2-ME, the spleen cells become more responsive, show normal kinetics, and are less dependent on particular lots of fetal calf serum. Furthermore, in the presence of 2-ME, these cells can be cultured at a much lower density than in the absence of 2-ME. Thus, although its mode of action is not clearly defined, 2-ME has proved valuable in enabling primary *in vitro* responses to occur under conditions that are otherwise unsatisfactory.

MATERIALS AND REAGENTS

Culture Medium

Fetal calf serum (FCS), pretested (Appendix A.1)†
Eagle's minimum essential medium for suspension cultures (MEM; Microbiological Associates, #12-126B) or RPMI 1640 (Grand Is-

---

* Similar immunological hypoactivity has been found in mice maintained under pathogen-free conditions.

† We at times test lots of FCS from various suppliers. Lots of FCS found satisfactory for use in this system are reserved by the companies for sale to those who specifically request them. The identification numbers of tested lots of FCS, if available, can be obtained from us by phone or mail.

land Biological, #320-1875) or equivalent medium from alternative supplier

Eagle's minimum medium nonessential amino acids, 100× solution

Sodium pyruvate, 100 mM solution

L-glutamine, 200 mM solution

2-mercaptoethanol (2-ME; Sigma Chemical, #M-6250; Appendix A.6)

Penicillin-streptomycin: 5000 units of penicillin, 5000 μg of streptomycin per ml

Graduated cylinder, 100 ml

Bottle, 100 ml, glass or plastic

Cell Culture

Spleen cell suspension (Section 1.2)

Sheep red blood cells (SRBC), pretested (see Comments)

Balanced salt solution (BSS; Appendix A.3)

Nutritive cocktail (Appendix A.5)

70% ethanol

Pasteur pipettes and rubber bulb

Pipettes, 1 ml, 5 ml, 10 ml

Graduated centrifuge tubes, conical (Bellco Glass, #3041-00012) with stainless steel closures (Bellco Glass, #2005-00016)

Tissue culture dishes, 35 × 10 mm (Falcon, #3001, Corning Glass Works, #25000-35, or similar)

Equipment for cell counts

Tissue culture chamber, fitted with trays (Bellco Glass, #7741-10005)

Rocker platform (Bellco Glass, #7740-20020)

Gas mixture: 7% O_2, 10% CO_2, 83% N_2

Cell Harvest

BSS

Teflon policeman (Scientific Products, #R5115-3)

Centrifuge tubes, 17 × 100 mm (Falcon, #2017 or similar)

PROCEDURE

Culture Medium

Prepare medium as follows and place on ice (volumes given are for 100 ml of medium): To a 100-ml graduated cylinder, add 1.0 ml of 100 mM sodium pyruvate, 1.0 ml of 200 mM L-glutamine, 1.0 ml of 100× solution of nonessential amino acids, 1.0 ml of 5×10^{-3} M 2-ME, and 5–10 ml of FCS. One milliliter of penicillin-streptomycin can be added if desired. Bring the volume to 100 ml with MEM or RPMI 1640 and transfer medium to a bottle.

Cell Culture

1. With a lint-free tissue, wipe culture chamber and trays with 70% ethanol and allow them to dry completely. Place culture dishes (a minimum of 2–3 per experimental line) on trays and label.

2. Wash SRBC twice in BSS (0.1 ml packed cells is ample for 100 ml of medium). If all cultures will receive the same antigen, resuspend the packed red cells to 10% (v/v) in BSS and add 0.3 ml to 100 ml of medium. Alternatively, the red cells can be resuspended to 1% and distributed directly to the culture dishes with a disposable Pasteur pipette (1 drop, approximately 30 μl, per dish). With either method, each culture will receive approximately 3×10^6 SRBC.

3. Remove spleens from mice and prepare a single-cell suspension in BSS. Pellet the cells and hold them on ice until placed in culture (see comment 2).

4. The cells can be placed in culture in a variety of ways, depending on experimental design. Three possibilities are offered:

   a. If all of the cultures contain the same serum, the same antigen, and the same concentration of spleen cells, resuspend the spleen cells in the complete medium containing the antigen and serum. The cells can then be rapidly distributed to the Petri dishes in 1-ml aliquots with a 10-ml pipette.

   b. If there are variations in antigen, serum, or cell concentration, it is often easier to place these constituents separately into the culture dishes. Note that this includes adding the medium but not the spleen cells. Any additional experimental reagents can be placed in the dishes at this time by adding 50 μl or 100 μl of 20× or 10× stocks, respectively. With this approach one can work leisurely, since, with no spleen cells in the culture dishes, it does not matter whether the medium changes to alkaline pH. When the culture dishes have received all additives, place them in the culture chamber and exchange the air in the chamber with the gas mixture to adjust the pH of the medium to about 7.2. Adjust the spleen cell concentration to 10× the desired final concentration in either BSS or medium. With a 1-ml pipette, distribute the spleen cells in 0.1-ml aliquots to the culture dishes. Return the culture dishes to the culture chamber and gas as above.

   c. When performing titrations of immunoregulatory substances, the following procedure is useful. Titrate by adding to a series of culture dishes the appropriate volumes of test material and sufficient *incomplete* medium (containing no additives) so that each dish contains 0.5 ml. Allow these mixtures to equilibrate with the gas mixture in order to bring the pH to 7.2 prior to the addition of cells. Prepare complete medium with 2× the standard concentrations of additives (pyruvate, nonessential amino acids, glutamine, 2-ME, and FCS) by adding the amount of supplements given under the procedure for culture medium to 50 ml instead of 100 ml of medium. Then combine spleen cells and red cells at twice the desired final concentration with the enriched medium. The appropriate final concentrations of cells and medium supplements are obtained by adding 0.5 ml of the enriched medium and cell suspension to the dishes containing 0.5 ml of the mixtures of incomplete medium and test substances.

In medium supplemented with 2-ME, the optimal concentration of nucleated cells is 4–8×10^6 cells/ml. As a guide for obtaining the appropriate cell concentration, assume that 0.1 ml of packed spleen cells contains 1–2×10^8 nucleated cells. Resuspend the cells to a higher concentration than required, count an aliquot, and adjust the concentration by adding additional medium. If the cell concentration initially made is too dilute for use, centrifuge the cells into a pellet again. When calculating the correct resuspension volume, expect a loss of cells from the additional centrifugation.

As the cells are being dispensed, the culture medium will immediately begin to shift toward alkaline pH (see comment 3); this shift is indicated by a change in color from pale orange to deep lavender. A slight shift is not harmful but it is essential to prevent a major change by placing the cultures in the chamber and exchanging the air with the gas mixture until the pH drops—before continuing to dispense the cells.

5. After preparing all of the cultures, place the trays of culture dishes into the culture chamber, secure the chamber lid, and exchange the air with the gas mixture. Adjust the gas regulator to a low flow rate and make sure that the culture chamber receives gas from the upper inlet to avoid blowing the lids off the dishes.

6. Place the culture chamber on a rocker platform in a 37°C incubator and rock at 7–14 cycles per minute.

7. Feed the cultures daily with nutritive cocktail and FCS in either of two ways:

   a. Prepare a feeding mixture consisting of 2 parts cocktail and 1 part FCS. Add 3 drops to each dish with a Pasteur pipette or 2 drops with a 5- or 10-ml pipette.

b. With Pasteur pipettes, add 1 drop of FCS and 2 drops of cocktail to each dish. Add the cocktail after the FCS has been added since the cocktail is alkaline.

Re-gas the cultures after each feeding. After thawing, store nutritional cocktail at 4°C; discard after two weeks.

Cell Harvest

Harvest the cultures after 4–5 days of incubation. Harvest them rapidly since they turn alkaline when removed from the gas mixture. Scrape the dishes with a policeman and transfer the contents of the cultures to 17 × 100-mm tubes. Pellet the cells by centrifugation ($200 \times g$, 10 min). Immediately remove the medium and replace it with an appropriate volume of BSS. Hold the pelleted cells on ice until ready to assay.

COMMENTS

1. After 4–5 days in culture, approximately 30–35% of the cells will be recovered if MEM is used, whereas 50–60% of the cells may be recovered if the cells have been cultured in RPMI 1640. Optimal responses range from 1000–12 000 plaque-forming cells (PFC) per culture in a primary response to SRBC.

2. We tease spleens at room temperature and keep the cells cold during all other steps in the procedure unless experimental design prevents this (e.g., treatment with rabbit anti–mouse brain serum). Some investigators claim that chilling the cells has a deleterious effect in some systems. We have compared cells handled in both ways and found no difference in response in the system described above.

3. Both MEM and RPMI 1640 are buffered to maintain pH 7.0–7.4 in a 5–10% CO_2 atmosphere; exposure to the lower CO_2 content of air results in a shift to alkaline pH. The surface area of the cultures described above is sufficiently large that the pH can shift quite rapidly. When the color of the cultures begins to change, immediately place them in the culture chamber and administer the special gas mixture. Continue with the procedure in progress only after adjusting the pH. The medium can be supplemented with 25 mM HEPES buffer to maintain the pH independent of the CO_2 content of the atmosphere. Commercially prepared media

buffered with HEPES are available but expensive. Considerable savings can be achieved by purchasing separately 1 M HEPES buffer and using it to supplement conventionally buffered media.

4. Unless dialysis tubing is specially prepared (Appendix D), dialyzed reagents can be very toxic to these cultures.

5. Certain inbred mouse strains respond strongly to an antigen(s) present on the red blood cells of some, but not all, sheep (McCarthy and Dutton 1975a, 1975b). To ensure maximum responses with these strains of mice, test red cells from different sheep to identify a donor that has the relevant red cell antigen(s).

6. In this system, the spleen cells from some strains of inbred mice respond less well than the spleen cells of others (regardless of the type of SRBC). C3H/HeJ, for example, generally respond poorly; BDF$_1$ hybrids (C57BL/6 × DBA/2) respond well.

7. All reagents must be prepared with nontoxic, double-distilled water and all glassware must be washed by methods appropriate for tissue culture (Appendix B).

8. At the end of the culture period, the cultures should be clear and red blood cells should be apparent. Cloudiness in a culture usually indicates microbial contamination. Contamination can occur even in the presence of antibiotics.

9. The cells may be cultured in the 16-mm wells of a 24-well tissue culture plate (Falcon, #3008 or Linbro, #FB-16-24-TC). The modifications are:

   a. Culture 2–5 × 10^6 cells per well in a volume of 0.25–0.5 ml of medium.

   b. Feed with approximately 30 μl (1 drop from a Pasteur pipette) of feeding mixture at 24-hour intervals.

   Our experience with the 16-mm wells suggests that optimal responses are obtainable only in a narrow spleen cell concentration range which varies with different cell preparations.

10. Occasionally, culture boxes fabricated in our shop and elsewhere have been toxic. The toxicity may be severe, resulting in the death of cells, or subtle, resulting in partial inhibition of the generation of primary immunity. We have generally found that such toxicity is due to either the glue or the plastic used in the construction of the boxes. Since the shortages in the world supply of plastics brought on by the oil embargo of 1973, we have found several lots of plastic to be insufficiently aged. Such plastics are toxic and may continue to release inhibitory volatiles for

several years. We recommend that samples of plastic to be used in the construction of boxes be incubated with cultures in culture boxes of known quality to determine if the plastics adversely affect responses. We also recommend that cultures from a single pool of spleen cells be established in both control and newly constructed boxes to test for subtle toxicity.

REFERENCES

Click, R. E., L. Benck, and B. J. Alter. 1972a. Enhancement of antibody synthesis *in vitro* by mercaptoethanol. *Cell. Immunol.* **3**:156.

Click, R. E., L. Benck, and B. J. Alter. 1972b. Immune responses *in vitro*. I. Culture conditions for antibody synthesis. *Cell. Immunol.* **3**:264.

Dutton, R. W., and R. I. Mishell. 1967. Cellular events in the immune response. The *in vitro* response of normal spleen cells to erythrocyte antigens. *Cold Spr. Harb. Symp. Quant. Biol.* **32**:407.

McCarthy, M. M., and R. W. Dutton. 1975a. The humoral response of mouse spleen cells to two types of sheep erythrocytes. I. Genetic control of the response to H and L SRBC. *J. Immunol.* **115**:1316.

McCarthy, M. M., and R.W. Dutton. 1975b. The humoral response of mouse spleen cells to two types of sheep erythrocytes. II. Evidence for gene expression in the B lymphocyte. *J. Immunol.* **115**:1322.

Mishell, R. I., and R. W. Dutton. 1966. Immunization of normal mouse spleen cell suspensions *in vitro*. *Science* **153**:1004.

Mishell, R. I., and R. W. Dutton. 1967. Immunization of dissociated spleen cell cultures from normal mice. *J. Exp. Med.* **126**:423.

Shiigi, S. M., and R. I. Mishell. 1975. Sera and the *in vitro* induction of immune responses. I. Bacterial contamination and the generation of good fetal bovine sera. *J. Immunol.* **115**:741.

Silverman, M. S., and M. F. La Via. 1976. Letters to the Editor, *J. Immunol.* **117**:2270.

2.3   PRIMARY IMMUNIZATION IN DIFFUSION CULTURES

John Marbrook

This method of culturing cells has been used to investigate the generation of antibody-producing cells, proliferative responses, and the development of cytotoxic lymphocytes. Many modifications of the original culture vessel have been devised and the simplest and most economical vessel is described here. The design of the system enables cells to grow as a layer of cells on a dialysis membrane that is immersed in a reservoir of culture medium. The design of the vessel allows the culture of cells under favorable nutritional conditions that do not require the repeated supply of additives.

MATERIALS AND REAGENTS

Preparation of Culture Vessels

EDTA
Glass tubing, 1-cm inside diameter, cut to 10-cm lengths
Round-bottom glass vessels, approximately 2.2 cm in diameter
Dialysis membrane
Silicon rubber tubing
Aluminum foil
Rubber band, standard type
Aluminum or stainless steel closures that fit loosely over the glass
   tubing

Culture Medium

RPMI 1640
Fetal calf serum (FCS)
2-mercaptoethanol (2-ME), 5×10^{-3} M (Appendix A.6)

Removal and Preparation of Spleen Cells

As described in Section 1.2 with the addition of:

FCS
HEPES-buffered balanced salt solution (Appendix A.4)

Cell Culture

Antigen
Culture vessels
CO_2 incubator (10% CO_2 in air)
FCS
Continuous dispensing syringe with a 16- or 18-gauge needle attached

PROCEDURE

Preparation of Culture Vessels

The size of the culture vessel can vary widely. The methods described here are for vessels assembled from the components given in
Figure 2.1.

1. Cut the inner vessel (glass tubing) to size and fire polish the edges.
   Wash the inner vessel and the reservoir (round-bottom glass vessel) as described in Appendix B.
2. Cut the dialysis membrane (approximately 2.5 × 2.5 cm) from
   standard rolls of dialysis tubing and boil two times in glass-
   distilled water. If toxic dialysis tubing is encountered, boil the
   membranes once in 0.1% EDTA and two times in glass-distilled
   water.

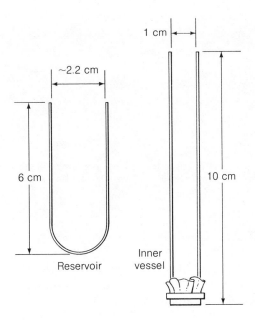

FIGURE 2.1
Dimensions of components for culture vessel.

3. Cut 3-mm sections from silicon rubber tubing of the appropriate diameter to prepare the silicon rubber bands. Boil the silicon rubber bands in glass-distilled water.

4. Clamp the dialysis membrane over the inner vessel with a silicon rubber band. This step is made easier if the membrane is first held in place by a loose-fitting collar made, for example, of Plexiglas. As shown in Figure 2.2, slip the collar off when the silicon rubber band is in place. Remove any wrinkles in the dialysis membrane by manipulating the edges. Use a piece of membrane slightly larger than is required and trim any excess with scissors after the band is in place.

5. Stand the assembled inner vessels upright in a beaker of glass-distilled water and discard any vessels that leak.

6. Place the vessel with membrane attached into the reservoir and roll a strip of aluminum foil around both the vessel and the reservoir with adequate overlap, as shown in Figure 2.3. Squeeze the top edge of the foil around the inner vessel and fix tightly in place with rubber band so that the tube is held in place. The level of the inner vessel can be adjusted later.

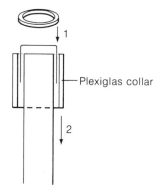

FIGURE 2.2
Method for holding membrane in place with a Plexiglas collar while securing silicone rubber band.

7. Place the closures on the inner vessels, as shown in Figure 2.3, and autoclave the assembled culture vessels (120°C, 20 min). Stand the culture vessels upright in a glass or stainless steel beaker during autoclaving. The sterile culture vessels can be stored for long periods under normal laboratory conditions.

Culture Medium

To prepare 100 ml of complete medium, mix 10 ml FCS with 1 ml 5 × 10^{-3} M 2-ME and bring up to a volume of 100 ml with RPMI 1640 (see

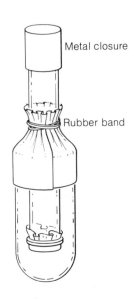

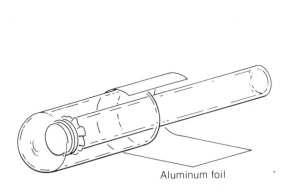

FIGURE 2.3
Assembly of culture vessel.

comment 4). If all the cultures are to receive the same antigen, add the antigen to the medium (e.g., add 0.4 ml of 10% v/v SRBC suspension to 100 ml medium). The final antigen concentration will be approximately 4×10^6 cells/ml.

Removal and Preparation of Spleen Cells

1. Remove and tease mouse spleens by the procedure described in Section 1.2, with the following modifications: Tease the cells in ice-cooled HEPES-buffered BSS (Appendix A.4) containing 5% FCS. After teasing, keep the cells cool in an ice bucket at each subsequent step.

2. Transfer the suspended cells from the teasing dish into a conical centrifuge tube and quickly underlayer the suspension with 0.5–1.0 ml FCS (use a Pasteur pipette). Allow the cell suspension to settle into the FCS for 5 minutes. Clumps of connective tissue and other debris settle into the FCS and are thus cleanly separated from the single-cell suspension.

3. Transfer the cell suspension to a graduated centrifuge tube, centrifuge ($200 \times g$, 10 min), discard supernatant, and resuspend cells to 1.4×10^7 cells/ml in FCS-supplemented medium (the optimum cell concentration will depend on the dimensions of the culture tube and the nature of the immune response under investigation).

Cell Culture

1. An outer reservoir of 8–10 ml is quite adequate with an inner vessel of the dimensions shown in Figure 2.1. Fill the reservoir with medium using a continuous dispensing syringe (see Figure 2.4): (a) Flame the surface of the foil. (b) Raise the inner vessel, insert the needle through the foil, and dispense 8–10 ml of medium into the reservoir. (c) Withdraw the needle and lower the inner chamber. (d) Flame the perforation made by the needle in the foil.

2. Place 1.0 ml of cell suspension (including antigen) into each of the inner vessels. Adjust the height of the inner vessels such that the level of the medium in the inner vessel is the same as that in the reservoir.

3. Place the cultures in a CO_2 incubator (10% CO_2 in air).

4. After a given period of culture (never longer than 7–8 days), remove the cells by resuspending them with a Pasteur pipette; then centrifuge the suspension. Although macrophage-like cells adhere to the membrane, all plaque-forming cells (and cytotoxic lymphocytes) can be harvested by fairly vigorous resuspension with a Pasteur pipette.

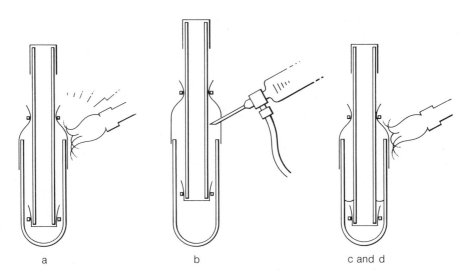

FIGURE 2.4
Filling the culture vessel.

COMMENTS

1. After 4 days in culture, about 50% of the cells can be recovered. The number of plaque-forming cells (PFC) is usually 100–500 PFC/10^6 cells placed into culture. The level of the responses depends, in part, on the age and strain of the mouse donor.

2. If a large number of cultures are set up, the medium may become alkaline. It is therefore best to gas the medium with CO_2 so that it is initially slightly acidic. Cells survive in slightly acidic conditions but quickly lose viability when the medium becomes slightly alkaline. (Never gas medium that contains cells with 100% CO_2; the pH changes too rapidly to be controlled.)

3. The size of the culture vessel can vary widely. However, since the optimal concentration of cells will depend on both the dimension of the inner vessel and the nature of the immune response under investigation, control experiments should be carried out to determine the optimal cell concentration (and suspension volume) for any particular size of culture vessel. Several sizes of vessels designed for use with this culture system are available from Bellco Glass.

4. The choice of medium will depend on the experimental system. For examining the generation of murine antibody-forming cells, we use RPMI 1640 with no additives, except FCS.

5. We have found that silicon rubber tubing is the best source of nontoxic rubber bands able to withstand repeated boiling and autoclaving. Many other types of tubing are cytotoxic even after prolonged boiling.

6. A modified culture vessel that uses the diffusion principle has been designed to fit inside a Petri dish (Maizels and Dresser 1977); the modified vessel enables experimenters to save tissue culture medium and facilitates the handling of large numbers of cultures. (A disposable version of this culture vessel is commercially available from Hendley Engineering, Victoria Rd., Buckhurst Hill, Essex, England.)

REFERENCES

Maizels, R. M., and D. W. Dresser. 1977. Conditions for the development of IgM and IgG antibody secreting cells from primed splenocytes *in vitro*. *Immunology* **32**:793.

Marbrook, J. 1967. Primary immune response in cultures of spleen cells. *Lancet* **ii**:1279.

Marbrook, J., and J. S. Haskill. 1974. The *in vitro* response to sheep erythrocytes by mouse spleen cells: Segregation of distinct events leading to antibody formation. *Cell. Immunol.* **13**:12.

2.4 SECONDARY IMMUNIZATION TO HETEROLOGOUS ERYTHROCYTES

Eva Lee Chan, Barbara B. Mishell, and Stanley M. Shiigi

Substantial secondary humoral responses to heterologous erythrocytes occur under less stringent culture conditions than those required to produce primary responses. For example, it is possible to induce large secondary responses in the presence of sera that will not support primary responses (Mishell and Dutton 1967; Watson and Epstein 1973; Shiigi and Mishell 1975) and with a wider range of cell concentrations. To obtain secondary responses to heterologous red cells *in vitro*, it is necessary to prime mice with an intravenous injection of red blood cells (RBC) and remove the spleens at various intervals after priming, depending on whether primarily IgM or IgG responses are the object of study.

When spleen cells from mice primed 3 days earlier are cultured, a response of 10 000 to 100 000 anti-RBC PFC per culture (mainly IgM) occurs on days 3 to 4 of culture. The *in vitro* response is considerably greater than that obtained *in vivo* with similar priming conditions. The reason for this is not known but may stem from the absence *in vitro* of inhibitory antibody feedback mechanisms (Mishell and Dutton 1967).

The responses of spleen cells obtained from mice primed with RBC 7–14 days prior to culture includes both IgM and IgG PFC. With standard *in vitro* doses of antigen, the IgM:IgG ratio ranges from 1:1 to 2:1. To study the IgG response, it is desirable to have a greater difference in the ratio of the responses. This can be achieved by lowering the dose of RBC *in vitro,* which reduces the IgM response while maintaining the IgG response.

MATERIALS AND REAGENTS

In Vivo Priming

Sheep red blood cells (SRBC) or other red blood cells
Balanced salt solution (BSS; Appendix A.3) or saline: 0.85% NaCl, w/v, sterile
Tuberculin syringe with 27-gauge needle
Conical, graduated centrifuge tube

Removal and Preparation of Spleen Cells

As described in Section 1.2

Cell Culture

As described in Section 2.2

PROCEDURE

In Vivo Priming

1. Wash SRBC 3 times in sterile BSS or saline (400 $\times$ g, 10 minutes) in a conical graduated tube. Resuspend to 1% (v/v).

2. Inject mice intravenously in one of the lateral tail veins with 0.2 ml of the red blood cell suspension. (For a description of this procedure, see Garvey et al. 1977, p.11).

Removal and Preparation of Spleen Cells

As described in Section 1.2.

Cell Culture

Culture the cells as described in Section 2.2, with the following modifications:

1. When using spleen cell suspensions from mice immunized 3 days prior to culture, harvest the cultures after 3–4 days of incubation instead of after 4–5 days.

2. To study IgG responses, use spleen cell suspensions from mice immunized 7–14 days prior to culture. In addition, reduce the *in vitro* antigen dose to $\frac{1}{20}$ the standard dose of 3×10^6 SRBC/ml. Add either 0.3 ml of a 0.05% (v/v) suspension of SRBC to 100 ml of medium or 30 μl of a 0.005% suspension to each 1-ml culture. Either way, each 1-ml culture will receive approximately 1.5×10^5 SRBC.

COMMENT

Secondary cultures frequently are acidic at the end of the incubation period.

REFERENCES

Garvey, J. S., N. E. Cremer, and D. H. Sussdorf. 1977. *Methods in Immunology,* W. A. Benjamin, Reading, Mass.

Mishell, R. I., and R. W. Dutton. 1967. Immunization of dissociated spleen cell cultures from normal mice. *J. Exp. Med.* **126**:423.

Shiigi, S. M., L. S. Fujikawa, and R. I. Mishell. 1975. Sera and the *in vitro* induction of immune responses. II. Inhibitory effects of newborn calf sera on primary humoral responses. *J. Immunol.* **115**:745.

Watson, J., and R. Epstein. 1973. The role of humoral factors in the initiation of *in vitro* primary immune responses. I. Effects of deficient fetal bovine serum. *J. Immunol.* **110**:31.

2.5 SECONDARY IMMUNIZATION TO NITROPHENYL HAPTENS

Linda M. Bradley and Stanley M. Shiigi, with contributions from John North

Secondary IgG responses can be generated *in vitro* using spleen cells from mice primed with the nitrophenyl haptens—trinitrophenyl (TNP) or dinitrophenyl (DNP)—coupled to protein carriers such as keyhole limpet hemocyanin (KLH). With suspension cultures, optimal responses are obtained when lymphocyte donor mice are immunized twice (Figure 2.5): first, with antigen and adjuvant; second, two to eight months later, with soluble antigen without adjuvant. Seven to 14 days after the second injection, spleen cells from the primed animals are challenged *in vitro* with antigen. After 5 days of culture, hapten-specific antibody-forming cells are measured. The secondary responses to DNP-KLH or TNP-KLH range from 500 to 1000 IgM antibody-forming cells per culture and from 2000 to 50 000 IgG antibody-forming cells per culture (under the experimental conditions described below). If the second booster injection is omitted, IgM responses predominate (North and Askonas 1976). However, in diffusion culture vessels, it is possible to elicit IgG responses of similar magnitude without a second immunization (North and Maizels 1977).

The TNP and DNP haptens are highly cross-reactive at the level of the antibody-forming-cell precursors and their progeny. For this reason, it is possible to immunize *in vivo* with, for example, DNP conjugates, but challenge *in vitro* with TNP conjugates. In addition, cells from animals that have been primed and boosted *in vivo* and challenged *in vitro* with either TNP or DNP conjugates can be assayed for antibody-forming cells using TNP modified red blood cells. (Direct coupling of DNP to red blood cells is not practicable.)

For many experimental purposes, it is desirable to manipulate hapten- and carrier-primed populations separately. For such experiments, spleen cells from mice primed with nitrophenyl-protein conjugates (as described above) provide a source of hapten-primed B cells. Splenic carrier-specific helper T cells can be generated by either one of two methods. Mice can be primed to the same carrier that is used to generate hapten-specific B cells (Figure 2.6). However, if this procedure is used, the hapten-primed population must be depleted of T cells prior to use in the *in vitro* phase of the experiment. Alternatively, mice can be immunized with a carrier unrelated to the hapten-carrier conjugate used to prime the B cells (Figure 2.7). (The unrelated carrier can be either heterologous red blood cells or protein.) The two separately generated spleen cell populations are combined *in vitro* and immunized with a conjugate consisting of the hapten to which the B cells are primed and the carrier to which the T cells are primed.

In general, immunization with the carrier induces both helper and suppressor T cell activities. Which activity is expressed depends upon such factors as the particular carrier, the immunization regimen, and the culture conditions used to elicit the response. In several systems, procedures that inhibit cellular proliferation (irradiation, Section 10.4; treatment with mitomycin C, Section 10.3) eliminate detectable T suppressor activity without significantly inhibiting T helper activity (e.g., Chan and Henry 1976; Swain et al. 1977). When KLH is used for carrier priming following the procedure described below for hapten-modified KLH, the T helper function is dominant. However, when sheep red blood cells (SRBC) are used for carrier immunization (Kettman and Dutton 1970) as described below, significant T cell suppression is generated. We therefore routinely use irradiation to remove suppressor cells in order to elicit maximum help from spleen cells primed to the SRBC carrier. When irradiated SRBC primed T cells are combined *in vitro* with DNP-KLH primed B cells and TNP-SRBC is used as antigen, the magnitudes of the secondary hapten-specific IgM and IgG responses are similar to the ranges indicated above for responses to DNP-KLH.

A. Anti-Nitrophenyl Responses Using TNP(or DNP)-KLH Primed Spleen Cells

MATERIALS AND REAGENTS

TNP(or DNP)-KLH Priming

Bordetella pertussis vaccine (Commonwealth of Massachusetts, Department of Public Health)

TNP-KLH or DNP-KLH, 5 mg/ml in phosphate-buffered saline (PBS; Appendix A.8; See Section 16.3 for preparation of TNP-KLH)

Aluminum potassium sulfate (alum), 9% (w/v) in water

Syringes, 1 ml

Needles, 25 gauge

Removal and Preparation of Spleen Cells

As described in Section 1.2

Cell Culture

As described in Section 2.2, substituting TNP(or DNP)-KLH as antigen

PROCEDURE (see Figure 2.5)

TNP(or DNP)-KLH Priming

1. Mix equal volumes of antigen and alum. Adjust mixture to pH 6.5 and let stand for 30 minutes to allow a maximum of precipitate to form. Pellet the precipitate by centrifugation ($750 \times g$, 5 min) and discard the supernatant.

2. Resuspend the pellet in a mixture of PBS and *B. pertussis* so that the protein concentration is 500–1000 μg/ml, with 1–2 $\times$ 10^{10} *B. pertussis* organisms/ml.

3. Inject 100 μg of protein and 2 $\times$ 10^9 *B. pertussis* organisms/mouse intraperitoneally in a volume of 0.1 to 0.2 ml.

4. Rest the mice 2–8 months. Boost mice with an intravenous or intraperitoneal injection of 20 μg of soluble TNP-KLH or DNP-KLH 7–14 days prior to culture.

5. As an alternative to the above priming procedure, emulsify the antigen in Freund's complete adjuvant (Appendix F), using the method described for Lac-KLH (Section 2.6). For the initial priming, inject 100 μg of antigen either intraperitoneally or distributed among the rear footpads; follow the initial priming by an i.v. or i.p. boost with 20 μg of soluble antigen 2–8 months later.

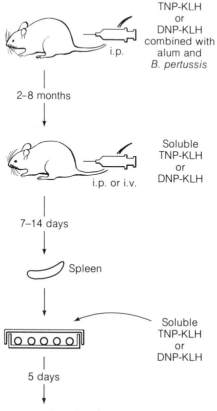

FIGURE 2.5
Anti-nitrophenyl responses using TNP(or
DNP)-KLH primed spleen cells (Procedure A).

Removal and Preparation of Spleen Cells

As described in Section 1.2.

Cell Culture

1. Procedures for culture are identical to those described in Section
   2.2. Batches of fetal calf serum that support responses to
   heterologous red blood cells usually also support responses to
   TNP-KLH or DNP-KLH. Culture the cells at $5–15 \times 10^6$ cells/ml.

2. Immunize the cultures with a predetermined optimal dose of soluble TNP(or DNP)-KLH dissolved in complete medium. We have found that 0.03 μg/culture is effective for highly conjugated KLH.

3. Harvest the cultures on day 5 and assay for anti-TNP plaqueforming cells by the procedure described in Section 3.8.

COMMENT

It is essential to assay plaque-forming cells with unmodified as well as hapten-modified target red blood cells, since "background" responses to unmodified red blood cells may be relatively high. The response to the unmodified targets is subtracted from that of the hapten-modified targets to provide a measure of the hapten-specific response.

B. Anti-Nitrophenyl Responses Using TNP(or DNP)-KLH Primed B Cells and KLH Primed T Cells

MATERIALS AND REAGENTS

TNP(or DNP)-KLH and KLH Priming

As described in Section 2.5A, with the addition of: KLH, 5 mg/ml in PBS

Removal and Preparation of Spleen Cells

As described in Section 1.2

Depletion of T Cells from TNP(or DNP)-KLH Primed Spleen Cells

As described in Section 9.2, with the following antiserum: Rabbit anti–mouse brain serum (RAMB; Section 11.1)

Cell Culture

As described in Section 2.2

PROCEDURE (see Figure 2.6)

TNP(or DNP)-KLH and KLH Priming

Prime one set of mice with TNP(or DNP)-KLH and another set with KLH as described in Section 2.5A. Use mice of the same strain, sex, and age.

Removal and Preparation of Spleen Cells

Remove spleens and prepare suspensions from both sets of mice as described in Section 1.2.

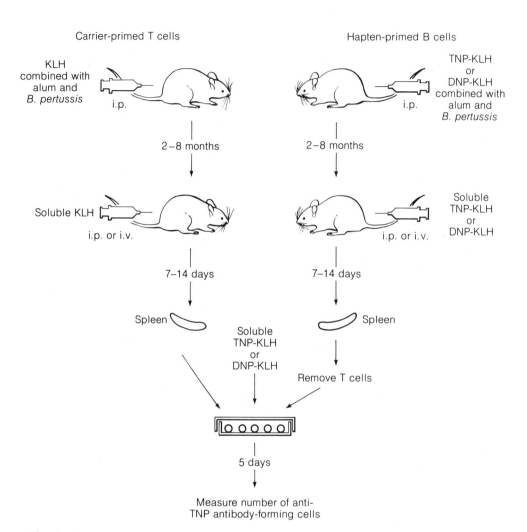

FIGURE 2.6
Anti-nitrophenyl responses using TNP(or DNP)-KLH primed
B cells and KLH primed T cells (Procedure B).

Depletion of T Cells from TNP(or DNP)-KLH Primed Spleen Cells

Remove T cells from the TNP(or DNP)-KLH primed spleen cell population by the procedure described in Section 9.2.

Cell Culture

1. Culture the cells by the procedure described in Section 2.2. Combine $5-8 \times 10^6$ hapten-primed B cells and an equal number (or

more) of carrier-primed T cells. Immunize cultures with 0.03 μg/culture of highly conjugated TNP(or DNP)-KLH.

2. Harvest cultures on day 5 and assay for anti-TNP plaque-forming cells by the procedure described in Section 3.8.

COMMENT

See comment 1 in Section 2.5A.

C. Anti-Nitrophenyl Responses Using TNP(or DNP)-KLH Primed B Cells and SRBC Primed T Cells

MATERIALS AND REAGENTS

Low-Dose Carrier Priming with SRBC

Sheep red blood cells (SRBC), 0.05% (v/v) in sterile BSS
Balanced salt solution (BSS; Appendix A.3), sterile
Syringes, 1 ml
Needles, 27 gauge

Heavy TNP Modification of SRBC
for Use as *In Vitro* Immunogen

Fetal calf serum (FCS), heat inactivated (56°C, 30 min)
2,4,6-trinitrobenzene sulphonic acid (TNBS), $M_r = 293$, (Sigma Chemical, #P-5878)
Cacodylate buffer, 0.28 M, pH 6.9 (Appendix A.13)
Glucose-phosphate-buffered saline (G-PBS), pH 7.6 (Appendix A.11)
Small plastic tube with cap
Rotator (Scientific Products, #R4193-1)

Removal and Preparation of Spleen Cells

As described in Section 1.2

Cell Culture

As described in Section 2.2

PROCEDURE (see Figure 2.7)

Low-Dose Carrier Priming with SRBC

Inject 0.2 ml of the 0.05% SRBC suspension per mouse, intravenously, 3 days prior to culture.

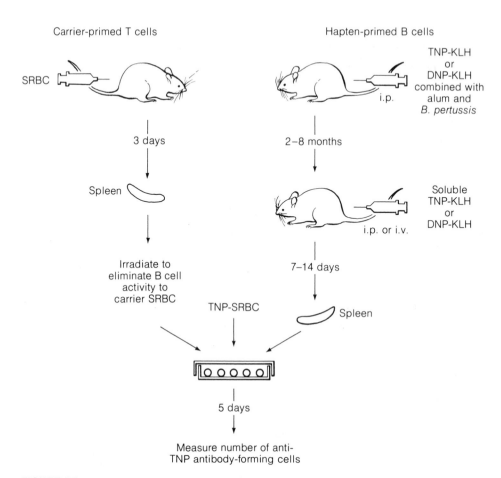

FIGURE 2.7
Anti-nitrophenyl responses using TNP(or DNP)-KLH primed
B cells and SRBC primed T cells (Procedure C).

Heavy TNP Modification of SRBC
for Use as *In Vitro* Immunogen

Note: Avoid skin contact with TNBS. To prevent sensitization and
contact dermatitis, wear disposable gloves. Cacodylate buffer is
poisonous; avoid skin contact and do not pipet by mouth.

1. Dissolve 75 mg of TNBS in 4 ml of cacodylate buffer at room
   temperature. Sterilize the solution by membrane filtration (Appendix C.2).
2. Wash SRBC 4 times with G-PBS (400 × g, 10 min).

3. Add 0.3 ml of packed SRBC drop by drop to 2.1 ml of sterile TNBS-cacodylate solution in a small, sterile plastic tube. Cap the tube tightly and wrap tube in foil to prevent photodecomposition of TNBS.

4. Tumble the mixture for 30 minutes at room temperature.

5. Wash the cells in cold G-PBS containing 1% heat-inactivated fetal calf serum until the supernatants are colorless; wash at least 4 times.

6. For *in vitro* immunization, use 30 μl of a 0.1% TNP-SRBC suspension per ml of culture.

Removal and Preparation of Spleen Cells

As described in Section 1.2.

Cell Culture

1. Culture the cells by the procedure described in Section 2.2. Irradiate the SRBC primed spleen cells (1000–2700 R) as described in Section 10.4. Combine 5–8 × 10^6 TNP(or DNP)-KLH primed spleen cells with an equal number (or more) of irradiated SRBC primed cells. Immunize the cultures with the TNP-SRBC suspension prepared by heavy modification.

2. Harvest the cultures on day 5 and assay for anti-TNP plaque-forming cells by the procedures described in Section 3.8. It is preferable to use TNP modified horse red blood cells (HRBC) as the indicator cells since a primary response to SRBC is also generated in the cultures.

COMMENTS

1. See comment 1 in Section 2.5A.

2. Primary IgM responses to TNP modified red blood cells are also readily obtainable *in vitro* (Kettman and Dutton 1970). TNP-SRBC prepared by the 'heavy' modification developed by Kettman and Dutton (see above) is used as immunogen. Because TNP specific primary responses tend to be low when spleens from normal unimmunized mice are cultured, many workers prefer to use cells from donors that have been primed to the red blood cell carrier. Alternatively, it is possible to mix cells from normal unimmunized mice with irradiated cells from carrier-primed mice to provide adequate T helper activity. Culture conditions are otherwise the same as those described in Section 2.2.

REFERENCES (for 2.5)

Chan, E. L., and C. Henry. 1976. Coexistence of helper and suppressor activities in carrier primed spleen cells. *J. Immunol.* **117**:1132.

Kettman, J., and R. W. Dutton. 1970. An *in vitro* primary immune response to 2,4,6-trinitrophenyl substituted erythrocytes: response against carrier and hapten. *J. Immunol.* **104**:1558.

Kettman, J., and R. W. Dutton. 1971. Radioresistance of the enhancing effect of cells from carrier immunized mice in an *in vitro* primary immune response. *Proc. Nat. Acad. Sci.* (USA) **68**:699.

North, J. R., and B. A. Askonas. 1976. IgG response *in vitro*. I. The requirement for an intermediate responsive cell type. *Eur. J. Immunol.* **6**:8.

North, J. R., and R. M. Maizels. 1977. B memory cells can be stimulated by antigen *in vitro* to become IgG antibody secreting cells. *Immunology* **32**:771.

Swain, S. L., P. E. Trefts, H. Y. S. Tse, and R. W. Dutton. 1977. The significance of T-B collaboration across haplotype barriers. *Cold Spr. Harb. Symp. Quant. Biol.* **XLI**:597.

2.6   SECONDARY IMMUNIZATION TO AZOPHENYL HAPTENS

Claudia Henry

Azophenyl haptens, in contrast to the nitrophenyls (TNP and DNP), are hydrophilic. Because hydrophobic interactions contribute significantly to the binding of antibodies and their ligands, hydrophobic determinants react with a relatively large number of structurally different antibody molecules, with affinities ranging from low to very high. Thus, nitrophenyls bind to and trigger a high frequency of cells. By comparison, hydrophilic determinants react with a relatively small number of structurally different antibodies and achieve only moderate binding affinities. Therefore, the hydrophilic azophenyl haptens are useful in studies of immune induction conducted by experimentalists who wish to study the interactions of immunogens and lymphocytes without the nearly ubiquitous binding of the nitrophenyls.

We have employed azophenyl lactoside (Lac) conjugated to keyhole limpet hemocyanin (KLH) or heterologous red blood cells in most of our work with the hydrophilic haptens. We describe our methods in detail below. Similar methods apply to the use of other azophenyl haptens, such as azophenyl glucoside (Glu), azophenyl arsonate (Ars), azophenyl sulfonate (Sulf), azobenzoyl glutamate (Glut), and azobenzoyl glycine (Gly). Since the reagents for preparing conjugates of Ars, Sulf, Glut, and Gly are inexpensive and readily available from commercial suppliers, these conjugates may be conveniently used by laboratories not prepared to do the organic syntheses usually required for the preparation of Lac and Glu conjugates. Although there is some cross-reactivity between Sulf and anti-Ars (see Section 13.2), the other haptens listed above react only with their specific antibodies.

Primary responses to the hydrophilic azophenyl haptens are small, probably reflecting the low frequency in unprimed mice of precursor cells whose surface immunoglobulins bind those determinants. Therefore, in most studies using azophenyl haptens, cells for *in vitro* experiments are obtained from mice that have been immunized. The *in vitro* responses of primed cells to azophenyl protein conjugates range from 8000 to 80 000 IgG antibody-forming cells per culture. IgM responses are small, accounting for only about 5% of the total plaque responses.

MATERIALS AND REAGENTS

Priming of Mice

Mice: $H-2^d$ and $H-2^k$ strains have been used with success; strains with other haplotypes have not been tested.

Horse red blood cells (HRBC)

Lac-KLH (Section 16.2), containing about 40 Lac groups per 10^5 daltons. Dilute a stock solution of 2–4 mg/ml immediately before use.

Glu-KLH (Section 16.2), containing about 40 Glu groups per 10^5 daltons. Dilute a stock solution of 2–4 mg/ml immediately before use.

Complete Freund's adjuvant (CFA). Note: Freund's adjuvant is a potentially hazardous agent (see Appendix F).

1-ml tuberculin syringe, Luer-lock, with a 24-gauge needle. Note: If Luer-lock syringes are not available, protective glasses should be worn (see Appendix F).

Removal and Preparation of Spleen Cells

As described in Section 1.2

Culture Medium

Fetal calf serum (FCS), pretested: Lots found satisfactory for a primary anti-SRBC response are not necessarily optimal for an anti-Lac response, but they provide a good starting point for testing (see Appendix A.1).

RPMI 1640 with 25 mM HEPES buffer

$100\times$ vitamins

100 mM sodium pyruvate

$100\times$ nonessential amino acids

$200\times$ L-asparagine stock: 4 mg/ml of RPMI 1640

Freshly prepared 5×10^{-3} M 2-mercaptoethanol (2-ME; Appendix A.6)

Cell Culture

As described in Section 2.2, plus Lac-KLH or Lac-HRBC (Section 3.8).

PROCEDURE

Priming with Lac-KLH

Lymphocytes from Lac-KLH primed mice are used for anti-Lac *in vitro* responses of unseparated cells or as a source of Lac-specific B cells after removal of T cells from the cell suspension by treatment with anti–T cell serum and complement (Section 9.2).

1. Emulsify equal volumes of Lac-KLH (1.0 mg Lac-KLH/ml of saline) and CFA as described in Appendix F.
2. Inject a total of 0.1 ml of the emulsion (equivalent to 50 μg Lac-KLH), distributing it among the rear foot pads.
3. Six to thirty weeks later, inject intravenously 50 μg of Lac-KLH in saline.
4. Use the spleens 3–8 weeks after the second injection. Although good responses can be obtained 1 week after the second injection, waiting 3 weeks precludes the addition of specific antibody-secreting cells to the cultures.

Priming with KLH or Glu-KLH

In studies of *in vitro* responses to Lac-KLH, mice primed with either unmodified KLH or KLH conjugated with Glu or Ars are good sources of KLH-specific primed T helper cells. (Since the azo-protein carrier of the hapten-KLH conjugates is more analogous to that of Lac-KLH, these conjugates are usually preferable to unmodified KLH.) The following immunization schedule produces good T helper cell activity and avoids the complication of adding cells that are secreting anti-KLH antibody to the cultures.

1. Emulsify equal volumes of Glu-KLH (1.0 mg/ml in saline) and CFA as described in Appendix F.
2. Inject 0.1 ml of emulsion, distributing it among the rear foot pads.
3. Six to thirty weeks later, intravenously inject 50 μg of Glu-KLH, Ars-KLH, or KLH in saline.
4. Use the spleens 2–3 days later.

Priming with HRBC

This procedure is used to prepare HRBC specific T helper cells for use with Lac-HRBC as the *in vitro* antigen. High priming doses of

HRBC generate less suppressor cell activity than low doses. However, suppressor cell activity can be removed by irradiation (as little as 500 R is effective). Substantial helper activity can be recovered from primed spleen cells that have been irradiated with doses of up to 2700 R (Henry 1975; Chan and Henry 1976).

1. Inject intravenously 2×10^6 HRBC (low dose) or 2×10^8 HRBC (high dose) in 0.2 ml of sterile saline.
2. Remove the spleens 2–3 days later, and irradiate suspensions with 1000–2700 R as described in Section 10.4.

Preparation of Culture Medium

For 100 ml of complete medium: 1.0 ml of nonessential amino acids, 1.0 ml of sodium pyruvate, 1.0 ml of vitamins, 1.0 ml of 5×10^{-3} M 2-ME, 0.5 ml of L-asparagine stock, and 8.0 ml of pretested FCS. Make up to 100 ml with RPMI 1640 containing 25 mM HEPES buffer.

Removal and Preparation of Spleen Cells

As described in Section 1.2.

Cell Culture

Procedures for culture are identical to those described in Section 2.2 with the following modifications:

1. A dose of 0.02 μg Lac-KLH per ml of culture is usually used (optimal responses to azophenyl-KLH conjugates modified as above occur with doses ranging from 0.002 μg to 0.2 μg per ml). Prepare a fresh solution of 0.2 μg of Lac-KLH per ml of complete medium and add 0.1 ml per ml of culture. For azophenyl-HRBC conjugates, use 0.1 ml containing 6×10^5 HRBC for each ml of culture.
2. Suspend spleen cells to a concentration of $8–12 \times 10^6$ cells/ml in complete medium and add 1.0 ml of the cell suspension to each culture dish.
3. Harvest the cultures after 5 days of incubation and assay the anti-hapten response by the methods described in Section 3.8, using Lac-SRBC as indicator cells.

COMMENTS

1. Like responses to other hapten-carrier conjugates, responses to azophenyl haptens conjugated to KLH or HRBC have the advantage that a B cell population responding to the hapten and a T cell population responding to the carrier (KLH or HRBC) can be ma-

nipulated separately. Dilution assays of such specific B and T cells
are also feasible. For responses to Lac-KLH or Lac-HRBC for
example, Lac-specific B cells are obtained by treating spleen cell
suspension from Lac-KLH primed mice with anti–T cell serum
and complement (Section 9.2). It is possible to establish dose response curves for the Lac-specific B cells by adding a range of
5×10^4 to 5×10^6 of such T-depleted hapten-primed "B" cells to
cultures containing a constant number of carrier-primed T cells.
Usually, maximum T helper activity occurs with 2.5–5×10^6
azo-KLH primed spleen cells or 8×10^6 HRBC primed spleen
cells. Since the carrier-primed donor populations contain insignifi-
cant numbers of Lac-reactive B cells, there is no need to remove B
cells from the carrier-primed populations.

To determine dose response curves for carrier-primed T cell
populations, add a range of 10^5 to 10^7 azo-KLH primed spleen
cells to cultures containing a constant number (4–8×10^6) of
hapten-specific B (T-depleted) cells.

No nutritional artifacts are observed with cell densities ranging
from 5×10^6 to 20×10^6 cells per ml of culture. If the concentration
is less than 5×10^6 cells/ml, use irradiated spleen cells from
unimmunized donors as "filler" cells.

2. The generation of *in vitro* responses to the azophenyl haptens appears to be much more dependent on the helper functions of both
   carrier-specific, antigen-primed T cells and antigen-independent
   "accessory" cells than is true for most other antigens. Responses
   to these haptens are therefore particularly useful in assaying the
   activities of these two cell types.

3. Secondary *in vitro* responses to azophenyl haptens have also been
   used to establish the existence of hapten-specific T helper cells
   (Henry and Trefts 1974). For these studies, B cells primed to one
   hapten (e.g., Lac) are combined with T cells primed to a different,
   non-cross-reacting hapten (Ars). The B cells are obtained by treating Lac-KLH primed spleen cells with anti–T cell serum and
   complement. To elicit Ars-specific T cells, mice are injected in the
   foot pads with an emulsion of CFA and Ars-*Mycobacterium* (Ars-
   Mb) conjugate. This conjugate is prepared as follows: Resuspend
   washed *Mycobacterium tuberculosis* in 0.125 M borate buffer, pH
   8.2 and react with *p*-diazonium phenylarsonate for 8 hours at 4°C
   at a concentration of 1 mM of the diazonium reagent per 200 mg of
   dry *M. tuberculosis*. Wash and resuspend in 0.15 M NaCl at a
   concentration of 1 mg/ml. Inject 50 μg of Ars-*Mb*, distributed
   among 2 to 4 pads. Six weeks to several months later, inject 50 μg

of Ars-HGG (human gamma globulin) intravenously. Harvest spleen cells 2 to 3 days later. *In vitro* anti-Lac responses with mixtures of the two cell populations are obtained when 0.02 μg of the double conjugate (Lac-KLH-Ars) is used as antigen in the cultures. When appropriate controls show that all KLH-specific T helper cells have been removed by the anti–T cell serum treatment of the Lac-KLH primed donors, anti-Lac responses indicate the presence of T cells specific for the Ars hapten.

REFERENCES

Chan, E. L., and C. Henry. 1976. Coexistence of helper and suppressor activities in carrier-primed spleen cells. *J. Immunol.* **117**:1132.

Henry, C. 1975. *In vitro* anti-hapten response to a lactoside-conjugated protein. *Cell. Immunol.* **19**:117.

Henry, C., and P. Trefts. 1974. Helper activity *in vitro* to a defined determinant. *Eur. J. Immunol.* **4**:824.

2.7 IMMUNIZATION IN MINIATURE SUSPENSION CULTURES (100 μl)

Douglas C. Vann

In recent years, modifications of the basic methods for preparing suspension and diffusion cultures have reduced the requisite volumes of the cultures as well as the required numbers of cells per culture. In a widely used modification, 10^5 to 10^6 cells are cultured in 100- to 300-μl volumes in microwell plates. In addition to conserving reagents, an advantage of this technique is that the hemolytic plaque assay can be performed directly in the wells (Section 3.6). These methods are particularly useful for experiments requiring a large number of assays (as in limiting dilution techniques) or when only a limited number of cells or other special reagents is available.

MATERIALS AND REAGENTS

As described in Section 2.2, with the following additions:

Microwell plates (Falcon, #3040) with lids (Falcon, #3041) or similar
Syringes, 5 ml, 2.5 ml, and 1 ml (Hamilton, #1005LT, #1002LT, and #1001LT, respectively) and repeating dispensers (Hamilton, #PB600-1 and #PB600-10)

PROCEDURE

1. In this procedure, cells are cultured in a total volume of 0.1 ml (see Comment 2). Depending on the experimental design, medium containing cells and antigen can be dispensed in 0.1-ml volumes or, alternatively, antigen and cells, each at 2× the desired final concentration, can be separately dispensed in 0.05-ml volumes.

2. Prepare culture medium as described in Section 2.2. If all wells are to receive the same antigen, prepare a 0.01% suspension of SRBC by adding 1 ml of a 1% (v/v) SRBC suspension in BSS per 100 ml of complete medium. Alternatively, prepare a 0.02% suspension of SRBC in medium and add 50 μl to individual wells. Either way, each well receives approximately 2×10^5 SRBC.

3. Remove and prepare spleen cells (Section 1.2). Suspend cells in medium such than $2–3 \times 10^5$ cells are contained in 100-μl aliquots ($2–3 \times 10^6$ cells/ml if cells and antigen are dispensed together) or 50-μl aliquots ($4–6 \times 10^6$ cells/ml if cells and antigen are dispensed separately).

4. Dispense appropriate volumes of cells and antigen so that each well contains a total volume of 100 μl.

5. Incubate cultures for 4–5 days in an atmosphere of 7% O_2, 10% CO_2, and 83% N_2 (5% CO_2 in air can also be used). Rock and feed daily as described in Section 2.2. Add 20 μl of the feeding mixture (2 parts cocktail and 1 part FCS) to each well with a 1-ml Hamilton syringe and dispenser.

6. Assay the humoral responses directly in the wells (Section 3.6) or harvest the cells with Pasteur pipettes and assay by other methods described in Chapter 3.

COMMENTS

1. Store Hamilton syringes used for sterile work filled with 70% ethanol to maintain sterility. Before use, rinse the syringes a number of times with sterile BSS, and rinse between different additions.

2. The method described above is for 100-μl volumes, but some investigators use up to 300 μl with success.

3. The medium described by Click et al. (1972a, 1972b) is used by some investigators.

REFERENCES

Click, R. E., L. Benck, and B. J. Alter. 1972a. Enhancement of antibody synthesis *in vitro* by mercaptoethanol. *Cell. Immunol.* 3:156.

Click, R. E., L. Benck, and B. J. Alter. 1972b. Immune responses *in vitro*. I. Culture conditions for antibody synthesis. *Cell. Immunol.* **3**:264.

Kappler, J. W. 1974. A micro-technique for hemolytic plaque assays. *J. Immunol.* **112**:1271.

Vann, D. C., and C. R. Dotson, 1974. Cellular cooperation and stimulatory factors in antibody responses: Limiting dilution analysis *in vitro*. *J. Immunol.* **112**:1149.

2.8 IMMUNIZATION IN MINIATURE DIFFUSION CULTURES (100 μl)

Erich F. Eipert and Luciano Adorini

We describe a practical miniaturized diffusion culture apparatus in which a single compact unit holds 24 individual cultures. The scale is one-tenth that of standard Marbrook-type cultures; each culture contains a volume of 0.1 ml and a reservoir of 1.0 ml. The optimal cell concentration of 2×10^6 spleen cells per culture allows the creation of at least 50 replicate cultures from a single mouse spleen. Once cells are in culture, the easy and simultaneous access to all cell chambers and reservoirs considerably simplifies experiments involving manipulations of cells or supernatants. Changes in reservoir medium can be carried out within seconds by simply exchanging the base unit for a fresh medium-filled base unit.

MATERIALS AND REAGENTS

Cell Chamber Assembly* (see Figure 2.8)

30-mm length of fire-polished glass tubing (8-mm outer diameter) with flange 20 mm from bottom (Figure 2.8a)

Rubber grommet through which 30-mm cell chamber fits to depth of the flange (Figure 2.8b)

Dialysis membrane or Nuclepore membrane (Nuclepore, #110606; Figure 2.8c)

Silicone rubber ring (5–6 mm) cut from tubing to fit tightly over glass tubing and hold membrane in place (Figure 2.8d)

Holding Frame for Cell Chambers* (See Figure 2.8f for dimensions and construction)

Materials include 4-mm thick polycarbonate (lexan) plastic and lex-grip adhesive (General Electric, Plastics Business Division)

---

* The cell chamber assembly and holding frame, adapted to Costar multiwell plates, are commercially available from Bellco Glass, Inc., Vineland, NJ, 08360.

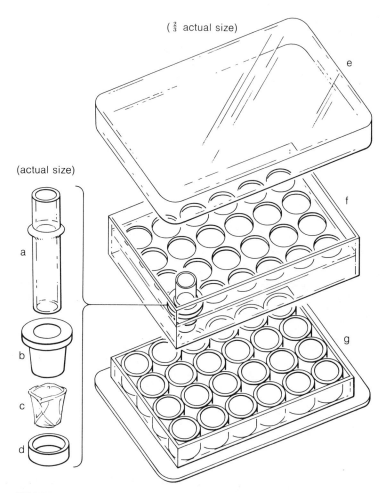

FIGURE 2.8
Schematic diagram of cell chamber assembly (a)–(d) and holding frame
(f), used with the cover (e) and plate (g) of the multiwell tissue culture plate.
(From Eipert, Adorini, and Couderc 1978. With permission from Elsevier/
North-Holland Biomedical Press.)

Culture Medium

RPMI 1640 medium, 100 ml, supplemented with:

  200 mM L-glutamine, 1 ml

  Fetal calf serum (FCS), 10 ml

  5×10^{-3} M 2-mercaptoethanol (Appendix A.6), 1 ml

  Penicillin-streptomycin (5000 units penicillin, 5000 μg streptomycin), 1 ml

  1 M HEPES buffer, pH 7.2, 1.5 ml (optional)

Spleen Cell Suspension

As described in Section 1.2.

Cell Culture

Antigen (e.g., SRBC)
Culture box* (Bellco Glass, #7741-10005)
Multiwell tissue culture plate (Falcon, #3008; see Figure 2.8e and g)
Cell counting equipment
Gas mixture: 7% O_2, 10% CO_2, 83% N_2

PROCEDURE

Assembly of Culture Vessels (see Figure 2.8)

1. Boil dialysis membrane in distilled water 2 times for 15 minutes. (Nuclepore membrane can be used without boiling.)
2. Cut membrane in squares (approximately 1.5 × 1.5 cm). Assemble the diffusion chambers and fit them in the holding frame (see Figure 2.8).
3. Put the frame in a surgical tray containing enough distilled water to submerge the membrane. Autoclave. (Nuclepore fitted chambers can be autoclaved and stored dry in surgical trays or sterilizing envelopes.)

Cell Culture

1. Prepare the ethanol-cleaned culture box, which will contain the miniature diffusion culture chambers during the culture period. The box must be free of ethanol fumes.
2. Prepare medium and place on ice. Generally, 200 ml is adequate for servicing 3–4 trays of cultures, including washing cells and diluting the antigen.
3. Prepare the antigen and dilute in medium to the concentration required in the cultures, using a volume sufficient for resuspending the packed lymphocytes. Resuspend control cultures in medium lacking antigen.
4. Prepare the cells to be cultured and dilute to 2×10^7 cells/ml. It is best to do this after centrifugation by resuspending the packed cells in the antigen-containing culture medium.

---

* Although this item is listed as a "culture chamber" in the Bellco catalogue, the words "culture box" are used in this section to avoid ambiguity.

5. Fill the multiwell plate with reservoir medium. If Nuclepore membrane is used in the culture wells and the antigen is able to pass through the membrane pores, include antigen in the reservoir medium.

6. Remove the support frame containing the diffusion chambers from the sterilizing tray or packet, maintaining the sterility of the individual cell chambers. For those chambers autoclaved in water, use a sterile Pasteur pipette connected to the vacuum source to remove any water from within the cell chamber as well as any water clinging to the underside of the cell chambers. Fit the apparatus onto the reservoir plate containing the medium. Wash the cell chamber with a small amount of culture medium to ensure that all water has been removed.

7. Dispense 0.1-ml aliquots of the cell suspension (containing antigen) in each cell chamber and cover each 24-well unit with the multiwell plate lid. Place the units in a culture box, flush with the gas mixture, and incubate. Rocking and feeding are not necessary.

8. Harvest cells by resuspending and then removing the contents of the cell chambers with a Pasteur pipette. Rinse each chamber with medium and repeat the operation.

COMMENTS

1. In our experience, C57BL/6 spleen cells generate primary responses to SRBC of 10 000 direct PFC/culture on day 6; the corresponding response of CBA spleen cells, however, is only 200 direct PFC/culture. Spleen cells from CBA mice primed and boosted with SRBC have given responses of 2000–3000 direct PFC and 10 000–15 000 indirect PFC/culture at a day 5–6 peak.

2. The cell recovery obtained late in the response on days 7 and 8 of culture ranges from 60–90% of the cells cultured and the cell viability ranges from 25–40% of the recovered cells.

3. Higher anti-SRBC responses were obtained when 0.2 μ Nuclepore membrane was used in lieu of dialysis membrane; however, Nuclepore membranes may not be suitable for all purposes because of the nonrestrictive pore size. If antigens of low molecular weight are used, Spectrapor membrane of the appropriate pore size may be employed (Spectrum Medical Industries, 60916 Terminal Annex, Los Angeles, CA 90054).

REFERENCE

Eipert, E. F., L. Adorini, and J. Couderc. 1978. A miniaturized *in vitro* diffusion culture system. *J. Immunol. Meth.* **22**:283.

2.9 IMMUNIZATION IN MICROSUSPENSION CULTURES (10 μl)

Claudia Henry and James Watson

The microculture system developed by Lefkovits (1972) uses 10-μl aliquots of lymphoid cells in the wells of microculture trays. The technique, originally developed for the anti-SRBC response, has since been used to generate responses to a large variety of antigens and mitogens.

Because each well in this culture system contains 2×10^5 or fewer lymphocytes, it is easy to achieve a situation where the number of specific cells per well becomes limiting. The technique is thus particularly well suited for studying the activity of single immunocompetent cells or the products synthesized by them. The ability to culture and assay many replicate cultures also makes the system very valuable for quantitating the number of B cells and T cells or estimating clone size (Section 5.3).

An important technical innovation was the development of the "replicator," an instrument that makes it possible to handle in a single operation the culture fluids of the 60 wells of a microculture tray (Lefkovits and Kamber 1972). The presence of specific antibody in the supernatants is determined by means of a hemolytic "spot" test on a layer of the appropriate indicator cells. Samples of the 60 wells of the culture trays are removed by means of the replicator and released onto assay plates that contain agar with embedded indicator red blood cells. Complement-dependent zones of lysis indicate cultures in which antibody has been produced. This test allows the quick screening of a large number of microcultures for their ability to respond.

The use of the microculture system for an IgM anti-SRBC response is described below to illustrate the basic experimental operations.

MATERIALS AND REAGENTS

Preparation of Spleen Cells

As described in Section 1.2

Cell Culture

Sheep red blood cells (SRBC)
Eagle's minimum essential medium for suspension cultures (MEM), 100 ml supplemented with:
    200 mM L-glutamine, 1.0 ml
    100 mM sodium pyruvate, 1.0 ml
    1 M HEPES, 2.0 ml
    Penicillin-streptomycin (5000 units penicillin, 5000 μg streptomycin), 1.0 ml
    2-mercaptoethanol, 5×10^{-3} M (Appendix A.6), 1 ml

Fetal calf serum, 5.5 ml
Nutritive cocktail (Appendix A.5)
Tissue culture plates (Falcon, #3034)
Tissue culture chamber, humidified by placing wet paper towels at
the bottom of the chamber (Bellco Glass #7741-10005)
Gas mixture: 7% O_2, 10% CO_2, and 83% N_2
Multisyringe dispensers:
  6 syringes holding 500 μl each and delivering 10 μl at a time
    (Hamilton, #83729)
  6 syringes holding 50 μl each and delivering 1 μl at a time (Hamilton, #83726)
  Note: Wash syringes with sterile medium 10 to 15 times for sterile
    work.

Spot Test for Antibody Production

SRBC
Guinea pig serum as a source of complement
Bacto agar (Difco)
Balanced salt solution (BSS; Appendix A.3)
DEAE dextran (Pharmacia Fine Chemicals)
Replicator, vacuum-operated instrument for simultaneous replication
of 60 2-μl samples (the replicator can be purchased by special
order from BIOTEC Aktiengesellschaft, Baselstrasse 59, CH-4124
Schoenenbuch/Basel, Switzerland.)
Petri dishes, 100 × 15 mm
Glass tubes
Waterbath at 45°C

PROCEDURE

Preparation of Spleen Cells

As described in Section 1.2. Adjust final concentration to 2×10^7
cells/ml in supplemented medium.

Cell Culture

1. Using a Pasteur pipette, add two drops (~50 μl) of 1% (v/v) SRBC
   per ml of spleen cell suspension.
2. Draw cell suspension into a multisyringe dispenser (#83729) and
   dispense 10 μl into each of the 60 wells of the culture plate.
3. Pipette about 0.4 ml of medium into the peripheral groove to maintain the humidity.

4. Cover plates and incubate in a humidifed tissue culture chamber perfused with the gas mixture of 7% O_2, 10% CO_2 and 83% N_2. Seal chamber and incubate at 37°C, without rocking, for 4 to 5 days.

5. Feed cultures on days 1, 2, and 3 with a mixture of 1 part FCS and 2 parts nutritive cocktail. Deliver 1.0 μl of the feeding mixture per well with the Hamilton #83726 dispenser.

Spot Test for Antibody Production

1. In advance, prepare Petri dishes containing bottom layers of about 10 ml 1.4% Bacto-Agar in BSS; dry at 37°C for 1 hour. (See Section 3.3 for detailed description.)

2. Prepare 0.7% Difco agar in MEM containing 1.0 mg/ml DEAE dextran, and distribute in 2-ml amounts to warmed tubes in a 45°C water bath (see Section 3.3). Add 0.1 ml 20% SRBC to each tube, pour onto a bottom layer, and distribute over the entire surface. Allow to solidify, and leave at room temperature for about a half-hour before using.

3. Place a microculture tray on the microscope stage attached to the replicator and take 2-μl samples with the replicator. Place an assay plate containing indicator cells under the dispensing unit and release the fluid, gently touching the plate with the droplets on the tips of the replicator.

4. When drops have soaked into the agar, add 1.5–2.0 ml of diluted guinea pig serum and incubate at 37°C for 45 minutes. Cultures producing specific antibody give spots of lysis. Count both strong and weak lytic zones as positive.

COMMENTS

1. The optimal cell density for mouse spleen lymphocytes is 2×10^5 cells per well. When fewer viable cells are used per microculture, for example in dilution assays, irradiated cells are added as "fillers" to maintain this density. Lymphocytes from other sources may have different optimal densities. For example, rabbit peripheral blood lymphocytes respond best with a cell input of $2-4 \times 10^4$ cells per well.

2. The microculture system can also be used to study responses to soluble hapten-protein conjugates. Since the optimal antigen dose for microcultures is generally found to be higher than that for 1-ml cultures, antigen dose response curves should be determined for each antigen.

REFERENCES

Lefkovits, I. 1972. Induction of antibody-forming cell clones in microcultures. *Eur. J. Immunol.* **2**:360.

Lefkovits, I., and O. Kamber. 1972. A replicator for handling and sampling microcultures in tissue culture trays. *Eur. J. Immunol.* **2**:365.

Luzzati, A. L., I. Lefkovits, and B. Pernis. 1973. Antibody response by rabbit peripheral blood lymphocytes in microcultures. *Eur. J. Immunol.* **3**:632.

Hemolytic Plaque Assays

3.1 INTRODUCTION

Claudia Henry

The hemolytic plaque method permits the visualization of the small amount of lytic antibody (10^3 to 10^6 molecules) released in the vicinity of a single lymphocyte. Lymphocytes and a dense suspension of indicator red blood cells are mixed and distributed in a thin layer. Secreted antibodies sensitize the indicator red blood cells around the lymphocyte. With the addition of complement, the red blood cells lyse and plaques appear. The technique has the advantage that it permits the counting, recognition, and study of individual antibody-forming cells even when they are a small minority of the lymphocyte population. The lymphoid cells and indicator cells can be incorporated into an agar support medium (Sections 3.2 and 3.3) or a fluid monolayer (Sections 3.5 and 3.6).

The hemolytic plaque method described above (direct method) measures the number of cells secreting high-efficiency IgM antibodies. The assumption that the direct method measures only cells secreting IgM antibody is based on (1) the greater efficiency of IgM in fixing complement (theoretically, one molecule of IgM is sufficient to trigger the lytic complement pathway if the antigenic-determinant density on the red cells is high enough); and (2) the finding that the increase in the number of cells that form plaques directly and the rise in the serum titer of specific IgM antibodies both peak four days after a primary immunization with a large dose of sheep red blood cells (SRBC) *in vivo*. Although the assumption that the direct method detects only cells secreting IgM antibody is probably valid for the primary immune response to SRBC, there are indications that for anti-NNP responses some of the direct plaques found with densely coupled indicator cells are caused by IgG (Pasanen and Makela 1969). It also appears that not all IgM-producing cells can form plaques directly (Plotz et al. 1968; Sell et al. 1970).

Plaques caused by cells secreting other classes of specific antibodies may be measured by indirect methods that use amplifying anti-Ig sera. The anti-Ig antibodies attach to the antibody molecules, which have already been fixed to the red blood cells during an initial incubation period. The presence of these Ig-anti-Ig complexes facilitates hemolysis upon subsequent treatment with complement. Polyvalent anti–mouse Ig antisera directed against various mouse Ig classes or allotypes can serve as amplifying sera (Plotz et al. 1968; Wortis et al. 1969; Sell et al. 1970; Weiler et al. 1965). An approximate determination of the number of cells that form plaques indirectly can be made by subtracting the number of direct plaques from the total number of plaques measured by the indirect method. It is possible to obtain a more precise measurement of the number of indirect-plaque-forming cells by inhibiting IgM plaques before performing the indirect assay (Section 3.7).

The hemolytic plaque method is applicable to more than the detection of cells secreting antibodies to red blood cell antigens. Cells secreting antibodies to polysaccharides, haptens, or heterologous proteins can be detected by attaching the polysaccharides, haptens, or proteins to the surfaces of the red cells (Sections 3.8 and 3.10). Furthermore, by employing Protein A-coated indicator red cells and the appropriate amplifying anti-Ig sera (Section 3.11), it is possible to use the hemolytic plaque method to enumerate all cells synthesizing immunoglobulins, irrespective of specificity (polyclonal responses).

As in most procedures, occasional artifacts that have the appearance of true hemolytic plaques may appear. In the description of individual procedures, we indicate the major reasons for the occurrence of such artifacts, the best ways to avoid them, and how to distinguish them from true plaques (most artifacts are readily distinguishable from true plaques by the absence of a lymphocyte in the center of the zone of lysis). In addition to the reasons mentioned in the following sections, the transfer of passively adsorbed antibody can generate artifactual plaques. This problem has been discussed by Lambert and Hanna (1973, 1974, 1975).

Also included in this chapter is a description of a complement-dependent plaque assay using nucleated cells as indicators instead of red blood cells (Section 3.13). This modification of the original hemolytic plaque assay has been used to study the primary antibody responses to cell surface antigens (such as H-2 and Thy-1) and tumor-associated antigens. As with the hemolytic plaque assay, this method is especially useful because of its great sensitivity and because it permits the enumeration of the number of cells secreting antibody against particular cell surface antigens.

REFERENCES

Jerne, N. K., and A. A. Nordin. 1963. Plaque formation in agar by single antibody-producing cells. *Science* **140**:405.

Jerne, N. K., A. A. Nordin, and C. Henry. 1963. The agar plaque technique for recognizing antibody-producing cells. In B. Amos and H. Koprowski (Eds.), *Cell-Bound Antibodies*. Wistar Institute Press, Philadelphia.

Jerne, N. K., C. Henry, A. A. Nordin, H. Fuji, A. M. C. Koros, and I. Lefkovits. 1974. Plaque forming cells: Methodology and theory. *Transplant. Rev.* **18**:130.

Lambert, W. C., and E. E. Hanna. 1973. Hemolytic antibody plaques from rabbit spleen cell cultures in the presence and absence of lymphoid cells. *Federation Proc.* **32**:994.

Lambert, W. C., and E. E. Hanna. 1974. Characteristics of the PFC antibody response in primed rabbit spleen cell cultures. *Federation Proc.* **33**:732.

Lambert, W. C., and E. E. Hanna. 1975. Origin of antibody-dependent, lymphoid cell-independent hemolytic plaques in rabbit spleen cell cultures. *Proc. Soc. Exp. Biol. Med.* **150**:636.

Pasanen, V. J., and O. Mäkelä. 1969. Effect of the number of haptens coupled to each erythrocyte on haemolytic plaque formation. *Immunology* **16**:399.

Plotz, P. H., N. Talal, and R. Asofsky. 1968. Assignment of direct and facilitated hemolytic plaques in mice to specific immunoglobulin classes. *J. Immunol.* **100**:744.

Sell, S., A. B. Park, and A. A. Nordin. 1970. Immunoglobulin classes of antibody-forming cells in mice. I. Localized hemolysis-in-agar plaque-forming cells belonging to five immunoglobulin classes. *J. Immunol.* **104**:483.

Weiler, E., E. W. Melletz, and E. Breuninger-Peck. 1965. Facilitation of immune hemolysis by an interaction between red cell-sensitizing antibody and γ-globulin allotype antibody. *Proc. Natl. Acad. Sci.* (USA) **54**:1310.

Wortis, H. H., D. W. Dresser, and H. R. Anderson. 1969. Antibody production studied by means of the localized haemolysis in gel (LHG) assay. III. Mouse cells producing five different classes of antibody. *Immunology* **17**:93.

3.2 SLIDE METHOD (GEL)

Barbara B. Mishell, Stanley M. Shiigi, and Robert I. Mishell

The hemolytic plaque assay, originally developed using Petri dishes (Jerne et al. 1963), can be done on microscope slides. This modification (Mishell and Dutton 1967) allows a large number of assays to be processed rapidly and easily with a minimum of reagents and with very simple preparative procedures. Sample volumes of up to 100 μl can be tested. Normally, the suspension volume of each sample is adjusted according to the expected number of plaque-forming cells (PFC), and duplicate slides that contain 100 μl, 25 μl, and 10 μl of the test sample are prepared. If the expected number of PFC cannot be estimated, the sample is suspended in a small volume and a 10- or 20-fold dilution is made. Three volumes (in duplicate) are tested from each concentrated and diluted sample. Procedural errors can be detected by a lack of correspondence between slides. Usually it is possible to obtain several slides that fall within an easy and accurate counting range of 20 to 120 PFC per slide. With experience, more than 120 PFC can be counted accurately by marking a grid on the back of the slide with a marking pen. The slides can be scored for PFC immediately after the incubation period or the following day after being held overnight at 4°C in a refrigerator or cold room. The slides can also be fixed and dried for longer storage if desired (Section 3.4).

MATERIALS AND REAGENTS

Precoating Slides

Agarose (Bio-Rad Laboratories, #162-0100)
95% ethanol
Microscope slides, 1 × 3 inches, frosted end, cheapest grade (VWR Scientific, #48312-080)
Good quality brush (2–4 in. wide)
Lint-free tissue
Slide-coating tray (Bellco Glass, #7701-50008)

Assay

Indicator red cells (SRBC are used as the example in the following description)
Guinea pig serum as a source of complement, absorbed (Appendix A.2)
Washed lymphocyte suspensions (from animals or cultures, with an appropriate volume of BSS added to the pellet), on ice
Agarose, pretested (see below; Bio-Rad, #162-0100)
Anti-Ig serum (for indirect assay), pretitrated (Section 11.4)

Balanced salt solution (BSS; Appendix A.3)
Precoated slides
Glass tubes, 12 × 75 mm, disposable (Scientific Products, T1293-3)
Graduated, conical centrifuge tube, 12–15 ml
Pipettes
    Micropipettes: 10μl, 25 μl, 100μl
    Dropping pipette: 50 μl (Bellco Glass, #1270-50003)
    Pasteur pipettes
    5-ml pipettes
    10-ml pipettes
Slide assay chambers (Bellco Glass, #7741-04005)
Slide assay racks (Bellco Glass, #7741-04000)
Water bath adjusted to 45–47°C
Incubator adjusted to 37°C

Counting Plaques

Saline, 0.85% NaCl (w/v)
Magnifying glass (3–4 in. in diameter)
Microscope spotlight or other source of strong light
Hand counter

PROCEDURE

Precoating Slides with Agarose

The microscope slides must be precoated with agarose to allow the gelled agarose-cell mixture to adhere. Only coat the clear portion of the slides. Coating the frosted ends encourages the agarose-cell mixture to flow onto the frosted ends when the slides are poured.

1. Place slides on laboratory bench or in the slide-coating trays with frosted ends in line and facing up. Cover the frosted ends with a strip of tape, or if using the slide-coating trays, with the cover provided.

2. Wipe the clear portion of the slides with a lint-free tissue moistened with 95% ethanol, and allow them to dry by evaporation.

3. Prepare a 0.1% solution (w/v) of agarose by boiling the agarose in double-distilled water. With a brush, coat the clear portion of each slide with the hot agarose solution. Let the slides dry completely.

4. Remove the tape or plastic strip from the frosted ends. With a pencil, run a line through all the frosted ends of the slides. This procedure identifies each slide as being coated and detects slides that have been inadvertently coated on the wrong side (frosted end facing down).

5. The coated slides may be stored in their original box and kept indefinitely at room temperature.

Agarose Solution for the Assay

The water content and gelling qualities of different batches of agarose vary. Test each new batch to determine the optimal concentration. The considerations are: number of plaques, size of plaques, and ease of handling the slide (fragility of the agarose). The concentration range that is usually optimal is 0.3% to 0.6% (w/v).

Complement

To remove any antibodies in the guinea pig serum that will react with the red blood cells being used in the assay, absorb the serum with the indicator cells (Appendix A.2); otherwise general lysis can occur. Although most guinea pig sera diluted at 1:5 or 1:10 can serve as a source of complement, many lots can be diluted even more. Dilute complement with BSS immediately before use. Note that if the complement solution is very cold when added to the slides, bubbles will form at 37°C and will interfere with the assay by causing pressure artifacts.

Direct Assay to Detect Cell-Producing IgM Antibody

1. Add the predetermined amount of agarose (see above) to the required volume of BSS (0.5 ml/slide) and allow the agarose to swell in the 45°C water bath. Use a flask sufficiently larger than the volume indicated to allow for boiling the agarose at a later stage.

2. Place the tubes in the water bath and allow them to warm at 45°C.

3. Using a conical graduated centrifuge tube, wash SRBC three times in BSS and resuspend to 6.6% (v/v) in BSS (a 1:15 dilution of the packed cell volume); 50 μl will be required for each slide.

4. Label agarose-coated slides and put them in order on the counter. Wipe surface of slides free of dust with a lint-free tissue.

5. Prepare immune cells, and hold them pelleted on ice until it is time to pour the slides. The number of PFC declines over time when spleen cells are held in suspension.

6. Place the flask in a beaker of water containing a few boiling chips and boil the water over a bunsen flame until the agarose has dissolved. (For added insurance, bring the agarose to a boil by heating the flask for 5–10 seconds over an open flame.) Place the flask in the water bath. When the agarose has cooled slightly, dispense it in 0.5-ml aliquots to the tubes. When the agarose has cooled to 45°C, add 1 drop of the red cell suspension to each tube with a

50-μl dropping pipette. To prevent lysis in the heated agarose, dispense red cells only to the tubes that will be used within 15 minutes (even this may be too long for modified cells, which are more fragile).

7. Resuspend the pelleted immune cells, and add a volume of the suspension (10 μl, 25μl, or 100 μl) to duplicate tubes of agarose. Immediately remove tubes from the water bath. Swiftly but thoroughly mix the contents of both tubes, and pour the contents onto the clear portion of the appropriate slides. To pour the slide, tip the tube onto the slide and quickly spread the agarose to cover the clear portion only. End the spreading in the center of the slide and lift the tube slowly. The cells seem to distribute more evenly if the pouring process ends at the center of the slide.

8. After pouring the slides, make the appropriate dilution of complement and add 7–8 ml to the well of each rack. Position the slides, agar side down, on top of the complement with a rolling motion, allowing bubbles to escape. Place the racks into the chamber, humidified with wet paper towels in the bottom, and incubate the slides at 37°C.

9. If the slides are to be scored on the day of the assay, incubate them for 3 hours. They can be read immediately after this time. If the slides are to be scored the following day, incubate them from $1\frac{1}{2}$ to 3 hours and then place them in the cold (4°C) overnight. To preserve the slides longer than overnight, fix them according to Section 3.4C.

Indirect Assay to Detect Cells Producing IgG Antibody

Slides treated with anti-Ig sera will have both IgM plaques and IgG plaques, unless the formation of IgM plaques is inhibited (Section 3.7). It is possible to calculate the number of plaques due to the IgG antibodies by subtracting the number of direct PFC (IgM) from the total of indirect PFC (IgM + IgG). It is therefore necessary to run duplicate assays, one treated with complement plus antiserum (indirect) and one treated with complement alone (direct). The indirect assay is performed similarly to the direct assay described above, except that a double set of slides must be poured. Follow the procedures for the direct assay up to and including step 7. Continue as follows:

8. After pouring the slides, incubate them, agar side *up*, on slide racks for 90 minutes at 37°C. The chamber must be well humidified.

9. After the initial incubation, invert the direct set of slides over the appropriate dilution of complement as described in the previous section. Invert the indirect set of slides over complement (diluted as above) containing that quantity of antiserum which will give the desired final concentration (Section 11.4). Incubate both sets of slides for an additional 90 minutes at 37°C. Count the plaques as usual.

Counting Plaques

Dip a slide in saline and drain off excess saline by pressing the edge of the slide to a paper towel. Wipe the back side of the slide on a paper towel to clarify the field. Count the plaques in a strong indirect light (for example, from a microscope spotlight) with the aid of a magnifying glass attached to a ring stand. Do not count any plaques in the small area that rested on the raised edges of the rack. Pressure on the gel causes artifacts. Questionable plaques can be verified by microscopic examination, which should reveal the antibody-releasing lymphocyte in the center of the true plaque. With experience, the identification of plaques comes easily. Note that the number of plaques obtained by assaying different samples of the same cell suspension must be proportional to the volumes plated. If there are more than 120 plaques on a slide, counting becomes easier and more accurate if a grid is marked on the back of the slide with a marking pen.

COMMENTS

1. Do not allow the agarose to evaporate excessively before placing the slides in the humid atmosphere. Excessive evaporation creates a hypertonic environment for the cells and seems to result in very small (and probably fewer) plaques. The slides should be in contact with the complement before any drying at the edges is observed.

2. There can be several explanations if the slides exhibit general lysis:
   a. The slides contain a very large number of cells producing antibody.
   b. The complement has not been absorbed with the indicator red cells.
   c. Antibody produced by the suspended cells has been transferred to the slide with the test volume. This can be avoided by washing the cells once just prior to assay.
   d. The racks contain residual detergent.

3. Bacto-Agar (Difco) with DEAE dextran can be used instead of agarose (Section 3.3). We prefer agarose because it is not anticomplementary and therefore does not require the use of DEAE dextran.

REFERENCES

Jerne, N. K., A. A. Nordin, and C. Henry. 1963. The agar plaque technique for recognizing antibody-producing cells. In B. Amos and H. Koprowski (Eds.), *Cell-Bound Antibodies*. Wistar Institute Press, Philadelphia.

Mishell, R. I., and R. W. Dutton. 1966. Immunization of normal mouse spleen cell suspensions *in vitro*. *Science* **153**:1004.

Mishell, R. I., and R. W. Dutton. 1967. Immunization of dissociated spleen cell cultures from normal mice. *J. Exp. Med.* **126**:423.

3.3 PLATE METHOD (GEL)

Claudia Henry

The plate method was the original procedure devised for the assay of antibody-secreting cells. Though other modifications using slides or omitting a gel support have subsequently been developed (each having its own advantage), the plate method still has its advantages in many situations. It also has disadvantages: A single assay requires greater amounts of reagents than slide methods, and this requirement may be critical when "facilitating" antisera (e.g., antiallotype sera) are in short supply or when the reagents used to modify red cells chemically are expensive. In addition, Petri dishes are more expensive than slides.

The plate method, however, extends the range of the volume of lymphocyte suspensions that can be assayed. The 2-ml agar-red blood cell indicator mixture can accomodate volumes of 0.005 ml to 0.8 ml, thus eliminating both the need to dilute the suspensions and the procedural error such dilution entails. This range of volumes also permits the plating of an entire culture (e.g., in limiting dilution assays). Further, the larger surface area makes it possible to count a larger range of plaques—any number up to 1000 per plate can be counted with reasonable accuracy, although we consider 700 plaques per plate to be the limit for reliability. Plaque counts on plates are therefore larger than those obtained by other methods. Since the variance associated with plaque counts is a composite of the Poisson variation and procedural errors, the plate assay gives more reliable estimations. Finally, plaques on plates with bottom layers are also readily stained to give improved definition (Section 3.4).

The first method described below is a direct method used to score lymphocytes synthesizing IgM antibodies to sheep red blood cells (SRBC). The second procedure outlined describes an indirect method for the recognition of cells that produce anti-SRBC antibodies of Ig classes other than IgM. Modifications of this method for additional applications are described at the end of this section.

MATERIALS AND REAGENTS

Preparation of Bottom Layers

Bacto agar (Difco Laboratories)
DEAE dextran, $M_r = 5 \times 10^5$ to 2×10^6 (Pharmacia Fine Chemicals)
2× balanced salt solution (BSS; Appendix A.3)
Petri dishes, 100 × 15 mm (cheapest grade)
Flat, cheap trays (obtained from a restaurant supplier)
Steamer or autoclave
Water bath adjusted to 45–47°C
Incubator at 37°C (either humidified or with a flat container of water)

Assays

Indicator red cells (SRBC are used as the example in the following description)
Guinea pig serum as a source of complement
Anti-Ig serum (for indirect assay), pretitrated (Section 11.4)
Washed lymphocyte suspensions (from animals or cultures, with an appropriate volume of BSS added to the pellet), on ice
Bacto agar (Difco Laboratories)
DEAE dextran (see above)
Glucose-phosphate-buffered saline (G-PBS), pH 7.6 (Appendix A.11)
2× and 1× balanced salt solution (BSS; Appendix A.3)
Petri dishes with bottom layers (see below)
Steamer or autoclave
Incubator (see above)
Vortex mixer
Sero-Fuge II (Clay Adams)
Polypropylene tubes with caps, 17 × 100 mm (Falcon, #2059), for use with Sero-Fuge
Pipettes, 5 μl to 1 ml

Counting Plaques

Dissecting microscope with a light source below stage
Automatic colony counter

PROCEDURE

Preparation of Bottom Layers

Most plastic Petri dishes are not flat and also repel water. Bottom layers of 1.4% agar in BSS provide an even, nonrepellent surface for spreading the soft agar. Such preparations are also easier to stain. Make the bottom layer 1 day to 2 weeks before the assay. The 1 liter of mixture described below yields 150–200 plates.

1. Add 14 g of Difco Bacto agar to 500 ml of water. Steam or autoclave (100°C) for 30 minutes or until agar is completely dissolved.
2. Warm 500 ml of 2× BSS containing 1 g of DEAE dextran to 45°C. This also requires about 30 minutes. (The DEAE dextran overcomes the anticomplementary properties of the Difco Bacto agar, presumably by binding to the sulphuric ester groups.)
3. Mix 1 and 2 above and keep at 45°C.
4. Remove the lids from about 150 Petri dishes.
5. Pour 5 to 8 ml of the mixture into the Petri dishes. *Quickly* flame the surface before the agar solidifies, to eliminate any bubbles on the agar surface.
6. When the agar has solidified, invert plates (without lids) and place them on trays. A large number can be placed on one tray if the plates are stacked with the rim of one leaning on the bottom of the adjacent plate (like fallen dominoes). Dry them in the humid 37°C incubator for 15 to 20 minutes.
7. Remove the dishes from the incubator, cover them with the lids, and stack in columns with the bottoms up. Store the dishes at 4°C in plastic bags. The plates can be used 1 day to 2 weeks later. Penicillin-streptomycin can be included in the agar if contamination becomes a problem with longer storage.

Direct Assay to Detect Cells Producing IgM Antibody

1. Allow plates to warm to room temperature. Number the bottoms of the dishes at one edge and place them in sequence on trays.
2. Prepare 0.7% Difco Bacto agar in BSS containing 1 mg/ml DEAE dextran for the top layers. The following recipe is for 100 ml (or 50 tubes): Add 0.7 g agar to 50 ml double-distilled water and steam (or autoclave) for 30 minutes. Prewarm 50 ml of 2× BSS containing 0.1 g of DEAE dextran to 45°C and add agar solution.
3. Put the tubes in the water bath and allow them to warm to 45°C.
4. With a 10-ml pipette, dispense 2 ml of the soft agar mixture into each tube.

5. Wash red cells with G-PBS at least 3 times. Remove the white blood cells (buffy coat) on the top of the packed red cells and resuspend the pellet to 15% (v/v) in G-PBS. In a Sero-Fuge, each wash takes 1–2 minutes.

6. Immediately before plating, resuspend the lymphocyte samples with a pipette or by gentle agitation with a vortex mixer.

7. Dispense 0.1 ml of the red cell suspension to about 10 tubes of soft agar in the water bath. Add 0.005–0.8 ml of a lymphocyte suspension to one tube. Rotate the tube between palms, and pour *rapidly* over the appropriate bottom layer, tilting the plate so the entire surface is covered. Although the cells must be well mixed before pouring, excessive handling causes the red cells to agglutinate. Allow the agar to solidify before moving the tray of plates. Prepare duplicate plates for each volume assayed. If the magnitude of the response is unknown, add volumes at 4-fold increments (a volume that contains 300 plaques is ideal). Cover dishes and incubate them on trays at 37°C for 1 hour in the humidified incubator. If many plates are poured, filling several trays, the trays can be stacked and only the dishes on the top tray need to be covered.

8. Add 1.5 ml of guinea pig serum, diluted 1 : 10 in 1× BSS, to each dish. Dilute the serum immediately before use and keep in an ice bucket.

9. Return the plates to the 37°C incubator for 1 hour. After this time, the plaques are visible as small round pale areas against a red cell background. Definition often improves if the plates stand at room temperature for an additional hour.

10. Pour off the complement and store the plates at 4°C overnight.

11. Stain the plates (Section 3.4) the following day and count at leisure.

Indirect Assay to Detect Cells Producing IgG Antibody

Plates treated with anti-Ig sera will have IgM plaques as well as plaques caused by other Ig classes (principally IgG) unless the formation of IgM plaques is inhibited (Section 3.7). Plaques due to specific IgG can be calculated by subtracting the number of direct PFC from the total of indirect PFC. It is therefore necessary to run duplicate assays, one treated with complement plus antiserum (indirect) and one treated with complement alone (direct).

1. Plate as for direct plaques (steps 1–7 above), but distribute aliquots to plates containing bottom layers for both direct and

indirect sets. The volume plated on each set will depend on the relative size of the IgM and IgG PFC response. Keep the direct and indirect sets on distinct trays since the subsequent treatment differs.

2. After 1 hour of incubation at 37°C, add to the indirect set 1.5 ml of anti-Ig serum diluted in BSS (previously titrated for optimal development of IgG plaques; see Section 11.4). The direct set should receive 1.5 ml BSS.

3. Incubate for 1 hour at 37°C. Pour off the anti-Ig serum from the indirect set and the BSS from the direct set. Add 1.5 ml of diluted complement (see above) to both sets. Process as for the direct assay of plaques (step 9–11 above).

Single (Thin) Layers

It is possible to pour the soft agar containing the lymphocytes directly into empty Petri dishes. This procedure is used when the plaques are counted unstained or if the released antibody is treated with 2-mercaptoethanol or dithiothreitol to inhibit the formation of IgM plaques (Section 3.7). The procedures for plating and plaque development are as outlined above.

Ultrathin Layers

Thinner layers are required for cytological or autoradiographic studies of single lymphocytes. The preparation of ultrathin layers requires a few changes in steps 1–7 of the direct technique described above:

1. The agar-cell mixture should contain 0.1 ml of 50% (v/v) indicator red cells and less than 3×10^6 lymphocytes. These two deviations guarantee a good red cell background and also ensure that each plaque contains only one lymphocyte.

2. Immediately after pouring the agar-cell mixture into empty Petri dishes, shake vigorously with one wrist flick to pour off about $\frac{4}{5}$ of the mixture; verify the amount by weighing or by counting plaques.

3. Incubate and treat with anti-Ig serum and complement as above.

4. To visualize with a microscope, break off the sides of the Petri dish. The central lymphocyte can be observed if it is stained with gentian violet or by fluorescence and autoradiography (Jerne et al. 1974).

5. Count plaques on thin and ultrathin layers on the following day, or fix preparations for counting at a later time (Section 3.4).

Counting Plaques

Counting is best done using a dissecting microscope with an indirect light source and an automatic colony counter. Use 7× magnification for routine counting; verify questionable plaques with higher magnification. Counting of plaques in plates with bottom layers is facilitated by staining the plates with benzidine or an equivalent stain (Section 3.4). The use of this stain is one of the advantages of the plate technique. The red blood cell background assumes a dark blue color thereby improving considerably the definition of the plaques.

Experience provides an advantage in counting plaques that range in size and morphology from small and fuzzy to large and clear; it also helps in recognizing spurious plaques. These may be due to air bubbles (sharp, darker edges), lumps of undissolved agar (usually not circular), tissue debris (hard, irregular spot in the plaque centers), or small bacterial colonies (dark spots in the center of the plaques). The bacterial colonies appear in the absence of complement. Long incubation (more than 6 hours) may also cause false plaques produced by the release of lysins from degenerating cells.

REFERENCE

Jerne, N. K., C. Henry, A. A. Nordin, H. Fuji, A. M. C. Koros, and I. Lefkovits. 1974. Plaque forming cells: Methodology and theory. *Transplant. Rev.* **18**:130.

3.4 STAINING AND FIXATION

Claudia Henry and Anne H. Good

The efficiency of counting plaques is improved by staining the indicator cells with benzidine or a similar compound. The plaques then appear as circular white areas in a blue lawn. We routinely find that the number of plaques counted after staining is 1.3 to 1.4 times that counted with unstained plates. The method is consistently successful only with preparations plated on bottom layers of agar in Petri dishes. It is more difficult to control the staining of slides or plates lacking a bottom layer because very thin layers of indicator cells tend to lyse. Stained plates can be kept at 4°C for at least 4 weeks without either deterioration of the plaques or microbial contamination.

A. Staining with Benzidine Dihydrochloride

MATERIALS AND REAGENTS

The following mixture will stain 50 plates:

0.2 g benzidine dihydrochloride, $M_r = 257.2$ (Sigma Chemical, #3383). Note: Benzidine dihydrochloride is a carcinogen. Use gloves when handling the solution and do not pipet by mouth.
10.0 ml glacial acetic acid
90.0 ml double-distilled water
1.0 ml of fresh 30% hydrogen peroxide (H_2O_2)

PROCEDURE

1. Mix reagents and stir the mixture in a chemical hood.
2. Add about 2 ml of benzidine solution to the plates. Check the stain by first staining one plate. Pale blue staining should occur within a few minutes. Slow staining is usually caused by old H_2O_2; if it occurs, add another 1 ml or use a fresh bottle.
3. When the plates have assumed a pale blue color, pour off the solution and rinse the plates with tap water. Since dark plates are more difficult to count, avoid overstaining.
4. Freeze the remaining stain.

COMMENT

See comment 4 in Section 3.4B.

B. Staining with O-tolidine

O-tolidine can be used in place of benzidine for staining plates if benzidine is not available.

MATERIALS AND REAGENTS

NaCl, $M_r = 58.4$
Tannic acid (J. T. Baker Chemical)
O-tolidine (4,4'-diamino-3,3'-dimethylbiphenyl), $M_r = 212.3$ (J. T. Baker Chemical). Note: O-tolidine is a suspected carcinogen. Wear plastic gloves when handling and do not pipet by mouth.

Glacial acetic acid
30% hydrogen peroxide (H_2O_2)
NaOH, $M_r = 40.0$
Disposable gloves

PROCEDURE

1. Prepare the following stock solutions:
    a. 0.85% (w/v) sodium chloride (saline)
    b. 1% (w/v) tannic acid in saline. This solution can be kept in the refrigerator for at least one month.
    c. 0.3% tannic acid in saline. This solution should be prepared fresh each day.
    d. 10% (w/v) O-tolidine in glacial acetic acid. Shield from light. This solution will keep for several months in a tightly closed container. O-tolidine dihydrochloride can be used in place of O-tolidine but will give a suspension rather than a solution in glacial acetic acid.
    e. 1% O-tolidine solution in saline. Prepare weekly from 10% stock solution and keep at room temperature shielded from light.
    f. 3 M NaOH.
    g. 5% hydrogen peroxide.
2. Prepare the following staining solution immediately before staining:
    - 25.0 ml 1% O-tolidine
    - 63.5 ml saline
    - 1.5 ml 3 M NaOH
    - 10.0 ml 5% H_2O_2 in saline.
3. Fix red cells by flooding each plate with 3 ml of 0.3% tannic acid solution in saline. After 5 minutes, decant tannic acid and rinse plate with 3 ml of saline.
4. Add staining solution rapidly to cover entire surface of plate and stain until plate is a deep blue color.
5. Decant stain and store plates inverted at 4°C until they are counted.

COMMENTS

1. The optimal concentration of tannic acid as well as the optimal time for fixation may need to be determined experimentally. The

erythrocytes will not stain if fixation is excessive, but insufficient fixation will result in hemolysis during the staining step.

2. The stain must be well mixed and is most conveniently added to the plates by decanting; slow addition by pipette sometimes results in uneven or mottled staining.

3. The color of the stained plates may turn from blue to brown during prolonged storage.

4. Preliminary experiments indicate that other benzidine substitutes, such as 3,3',5,5'-tetramethylbenzidine (available from Aldrich and Tridom Chemical, Inc.), can be used in procedures basically similar to those for benzidine or O-tolidine in the event that O-tolidine and benzidine become unavailable. The concentration of benzidine substitute to be used and in particular the pH required to obtain a satisfactory blue color must be determined experimentally for each system.

C. Fixation of Plates and Slides

If it is impractical to count plaques on slides or single-layered plates on either the day of assay or the following day, the slides or plates may be fixed and dried for scoring at a later time. The indicator cells in unfixed preparations lyse. Glutaraldehyde fixation can be used to fix both slides and single-layered plates.

MATERIALS AND REAGENTS

Saline, 0.85% NaCl (w/v) or phosphate-buffered saline (PBS; Appendix A.8)
Glutaraldehyde, 0.25% (v/v) in saline or PBS. Caution: Do not mouth pipet glutaraldehyde or splash solution into the eyes.
Petri dishes, 100 mm
Microscope slide-staining racks and baths for immersion

PROCEDURE

Petri Dishes

1. Pour 5–8 ml of glutaraldehyde solution into each 100-mm dish.

2. Store at 4°C and pour off excess fluid before counting.

Microscope Slides

1. Load slides into slide-staining racks, placing them back to back for economy of space.

2. Immerse in glutaraldehyde solution for 10 minutes at room temperature.

3. Wash the slides by immersing them in tap water for 10–20 minutes, followed by distilled water for 10 minutes. This step washes salt from the slides in preparation for drying.

4. Dry the slides on paper towels on the bench (agar side up). Avoid subsequent wetting of the dried layer.

REFERENCES

Staining with Benzidine

Jerne, N. K., C. Henry, A. A. Nordin, H. Fuji, A. M. C. Koros, and I. Lefkovits. 1974. Plaque forming cells: Methodology and theory. *Transplant. Rev.* **18**:130.

Staining with O-tolidine

Segre, D., and M. Segre. 1976. Visualization of plaque forming cells in agar plates stained with O-tolidine. *J. Immunol. Meth.* **12**:197.

Other Benzidine Substitutes

Holland, V. R., B. C. Saunders, F. L. Rose, and A. L. Walpole. 1974. A safer substitute for benzidine in the detection of blood. *Tetrahedron* **30**:3299.

Lomholt, B., and N. Keiding. 1977. Tetrabase, an alternative to benzidine and ortho-tolidine for detection of haemoglobin in urine. *Lancet* **1**:608.

3.5 LIQUID MATRIX (SLIDE METHOD)

John Marbrook

It is not necessary to use a supporting gel, such as agar, for plaque assays. Cunningham initially proposed a modification in which lymphoid cells and indicator red blood cells are placed in a microchamber and allowed to settle as a monolayer on the base of the chamber (Cunningham 1965; Cunningham and Szenberg 1968). The method is simple, economical, and sensitive. The conditions it engenders are the most favorable for microscopic examination of the plaque-forming cells (PFC) and permit the observation of rosette and plaque formation by the same cell. Generally considered to be the most sensitive of the hemolytic plaque assays, this method can also be adapted for micromanipulation studies.

MATERIALS AND REAGENTS

Construction of Microchambers

Microscope slides
Double-sided Scotch tape, 2–5 mm wide
Molten mixture of equal parts of paraffin wax and vaseline

Assay

Washed indicator red cells
Guinea pig serum as a source of complement
Lymphoid cell suspension containing PFC
HEPES-buffered balanced salt solution (Appendix A.4) containing
    5% fetal calf serum (FCS)
95% ethanol
Small tubes (or microwell plates)
Pipette capable of delivering a small volume accurately (Eppendorf
    or similar)

PROCEDURE

Construction of Microchambers

1. Clean the microscope slides by immersing them in 95% ethanol. Polish them with a clean cloth.
2. Place 10–20 clean slides in a row.
3. Place 2 strips of double-sided Scotch tape across both ends of the row of slides.
4. Place cleaned slides on top of the taped slides in such a way that a microchamber is formed between the two slides. The depth of the chamber is the thickness of the tape at each end of the slide. The capacity of the chamber is approximately 0.15 ml. The volume of the chambers is reasonably constant if care is taken in placing the double-sided tape to the slides.
5. Separate the slides in the row from each other by flexing adjacent slides to break the tape.

Assay

1. Suspend lymphoid cells containing PFC in the buffered BSS containing 5% FCS and keep the suspension on ice. Suspend the cells to a concentration that gives 75–100 PFC/chamber. It is difficult to count more than 150 PFC/chamber. Also, too many white blood cells in the chamber will obscure the plaques.

2. Prepare a suspension of indicator red cells (e.g., SRBC) in buffered balanced salt solution (5% FCS) containing guinea pig serum as a source of complement. This suspension consists of:

> 0.5ml 10% (v/v) washed SRBC
> 0.3 ml guinea pig serum
> 2.0 ml buffered balanced salt solution containing 5% FCS.

If necessary, adjust these concentrations to obtain a single monolayer in the chamber and the optimal concentration of guinea pig serum to cause hemolysis. Maintain the suspension in an ice water bath.

3. To a series of small tubes (or microwell plates) at room temperature, dispense 0.2 ml of suspension 1 (lymphoid cells) and 0.2 ml of suspension 2 (indicator red cells). Agitate to mix.

4. With an appropriate pipette, place a measured volume into the chamber such that the chamber is not quite filled to overflowing.

5. Dip the edges of the microscope slide chambers in a bath of molten wax to seal the chambers and incubate the slides at 37°C for 1 hour.

6. The hemolytic plaques are quite visible by naked eye but should be counted under low power microscope with oblique illumination.

COMMENTS

1. Slightly warm the cold suspensions towards room temperature before filling the chamber; this precaution will prevent a number of air bubbles from forming in the chamber during the incubation step. Excess air bubbles can obscure plaques but are easily distinguishable from plaques under a microscope.

2. The vaseline in the molten wax mixture softens the paraffin so that it does not crack and allow medium to evaporate from the chamber.

3. If IgG plaques need to be assayed, include anti-IgG developing serum in the assay mixture.

4. The assay slides can be moved freely but carefully. Any kind of tapping will cause the plaques to disappear, but it is possible to hold the slides briefly in a vertical position without disturbing the monolayer. Always hold them at the edges to preclude compression of the chambers.

5. There is a restriction on the number of cells that can be plated,

since plaques are masked by autologous cells. It is thus important to check that the number of plaques decreases proportionally with dilution of the lymphocyte suspension.

REFERENCES

Cunningham, A. J. 1965. A method of increased sensitivity for detecting single antibody-forming cells. *Nature* (London) **207**:1106.

Cunningham, A. J., and A. Szenberg. 1968. Further improvements in the plaque technique for detecting single antibody-forming cells. *Immunology* **14**:599.

3.6   LIQUID MATRIX (MICROWELL METHOD)

Douglas C. Vann

Hemolytic plaque assays can be performed in microwell plates (Kappler 1974). This obviates the need of transferring cultured cells out of the plates to perform the assay. At the time of assay, sheep red blood cells (SRBC), or other indicator red blood cells, and complement are mixed with the culture lymphocytes directly in the wells. The SRBC settle to form a monolayer on the flat bottom of the wells. Incubation at 37°C results in the development of hemolytic plaques. This technique has the additional advantage that a single well can be assayed sequentially with different antigens (Marrack and Kappler 1975).

MATERIALS AND REAGENTS

SRBC or other indicator red cells

Guinea pig serum as a source of complement, absorbed previously with indicator cells (Appendix A.2)

Balanced salt solution (BSS; Appendix A.3)

Vortex mixer

50-μl dispensing device (Hamilton syringe or calibrated dropping pipette)

Microwell plates, flat bottom (Falcon, #3040)

Refrigerated centrifuge (Damon/IEC Division, IEC #276 head)

IEC #353 cups (block bottom of cup so that trays ride at approximately a 45° angle) or Cooke #220-82 carrier (place two #9 stoppers on one side of carrier to tilt tray during centrifugation)

PROCEDURE

1. Wash SRBC three times in BSS and prepare a 0.5% (v/v) suspension in BSS.

2. Dilute complement to twice the desired final concentration in BSS. Mix equal volumes of complement with the SRBC suspension. Each tray requires 5 ml of this mixture.

3. Centrifuge trays containing lymphocytes (10 minutes at $250 \times g$) at an angle so that the cells will pellet at the sides of the wells. Invert the trays over a sink and give one brisk shake to expel the culture medium from the wells. Blot the tops of the trays on a pad of paper towels or soft tissue.

4. Place each tray on top of a vortex mixer (holding it in place with one index finger positioned in the center of the tray) and bring the mixer up to high speed to resuspend the pelleted lymphocytes.

5. Dispense 50 μl of the SRBC-complement mixture to each well. Mix the contents of the tray gently with the vortex mixer. Then refrigerate the tray at 4°C for at least one hour. The cells will settle into a monolayer at this stage.

6. Remove the tray from the refrigerator and warm it to room temperature by carefully placing it on a laboratory bench for 15–20 minutes. This step reduces the likelihood that convection currents resulting from rapid warming will disturb the monolayer.

7. Incubate the trays at 37°C for 1 to $1\frac{1}{2}$ hours. Score the trays, using a bright light shining obliquely from the bottom of the plate, with the aid of a magnifying glass or dissecting microscope.

COMMENTS

1. This method is especially convenient for determining PFC yields in limiting dilution experiments. The small surface area of the wells limits the number of plaques that can be counted but the cells can be removed from wells containing too many PFC and assayed on slides (Section 3.2) if necessary.

2. The lymphocyte concentration should not exceed 10^6 cells per well; higher numbers will interfere with the clarity of the plaques.

3. Different indicator red cells can be used sequentially. Determine the number of PFC with the first indicator cells. Then add 10 μl of previously titrated antiserum directed against the indicator red blood cells and 10 μl of complement diluted 1 : 3 in BSS. Incubate at 37°C for 20 minutes to lyse the red blood cells. Centrifuge the

plates, remove the supernatants (as above), and repeat the assay with the second type of indicator red blood cell.

REFERENCES

Kappler, J. W. 1974. A micro-technique for hemolytic plaque assays. *J. Immunol.* **112**:1271.

Marrack (Hunter), P. C., and J. W. Kappler. 1975. Antigen-specific and nonspecific mediators of T cell/B cell cooperation. I. Evidence for their production by different T cells. *J. Immunol.* **114**:1116.

3.7 ESTIMATION OF IgG RESPONSES BY ELIMINATION OF IgM PLAQUES

Claudia Henry

The number of IgG plaques is usually computed by subtracting direct plaque counts from indirect plaque counts obtained with similar aliquots of lymphocyte suspensions. This method is not precise for two reasons. First, most of the anti-Ig sera used to develop indirect plaques inhibit IgM plaques to some extent. The degree of inhibition must be checked by testing the antiserum on lymphocyte suspensions known to contain only IgM PFC (e.g., mouse spleen cells 2 to 3 days after injection with SRBC). It is best if the anti-Ig serum inhibits the development of all IgM plaques; indirect plaque counts then give a straightforward estimation of IgG PFC. Unfortunately, with most sera inhibition is partial and it is necessary to make the appropriate correction before subtracting the direct plaque count. Second, the variance associated with a number obtained by subtraction is the sum of the variances of the direct and indirect plaque counts.

It is therefore preferable to abolish IgM plaques and determine the number of IgG plaques directly. Three methods serve this purpose: reduction with 2-mercaptoethanol (2-ME), reduction with dithiothreitol (DTT) followed by alkylation, and treatment with concanavalin A (Con A). As noted above, these methods are not required if the anti-Ig serum *totally* inhibits the formation of IgM plaques. They are also unnecessary in assays of avian lymphocytes. Since avian Ig does not bind guinea pig complement, direct plaques must be developed with chicken complement; for indirect plaque formation with rabbit anti–avian Ig, guinea pig complement is effective. Thus, IgM plaques are measured after the addition of avian complement, IgG plaques after the addition of anti–avian Ig and guinea pig complement.

A. Elimination of IgM Plaques with 2-Mercaptoethanol

MATERIALS AND REAGENTS

2-mercaptoethanol (2-ME), M_r = 78.1, ρ = 1.114 (Sigma Chemical)
Saline, 0.85% NaCl (w/v)
Reagents for direct and indirect assay: using plates (Section 3.3) or
    using slides (Section 3.2)
Plastic bags large enough to contain the trays of Petri dishes or slide-
    rack chambers
0.15 M 2-ME in saline: Add 1.05 ml 2-ME to 99 ml saline. Caution:
    2-ME fumes are toxic. Prepare this solution in a fume hood and
    do not pipet by mouth.

PROCEDURE

1. Warm 0.15 M 2-ME in saline to 37°C.
2. Plate as usual on empty Petri dishes (i.e., no bottom layers) or plate
   on slides. Make two sets for direct plating and one for indirect
   plating. Incubate for 1 hour.
3. Add 4 ml of prewarmed 0.15 M 2-ME solution to *one* set of direct
   plates as well as to the set that will be processed for indirect
   plaques. Add warmed saline to the other direct set. For slide
   assays, invert in the appropriate solutions. Enclose in large plastic
   bags to contain toxic 2-ME fumes and incubate for 30 minutes at
   37°C.
4. Decant the fluid and wash thoroughly with saline to remove the
   2-ME which otherwise would subsequently inactivate the complement. For a few trays of Petri dishes it is sufficient to give 5
   generous saline washes spaced over 30 minutes. For large numbers of dishes it is more convenient to place the uncovered trays in
   racks that are submerged in a large volume of saline. Agitate
   occasionally over a 30-minute period and rinse once with fresh
   saline. Similarly, the best way to wash slides is to place them in
   microscope slide racks and submerge them.
5. Process the two direct sets and the single indirect set according to
   the procedures outlined in Section 3.3.

COMMENTS

1. All direct (IgM) plaques should be susceptible to 2-ME; the
   plaques surviving 2-ME treatment on the indirect set represent

IgG plaques. Any IgM plaques found after treatment with 2-ME should be subtracted from the indirect plaque count.

2. The 2-ME technique for eliminating IgM plaques is the procedure least demanding of expensive reagents. Its disadvantage is the toxic fumes. Using a hood for the preparation of solutions and large plastic bags to contain the samples can prevent most of the harmful effects of the fumes.

3. It has been reported that in the early stages of the IgG response, mouse IgG is sensitive to reduction. Calculations based on the 2-ME method may therefore underestimate the number of IgG plaques in the early stages of assays with mouse IgG.

B. Elimination of IgM Plaques with Dithiothreitol

MATERIALS AND REAGENTS

Dithiothreitol, M_r = 154.3 (Sigma Chemical, #D-0632)
Tris base, M_r = 121.1 (Sigma Chemical, #T-1503)
Saline, 0.85% NaCl (w/v)
1 M NaOH, M_r = 40.0
Iodoacetamide, M_r = 184.9 (Eastman Kodak, #1371)
1 M HCl
Reagents for direct and indirect assay: using plates (Section 3.3) or using slides (Section 3.2)
Solutions
      0.005 M dithiothreitol (DTT): Mix 100 ml of 0.1 M DTT with 100 ml 2 M Tris. Add saline to 2 liters. Adjust to pH 8.6–8.8 with 1 M NaOH. Store by freezing.
      0.011 M iodoacetamide: Mix 200 ml 0.11 M iodoacetamide with 100 ml 2 M Tris. Add saline to 2 liters and adjust to pH 7.3 with 1 M HCl. Store by freezing.

PROCEDURE

1. Plate as for 2-ME technique. Incubate for 1 hour at 37°C.

2. Add DTT solution to appropriate plates or invert appropriate slides in DTT. Incubate at room temperature for 30 minutes.

3. Pour off DTT and add iodoacetamide solution. Incubate at room temperature for 30 minutes.

4. Pour off iodoacetamide, wash in saline, and process for direct and indirect plaques.

COMMENTS

1. All direct (IgM) plaques should be susceptible to DTT; the plaques surviving DTT treatment on the indirect set represent IgG plaques. Any IgM plaques found after treatment with DTT should be subtracted from the indirect plaque count.

2. Because DTT is used at a lower concentration than 2-ME there is much less of a problem with toxic fumes. However, the DTT procedure does involve the additional step of alkylation and requires more expensive reagents.

C. Elimination of IgM plaques with Concanavalin A

MATERIALS AND REAGENTS

Solution of concanavalin A (Con A), obtained from Miles Research Products at a concentration of about 40 mg/ml in saturated NaCl. Dilute in PBS, pH 7.2 (Appendix A.8), to a final concentration of 0.3 mg/ml (see Comments).
Reagents for direct and indirect assay, slides only (Section 3.2)

PROCEDURE

1. Plate on slides using the same three sets as for 2-ME and DTT techniques. Incubate for 1 hour at 37°C (agar side up).

2. Invert appropriate slides in Con A solution and incubate for 1 hour at 37°C.

3. Wash slides with 5 to 6 rinses in PBS, draining off excess fluid on a paper towel.

4. Process for direct and indirect plaques.

COMMENTS

1. Since Con A is expensive, it is only feasible to use this method with the slide assay.

2. The selective sensitivity of IgM to the action of Con A depends on the fact that IgM possesses more carbohydrate groups than IgG. Although the concentration of 0.3 mg/ml is a good starting point, the concentration that will eliminate IgM plaques and not affect IgG plaques must be established for each lot of Con A.

REFERENCES

2-Mercaptoethanol

Jerne, N. K., C. Henry, A. A. Nordin, H. Fuji, A. M. C. Koros, and I.
Lefkovits. 1974. Plaque forming cells: Methodology and theory. *Transplant. Rev.* **18**:130. (H. Fuji is responsible for the work on 2-ME.)

Dithiothreitol

Plotz P. H., N. Talal, and R. Asofsky. 1968. Assignment of direct and facilitated hemolytic plaques in mice to specific immunoglobulin classes. *J. Immunol.* **100**:744.

Concanavalin A

Nordin, A. A., H. Cosenza, and W. Hopkins. 1969. The use of concanvalin A for distinguishing IgM from IgG antibody-producing cells. *J. Immunol.* **103**:859.

3.8 ANTI-HAPTEN PLAQUES

Claudia Henry

The procedures described in Sections 3.2–3.7 can be easily adapted to detect cells secreting anti-hapten antibodies. The only change consists in coating the red blood cells with an adequate density of hapten determinants without either causing excessive fragility of the red cells or changing their susceptibility to lysis by complement.

Two general approaches to coupling are used: direct chemical complexing to the red blood cells and indirect immunological coupling in which haptens are first conjugated to anti–red blood cell antibodies that can attach to red blood cells. To prevent the hapten-antibody conjugates from themselves causing lysis in the presence of complement, it is necessary to use Fab or F(ab')$_2$ fragments of mammalian anti–red blood cell antibodies or avian anti–red blood cell antibodies, which do not fix mammalian complement.

The number of plaques obtained with uncoated indicator cells must be subtracted from the number obtained with coated indicator cells. It is also necessary to do both direct and indirect assays because anti-hapten responses are predominantly IgG. A large variety of haptens have been successfully coupled to red blood cells to permit efficient detection of cells secreting specific anti-hapten antibodies. We have included only methods of coupling azophenyl and nitrophenyl haptens, since we study primarily these responses.

Anti-hapten plaque formation can be inhibited by incorporating free hapten or antigen in the cell-agar mixtures. This confirms the specificity of the plaques. The avidity of the antibodies released by the anti-hapten PFC can be analyzed by measuring the inhibition by free hapten (Section 3.9).

A. Modification of Red Blood Cells with Azophenyl Haptens

The preparation of reagents and the coupling procedures for a variety of azophenyl haptens are very similar. An outline of the procedure for azophenyl lactoside (Lac) is followed by short descriptions of the departures required for the other haptens.

1. Azophenyl Lactoside (Lac)

MATERIALS AND REAGENTS

Preparation of Diazonium Phenyl Lactoside

p-aminophenyl-β-D-lactoside,* $M_r = 433$
0.1 M HCl
NaNO$_2$, $M_r = 69.0$: 15 mg/ml in water
Ethanol-dry ice mixture

Modification of Red Blood Cells

Red blood cells
Fetal calf serum (FCS), heat inactivated (56°C, 30 min)
Glucose-phosphate-buffered saline (G-PBS; Appendix A.11)
1 M phosphate buffer, pH 7.6 (Appendix A.10)

PROCEDURE

Preparation of Diazonium Phenyl Lactoside, 4.6 × 10^{-3} M

It is critical to have all reagents completely chilled in an ice bath. Cold room temperature (4°C) is not satisfactory.

1. Dissolve 140 mg p-aminophenyl-β-D-lactoside in 12 ml of ice cold 0.1 M HCl.
2. Add 1.6 ml freshly prepared NaNO$_2$ solution.
3. Allow to react for 10 minutes on ice, swirling periodically.

---

* p-aminophenyl-β-D-lactoside can be synthesized as described by Babers and Geobel (1934).

4. Add 23 ml of ice cold water and react for an additional 40 minutes.

5. Dilute further with 34 ml of ice cold water.

6. Divide into 2-ml aliquots and freeze in ethanol-dry ice. Store at $-20°C$ to $-80°C$.

Modification of Red Blood Cells

1. Wash red blood cells 4 times in G-PBS ($400 \times g$, 10 min).

2. Resuspend red blood cells to 50% (v/v) in G-PBS.

3. Mix 1 ml of 1 M phosphate buffer and 2 ml of 4.6×10^{-3} M diazonium phenyl lactoside. Rapidly add this mixture to 2 ml of 50% red blood cells.

4. Tumble at room temperature for 1 hour.

5. Wash cells at least 4 times in G-PBS containing 1% heat-inactivated FCS. (Serum facilitates the removal of non–covalently bound reaction by-products.)

6. Resuspend to 15% (v/v) for use with the hemolytic plaque assay.

2. Azophenyl Glucoside (Glu)

The reagents and coupling procedures are the same as for Lac, except that diazonium phenyl glucoside is used. The preparation of the glucoside is like that of diazonium phenyl lactoside except that Step 1 should read:

1. Dissolve 87 ml of p-aminophenyl-β-D-glucoside ($M_r = 271$) in 12 ml of ice cold 0.1 M HCl.

3. Azophenyl Arsonate (Ars)

The coupling of Ars to red blood cells requires both a modification in the preparation of the diazonium reagent and a shortening of the coupling time.

MATERIALS AND REAGENTS

Preparation of Diazonium Phenyl Arsonate

Arsanilic acid, $M_r = 217.1$ (Sigma Chemical, #A-9258)
1 M HCl
$NaNO_2$, $M_r = 69.0$: 15 mg/ml in water
Ethanol-dry ice mixture

Modification of Red Blood Cells

Red blood cells
Fetal calf serum (FCS), heat inactivated (56°C, 30 min)
Glucose-phosphate-buffered saline (G-PBS; Appendix A.11)
1 M phosphate buffer, pH 7.6 (Appendix A.10)

PROCEDURE

Preparation of Diazonium Phenyl Arsonate

1. Dissolve 70 mg arsanilic acid in 1.2 ml of ice cold 1 M HCl.
2. Add 1.6 ml ice cold NaNO$_2$ solution. Mix.
3. Allow to react for 10 minutes on ice, swirling periodically.
4. Add 34 ml of ice cold water, and react for an additional 40 minutes.
5. Dilute further with 34 ml of ice cold water.
6. Divide into 2-ml aliquots, freeze in ethanol-dry ice and store at −20°C to −80°C.

Modification of Red Blood Cells

Follow the procedure outlined for azophenyl lactoside, but reduce the coupling time to 20 minutes (coupling for 1 hour causes fragility of the red blood cells).

B. Modification of Red Blood Cells with Nitrophenyl Haptens

1. Trinitrophenyl (TNP), Light Modification

MATERIALS AND REAGENTS

Red blood cells
Fetal calf serum (FCS), heat inactivated (56°C, 30 min)
2,4,6-trinitrobenzene sulphonic acid (TNBS), $M_r = 293$ (Sigma Chemical, #P-5878). Note: Avoid skin contact with TNBS to prevent sensitization and contact dermatitis. Wear disposable gloves.
Glucose-phosphate-buffered saline (G-PBS), pH 7.6 (Appendix A.11)
Balanced salt solution (BSS; Appendix A.3)
0.28 M cacodylate buffer, pH 6.9 (Appendix A.13). Note: Cacodylate buffer is poisonous; avoid skin contact and do not pipet by mouth.

PROCEDURE

Note: The hapten modification reaction and subsequent washing should be done in foil-wrapped glassware to protect against photodecomposition.

1. Wash red blood cells 4 times in G-PBS (400 × g, 10 min).
2. Dissolve 20 mg of TNBS in 7 ml of cacodylic buffer.
3. Add 1 ml of packed red blood cells dropwise and tumble the mixture for 10 minutes at room temperature (alternatively, mix slowly with a magnetic bar). Cover reaction mixture with foil.
4. Wash the cells in cold G-PBS that contains 1% heat-inactivated FCS until the supernates are colorless (a minimum of 4 washes).
5. Resuspend to 15% (v/v) in BSS for use in the hemolytic plaque assay.

2. Dinitrophenyl and Nitro-iodophenyl (DNP and NIP)

Direct coupling of SRBC with DNP or NIP epitopes, using dinitrobenzene sulphonic acid or nitro-iodophenyl azide, respectively, has generally been found unreliable. A more reproducible method is to couple the epitope to fowl anti-SRBC antibody or to Fab or F(ab')$_2$ fragments of rabbit or pig anti-SRBC antibody and subsequently coat target SRBC with the hapten-modified antibody.

PROCEDURE

1. Prepare anti-RBC antiserum (Garvey et al. 1977).
2. If necessary, prepare Fab or (Fab')$_2$ fragments of the IgG fraction (Section 12.5). For fowl anti-RBC, prepare a 40% saturated ammonium sulfate (SAS) cut (Section 12.2).
3. Conjugate with the appropriate hapten using conventional methods (Section 16.4, for DNP conjugates). From 6 to 26 haptenic groups per molecule of fowl IgG have been found to sensitize target cells well. Fewer than 6 groups per IgG molecule may be ineffective.
4. Couple hapten-antibody conjugates to washed RBC for 1 hour at 37°C at a final concentration of 8–10% RBC (v/v) in phosphate-buffered saline (PBS). Wash three times in PBS. (The amount of conjugated antibody required for optimal sensitization under standard conditions is determined by testing.)

REFERENCES

Babers, F. H., and W. F. Geobel. 1934. The synthesis of maltose, cellobiose, and genteobiose. *J. Biol. Chem.* **105**:473.

Garvey, J. S., N. E. Cremer, and D. H. Sussdorf. 1977. *Methods in Immunology.* W. A. Benjamin, Reading, MA.

Henry, C., and P. Trefts. 1974. Helper activity *in vitro* to a defined determinant. *Eur. J. Immunol.* **4**:824.

Ingraham, J. S. Specific, complement-dependent hemolysis of sheep erythrocytes by antiserum to azo hapten groups. *J. Infect. Dis.* **91**:268.

Rittenberg, M. B., and K. L. Pratt. 1969. Antitrinitrophenyl (TNP) plaque assay. Primary response of Balb/c mice to soluble and particulate immunogen. *Proc. Soc. Exp. Biol. Med.* **132**:575.

Silver, H., J. F. A. P. Miller, and N. L. Warner. 1971. A simple hemolytic plaque technique for the enumeration of anti-hapten antibody forming cells. *Int. Arch. Allergy* **40**:540.

Strausbauch, P., A. Sulica, and D. Givol. 1970. General method for the detection of cells producing antibodies against haptens and proteins. *Nature* (London) **227**:68.

Truffa-Bachi, P., and L. Wofsy. 1970. Specific separation of cells on affinity columns. *Proc. Natl. Acad. Sci.* (USA) **66**:685.

3.9 AVIDITY MEASUREMENTS WITH PLAQUE ASSAYS
Claudia Henry

The sensitivity of plaque formation to inhibition by free hapten provides a measure of the avidity of the antibodies secreted by the plaque-forming cells (PFC). Plaques due to high-avidity antibodies can be inhibited by low concentrations of free hapten while those due to low-avidity antibodies require high concentrations of hapten for inhibition. The avidity of the antibodies produced by PFC can be expressed as the molar concentration of hapten required to inhibit 50% of the plaque number (H_{50}). An estimate of the median association constant (K) of the released antibody can be obtained from the simple relationship, $K = 2/H_{50}$. It should be noted that theoretical considerations show this relationship holds only when the density of antigenic determinants (epitopes) on target red cells is high (De Lisi and Goldstein 1974). Disparities have also been reported between affinities measured by plaque inhibition and those measured by assays using antibody and antigen in solution (North and Askonas 1974). Nevertheless, if it is possible to achieve the condition of high epitope density, the technique has value because it provides a simple and rapid measurement of antibody affinity. For instance, values for the avidities of both IgM and IgG anti-Lac PFC obtained with the method outlined below correlate well with those of serum anti-Lac antibodies. The procedure makes use of plate assays of PFC, but slide assays can be performed as well.

MATERIALS AND REAGENTS

Same as for direct and indirect plate assay (Section 3.3), plus the following haptens:

For anti-Lac PFC: p-nitrophenyl lactoside, $M_r = 463$ (Accurate Chemical & Scientific)

For anti-TNP PFC: ϵ-TNP-L-lysine HCl $\cdot$ H$_2$O, $M_r = 412$ (ICN Nutritional Biochemicals, #104793)

PROCEDURE

1. Dissolve 23.15 mg of p-nitrophenyl lactoside in 10 ml of G-PBS (5×10^{-3} M). Make 10-fold dilutions in G-PBS to 5×10^{-7} M.
2. Prepare bottom layers as described in Section 3.3, but distribute only 1.7 ml of 0.7% agar into tubes.
3. Make two direct plates and four indirect control plates without hapten, delivering 0.1 ml of lymphocyte suspension, 0.1 ml of Lac-modified red blood cells, and 0.1 ml of G-PBS.
4. Make two direct and four indirect plates for each hapten dilution, delivering 0.1 ml of lymphocyte suspension, 0.1 ml of Lac-modified red blood cells, and 0.1 ml of each hapten dilution.
5. Make plates with uncoupled red cells with and without free hapten. Process for direct and indirect plaques as described in Section 3.3 or 3.7.

COMMENTS

1. Plot the fraction of the control PFC value for each hapten concentration. (Note that the range of effective concentration is now 2.5×10^{-4} to 2.5×10^{-8} M). Draw the best fitting line and find the concentration of hapten required for 50% inhibition.
2. Greater precision is obtained by making 0.5 $\log_{10}$ dilutions of free hapten rather than $\log_{10}$ dilutions as above.
3. The procedure for anti-TNP PFC is similar to that for anti-Lac PFC, except that ϵ-TNP-lysine is used to inhibit plaque formation. Anti-TNP PFC are of higher avidity than anti-Lac plaques which usually have a K of about 10^6 M^{-1}. The initial dilution range of

ε-TNP-lysine should be 5×10^{-8} to 5×10^{-4} M (final concentration: 5×10^{-9} to 5×10^{-5} M).

REFERENCES

Andersson, B. 1970. Studies on the regulation of avidity at the level of the single antibody-forming cell. The effect of antigen dose and time after immunization. *J. Exp. Med.* **132:**77.

De Lisi, C., and B. Goldstein. 1974. On the mechanism of haemolytic plaque inhibition. *Immunochemistry* **11:**661.

Jerne, N. K., C. Henry, A. A. Nordin, H. Fuji, A. M. C. Koros, and I. Lefkovits. 1974. Plaque forming cells: Methodology and theory. *Transplant. Rev.* **18:**130.

Miller, J. F. A. P., and N. L. Warner. 1971. The immune response of normal, irradiated, and thymectomized mice to fowl immunoglobulin G as detected by a hemolytic plaque technique. *Int. Arch. Allergy* **40:**59.

North, J. R., and B. A. Askonas. 1974. Analysis of affinity of monoclonal antibody responses by inhibition of plaque forming cells. *Eur. J. Immunol.* **4:**361.

3.10 ANTI-PROTEIN PLAQUES

To measure immune responses to protein antigens with the hemolytic plaque assay, the indicator red blood cells are coated with the protein. In selecting the optimal degree of modification, it is necessary to seek a balance between the degree of modification and the resulting fragility of the cells. The cells must be sufficiently modified to lyse in the presence of specific antibody and complement, but not so fragile that they lyse spontaneously or during routine handling. In developing techniques to couple proteins other than the ones described here, these procedures can serve as guides. The precise conditions, however, must be determined experimentally. We have included the method of Golub et al. (1968) as well as a modification of it (Kipp and Miller, unpublished). Although the procedure developed by Golub et al. works well, it requires considerably more protein than the modification by Kipp and Miller. However, the modified procedure has been used to date with only a limited number of proteins.

A. Preparation of Protein-Conjugated Red Blood Cells with ECDI

Barbara B. Mishell

This procedure has been used successfully to couple human gamma globulin, albumins, human transferrins, and bovine thyroglobulins to indicator red blood cells for use in the hemolytic plaque assay (Golub et al. 1968). The procedure works well but may not be suitable if the protein of choice is in short supply. Goat red blood cells (GRBC), perhaps because they are smaller than sheep red blood cells (SRBC), were found empirically to yield somewhat clearer plaques than the SRBC.

MATERIALS AND REAGENTS

Goat red blood cells (GRBC)

Human gamma globulin (HGG; Miles Research Products, #82-310): Dissolve in phosphate buffer (see below) to a final concentration of 20 mg/ml.

NaCl, M_r = 58.4

KH_2PO_4, M_r = 136.1

Anhydrous Na_2HPO_4, M_r = 142.0

Balanced salt solution (BSS; Appendix A.3)

1-ethyl-3-(3-dimethylaminopropyl)-carbodiimide HCl (ECDI; Sigma Chemical, #E-7750)

Materials and reagents for slide plaque assay (Section 3.2)

Phosphate buffer: Mix 34.8 g NaCl, 19.2 g KH_2PO_4, and 84.0 g Na_2HPO_4 and bring to 8 liters with double-distilled water. Adjust to pH 7.2 with the appropriate 0.15 M phosphate salt.

PROCEDURE

1. Wash GRBC three times in phosphate buffer and resuspend to 50% (v/v) in the same buffer.

2. To 0.1 ml of the 50% suspension, add 3 ml of HGG at a concentration of 20 mg/ml and mix.

3. Prepare ECDI immediately before use (100 mg/ml in phosphate buffer). While mixing, add 0.5 ml of the ECDI solution to the protein-red blood cell suspension. Allow the reaction to continue at 4°C for 1 hour, mixing or rotating the container all the while.

4. Remove cells from the reaction mixture by centrifugation (200 × g, 10 min) and wash the cells twice with phosphate buffer. Resuspend to 5% (v/v) in BSS for the slide hemolytic plaque assay.

B. Preparation of Protein-Conjugated Red Blood Cells with ECDI (Modification)

Dale Kipp and Alexander Miller

A modification of the method of Golub et al. (1968) results in a more efficient coupling of protein to red blood cells. Firstly, coupling is carried

out in saline rather than phosphate buffer because phosphate reacts with
ECDI. Secondly, the red blood cells are placed in a low ionic solute (0.35
M mannitol, 0.01 M NaCl), which greatly increases their effective acidic
charge. Under these conditions, proteins (and particularly basic proteins)
are strongly bound by red blood cells. This allows efficient conjugation with
initial concentrations of protein as low as 10 to 100 μg per ml and makes
it feasible to induce coupling with fairly precious materials. This modified
method has been used successfully to couple lysozyme, ribonuclease,
collagen, and cytochrome C to red cells and might be useful for conjugating other proteins.

MATERIALS AND REAGENTS

Goat red blood cells (GRBC)
Lysozyme
NaCl, $M_r = 58.4$
Mannitol, $M_r = 182.2$ (Sigma Chemical, #M-4125)
1-ethyl-3(3-dimethylaminopropyl)-carbodiimide HCl (ECDI; Sigma
  Chemical, #E-7750)
Balanced salt solution (BSS, Appendix A.3)
Solutions
  0.35 M mannitol, 0.01 M NaCl: Dissolve 63.7 g mannitol and
    0.58 g NaCl in water and bring to 1000 ml with double-
    distilled water.
  Lysozyme: Dissolve 1 mg/ml (approximately 7×10^{-5} M) in
    water or mannitol solution, pH 7.0–8.0.

PROCEDURE

1. Wash GRBC four times ($400 \times g$, 10 min, 4°C) in cold saline.

2. Wash GRBC once in cold mannitol solution. From this step on,
   there may be some clumping of the GRBC until the cells are
   placed in medium, where they will dissociate again. The clumping
   does not seem to affect the coupling of lysozyme to the red blood
   cells.

3. Resuspend the cells to 10% (v/v) in cold mannitol solution.

4. Add 1.0 ml of 10% red blood cell suspension to 0.1 ml of the
   lysozyme solution. Mix well and rock or rotate in the cold for 10
   minutes.

5. Add 0.1 ml of a 100 mg/ml solution of ECDI in mannitol solution.
   Rock or rotate in the cold for 30 minutes. The ECDI should be
   placed into solution just prior to use since it is not very stable.

6. Wash coupled cells two times in the medium of choice. To use cells in the hemolytic plaque assay, resuspend them to 6–10% (v/v) in BSS.

COMMENTS

1. Although the mannitol solution is not buffered, this does not seem to have an adverse effect on the coupling of the lysozyme to either goat or sheep red blood cells. However, if burro red blood cells are used, irreversible clumping can occur. This clumping can be prevented by adding 1 drop of 0.1 M NaOH for each 1.0 ml of 10% RBC just prior to adding lysozyme.

2. Executing all steps in the cold helps to decrease the clumping; allowing the cells to reach room temperature results in definite clumps and some degree of lysis.

C. Preparation of Protein-Conjugated Red Blood Cells with Bis-Diazotized Benzidine

Mary L. Rodrick

In the following method, protein is coupled to sheep red blood cells (SRBC) using bis-diazotized benzidine (BDB). Erythrocytes coated by this method with a wide variety of protein antigens have been used for many years in passive hemagglutination assays. With minor modifications, the procedure is useful for preparing coated erythrocytes for the detection of cells producing antibody to protein antigens.

MATERIALS AND REAGENTS

Preparation of Bis-Diazotized Benzidine (BDB)

Benzidine, free base, $M_r = 184.2$ (Sigma Chemical, #B-3503). Note: Benzidine is a carcinogen. Wear disposable gloves when handling and do not pipet by mouth.

0.2 M HCl

$NaNO_2$, $M_r = 69.0$

Acetone

Dry ice

Small tubes and stoppers; 10 × 75-mm Pyrex tubes will withstand rapid freezing and storage at −70°C

Ice-salt bath to maintain temperature at 0°C

Thermometer

Beaker, 200–300 ml

Propipette or similar device

Disposable gloves

Preparation of Protein-Coupled Red Blood Cells

Sheep blood in Alsever's solution (must be no more than 1 week old); 0.5 ml of packed sheep red blood cells (SRBC) is required for the following procedure

BDB

0.15 M phosphate buffer, pH 7.3 (Appendix A.12)

Phosphate-buffered saline (PBS), pH 7.3 (Appendix A.8)

Gelatin diluent: 0.1% gelatin in phosphate buffer, pH 7.3. Prepare a 10% (w/v) stock solution in distilled water. Dissolve by boiling or steaming. (The 10% stock will keep about 2 weeks at 4°C; the 0.1% gelatin solution will keep about 1 week at 4°C.)

Bovine serum albumin (BSA), 10 mg/ml in phosphate-buffered saline, pH 7.3

PROCEDURE

Preparation of Bis-Diazotized Benzidine (BDB)

The following description is for 50 ml of BDB.

1. Since the reaction must be performed in the cold and the BDB must be frozen quickly, prepare the ice-salt bath and 50 cold tubes for freezing BDB.

2. In the beaker, dissolve 0.23 g benzidine in 45 ml of cold 0.2 M HCl. Place the beaker in the ice-salt bath and bring the temperature of the solution to 0°C.

3. Add 0.175 g $NaNO_2$ dissolved in 5.0 ml cold distilled water.

4. Allow the reaction to proceed for 30 minutes with intermittent stirring. Maintain the temperature of the reaction mixture at 0°C.

5. At the end of the reaction period, distribute the BDB in 1-ml aliquots to the chilled tubes. Do not pipet by mouth. Stopper the tubes and quickly freeze a few at a time in the bath of dry ice and acetone. Immediately place the tubes in a suitable container and store at −70°C.

Preparation of Protein-Coated Red Blood Cells

1. In a conical graduated tube, wash SRBC three times in phosphate-buffered saline, pH 7.3 (400 × *g*, 10 min, 4°C), using 10 volumes per wash. After the last wash, resuspend the cells in an equal volume of phosphate-buffered saline (50% v/v).

2. *Protein-coupled cells*
   In a 50-ml, round-bottom centrifuge tube place:
   > 10.0 ml phosphate buffer, pH 7.3
   > 1.0 ml (10 mg) BSA
   > 4.0 ml PBS
   > 0.5 ml 50% SRBC

   Control cells
   In a second 50-ml, round-bottom tube place:
   > 10.0 ml phosphate buffer, pH 7.3
   > 5.0 ml 0.1% gelatin diluent
   > 0.5 ml 50% SRBC

   Mix both tubes well by swirling.

3. Thaw 1 tube of BDB (1 ml). As soon as it has thawed, add it to 14 ml of phosphate buffer (1:15 dilution). Mix and *immediately* add 2.5 ml to each of the two centrifuge tubes. Mix the tubes well by swirling and let the reaction proceed for 10–12 minutes at room temperature.

4. Centrifuge the tubes at $500 \times g$ for 5 minutes (4°C). Immediately remove the supernatant, resuspend the cells in 15 ml of 0.1% gelatin diluent, and centrifuge as before. Wash the cells 2–3 additional times with 15-ml volumes of the gelatin diluent.

5. Cells prepared in this manner can be used for about 1 week if stored at 4°C. If the cells are not used immediately, store at 4°C in about 15 ml of the gelatin diluent. Before use, wash the cells 1 or 2 times.

6. For use in the hemolytic plaque assay, resuspend cells in the gelatin diluent to the appropriate concentration. All assays with protein-coupled cells should be compared to those with control cells.

7. Protein-coupled cells may be tested for sensitization by passive hemagglutination in which the cells are diluted 1:160 in gelatin diluent or by passive immune hemolysis with specific antibody and complement.

COMMENTS

1. The preparation of BDB is critical and once made should be tested with cells to determine that adequate coupling occurs. Protein-coupled SRBC should resuspend easily and should not spontaneously lyse or agglutinate. If any of these difficulties occur, a titration of the BDB:protein ratio should be made. Once the optimal ratio has been determined, the titration need not be repeated until

either a new lot of BDB is prepared or a new lot of protein is used. The BDB can be stored as described for approximately 1 year.

2. It is very important to mix the protein or gelatin diluent with SRBC and buffer *before* adding BDB. The cells are more stable in the presence of the gelatin diluent. Serum would probably serve the same function but is much more expensive as a 1% concentration must be used.

3. To use BDB to couple proteins other than BSA to red cells, the optimal BDB : protein ration must be determined experimentally.

D. Preparation of Protein-Conjugated Red Blood Cells with Chromic Chloride
John North

The following general procedure can be used as a guide to couple proteins to red blood cells. The optimal conditions for a particular protein or species of red blood cell must be determined experimentally.

MATERIALS AND REAGENTS

Red blood cells (RBC)
Protein in saline, (5 mg/ml)
Saline, 0.85% NaCl (w/v)
Phosphate-buffered saline (PBS; Appendix A.8)
$CrCl_3·6H_2O$, $M_r = 266.5$ (J. T. Baker Chemical)
Sero-Fuge II (Clay-Adams)
Polypropylene tube, 17×100 mm (Falcon, #2059) for use with Sero-Fuge
Rotator

PROCEDURE

1. Wash RBC 5 times in saline ($400 \times g$, 10 min; or, 2 min in Sero-Fuge).

2. Immediately before use, prepare a solution of $CrCl_3·6H_2O$ in saline at a concentration of 6.6 mg/ml. Dilute 1 : 100 in saline for coupling.

3. To 0.1 ml packed RBC, add 0.1 ml of protein (5 mg/ml). Mix. Add 1.0 ml of the 1 : 100 dilution of $CrCl_3·6H_2O$. Rotate 1 hour at 30°C.

4. Add 6 volumes of PBS (phosphate inhibits the reaction) and cen-

trifuge cells (400 $\times$ g, 10 min). Wash two additional times in PBS. Resuspend RBC for plaque assay.

REFERENCES

ECDI

Golub, E. S., R. I. Mishell, W. O. Weigle, and R. W. Dutton. 1968. A modification of the hemolytic plaque assay for use with protein antigens. *J. Immunol.* **100:**133.

Kipp, D. E., and A. Miller. Unpublished notes.

Bis-Diazotized Benzidine

Gordon, J., B. Rose, and A. H. Sehon. 1958. Detection of "non-precipitating" antibodies in sera of individuals allergic to ragweed pollen by an *in vitro* method. *J. Exp. Med.* **108:**37.

Ivanyi, J., T. Hraba, and J. Cerny. 1964. Immunological tolerance to human serum albumin (HSA) in chickens of adult and juvenile age. *Folia. Biol.* **10:**198.

Tempelis, C. H., and M. L. Rodrick. 1972. Passive hemagglutination inhibition technique for the identification of arthropod blood meals. *Amer. J. Trop. Med. and Hyg.* **21:**238.

Tempelis, C. H., and M. L. Rodrick. 1969. The production in chickens of antibody by spontaneous escape following immunologic tolerance. *J. Immunol.* **103:**1254.

Chromic Chloride

Kishimoto, S., I. Tsuyuguchi, and Y. Yamamura. 1968. The immune response to hapten-azo bovine serum albumin as detected by hemolytic plaque technique. *Int. Arch. Allergy* **34:**544.

Sweet, G. H., and F. L. Welborn. 1971. Use of chromium chloride as the coupling agent in a modified plaque assay. Cells producing anti-protein antibody. *J. Immunol.* **106:**1407.

3.11   MEASUREMENT OF POLYCLONAL RESPONSES

Claudia Henry and John North

In experiments where a large proportion of lymphocytes have been activated to secrete immunoglobulin (polyclonal activation), the conventional hemolytic assay is inappropriate because most of the activated clones will not be secreting antibody directed against any single antigen. However, the plaque assay procedure has been modified to enumerate cells producing immunoglobulins of all specificities. We describe two procedures for measuring plaques arising after polyclonal activation (e.g., after exposure to lipopolysaccharide or other agents that induce both B cell proliferation and differentiation).

The *Staphylococcus aureus* protein A assay depends on the ability of protein A to bind to the Fc portions of the IgG of some species. After sheep red blood cells coated with protein A are plated in agar with lymphocytes, anti-Ig and complement are added (Gronowicz et al. 1976). Complexes of secreted Ig and the anti-Ig bind to protein A on the red cells and activate complement lysis. This method can be used to score all cells secreting Ig by using polyvalent anti-Ig sera containing antibodies to all Ig classes. Measurement of the number of cells secreting Ig of a given class may be made by using class-specific anti-Ig sera.

The alternative use of indicator red cells conjugated with a very high density of haptenic determinants (Coutinho and Möller 1975) depends on two factors. First, the dense presentation of hydrophobic haptenic groups permits cross-reacting antibody with relatively low anti-hapten affinity to bind bivalently, thus increasing the proportion of clones that secrete detectable antibody. Second, because the highly conjugated red cells are more labile, fewer complement-binding sites may be required for their lysis. This increased susceptibility to lysis may increase the effectiveness of antibody with otherwise unfavorable binding equilibrium.

Whereas the protein A assay may be expected to detect all Ig-secreting cells, the highly conjugated red cell system detects only those cells secreting Ig with some affinity for the hapten or red cell in question. Assuming such cells are a constant proportion of the population, the latter procedure provides an indication of the relative size of a polyclonal response but not of its absolute magnitude.

A. Staphylococcal Protein A Assay

MATERIALS AND REAGENTS

Coupling of Staphylococcal Protein A to Red Cells

Sheep red blood cells (SRBC)

Protein A (Pharmacia Fine Chemicals): Dissolve in saline to a final concentration of 0.5 mg/ml.

Saline, 0.85% NaCl (w/v)

$CrCl_3 \cdot 6H_2O$, $M_r = 266.5$ (J. T. Baker Chemical)

Rotator

Sero-Fuge II (Clay Adams)

Polypropylene tube, 17×100 mm (Falcon, #2059) for use with Sero-Fuge

Tube with tight-fitting cap

Assay

Rabbit anti–mouse Ig, polyvalent or class specific (Section 11.4 or 11.5)

Reagents and materials for the plate method (Section 3.3)

PROCEDURE

Coupling of Staphylococcal Protein A to Red Blood Cells

1. Wash SRBC four times in saline (400 $\times$ g, 10 min; or, 2 min in Sero-Fuge).

2. Immediately before use, prepare a solution of $CrCl_3 \cdot 6H_2O$ in saline at concentration of 6.6 mg/ml. Dilute this solution 1 : 100 in saline for coupling.

3. In a tube that can be tightly capped, mix together 1 part of packed SRBC and 1 part of protein A solution. While mixing, add 10 parts of dilute $CrCl_3 \cdot 6H_2O$ solution. Incubate with continuous rotation for 1 hour at 30°C (37°C for 45 minutes is also satisfactory).

4. Wash four times with saline and dilute to 15% by volume. (Assume no loss of red cells due to lysis, unless very obvious).

Assay

The following describes the use of the protein A-red cells by the plate method. (The slide method can also be used after proper dilution of the lymphocyte suspension.)

1. To 2 ml of 0.5% Bacto Difco agar in BSS containing 1 mg/ml DEAE dextran, add 0.1 ml of staph protein A-red cell suspension and the appropriate volume of washed lymphocytes. (We find that 5–10% of the cells score as Ig secretors after four days of incubation in RPMI 1640 containing 2-mercaptoethanol, lipopolysaccharide (LPS), and fetal calf serum. Cultures without LPS have about $\frac{1}{10}$ that number.)

2. Plate as usual in plates over bottom layers.

3. Incubate plates for one hour at 37°C. Then add 1.5 ml of an optimal concentration of rabbit anti-Ig and incubate for an additional hour.

4. Pour off antiserum and add 1.5 ml of guinea pig complement.

5. Incubate for one more hour. The plates can then be stained and scored for plaque-forming cells (Section 3.4).

COMMENTS

1. In the original method (Gronowicz et al. 1976), the antiserum and complement were incorporated into the agar-protein A-red blood

cell-lymphocyte mixture and plates were incubated for 6 hours. We find that the sensitivity of detection is increased by sequential addition of reagents as described above. The total of 3 hours incubation is then sufficient.

2. When using polyvalent anti-Ig serum, we find the same number of plaques when diluted antiserum is added above the agar layer immediately after plating. In this instance the plates are incubated for 2 hours prior to the addition of complement. However, when using monospecific antiserum of lower titer, delayed addition of antiserum may be advantageous.

3. Anti-Ig sera often exhibit a prozone effect in this assay; that is, they give submaximum numbers of plaques when used at concentrations that are too high. Therefore, each antiserum should be titrated to determine its optimal concentration. The absolute efficiency of individual antisera for each class of Ig cannot be determined readily; this shortcoming should be considered in the interpretation of results.

4. Since rabbit antibodies bind to protein A much more efficiently than goat antibodies and since rabbit antisera are less likely to contain noncomplement-fixing antibodies, rabbit anti-Ig sera are more satisfactory than goat antisera in this procedure.

B. Highly Conjugated TNP-SRBC

MATERIALS AND REAGENTS

Preparation of Highly Conjugated TNP-SRBC

Sheep red blood cells (SRBC)

2,4,6-trinitrobenzene sulfonic acid (TNBS), M_r = 293 (Sigma Chemical, #P-5878). Note: Avoid skin contact with TNBS to prevent sensitization and contact dermatitis. Wear disposable gloves.

0.28 M cacodylate buffer, pH 6.9 (Appendix A.13). Note: Cacodylate buffer is poisonous; avoid skin contact and do not pipet by mouth.

Glycylglycine, M_r = 132.1 (ICN Nutritional Biochemicals, #101856)

Phosphate-buffered saline (PBS; Appendix A.8)

Assay

As described for plates (Section 3.3) or slides (Section 3.2)

PROCEDURE

Preparation of Highly Conjugated TNP-SRBC

1. Wash SRBC three times in PBS (400 × g, 10 min).

2. Mix 1 ml packed SRBC, 7 ml cacodylate buffer, and 100 mg TNBS. Stir very gently at room temperature for 30 minutes.

3. Centrifuge and wash modified SRBC once with PBS.

4. Resuspend SRBC in 3 ml PBS and add 60 mg glycylglycine. Let stand at room temperature for 10 minutes.

5. Wash three times with PBS.

Assay

Use either the slide (Section 3.2) or Petri dish (Section 3.3) method to determine the number of plaques with the highly conjugated TNP-SRBC.

REFERENCES

Coutinho, A., and G. Möller. 1975. Thymus-independent B-cell induction and paralysis. *Adv. Immunol.* **21**:113.

Gronowicz, E., A. Coutinho, and F. Melchers. 1976. A plaque assay for all cells secreting Ig of a given type or class. *Eur. J. Immunol.* **6**:588.

3.12 DUPLICATE PLATING

Claudia Henry

The hemolytic plaque assay done on microscope slides can be modified to allow duplicate sampling of the products of a single cell. Duplicate plating can be used to determine if a single cell is producing antibodies of more than one Ig class and more than one specificity or to establish the reactivity of the antibody to two antigens.

MATERIALS AND REAGENTS

As described in Section 3.2.

PROCEDURE

1. Prepare an ultrathin layer of lymphocytes and indicator red blood cells in agarose by touching the edge of the slide to an absorbent towel and draining off the excess as soon as the slide is poured.

2. Prepare a similar slide containing only indicator red blood cells (without lymphocytes). Place the two slides together with a few drops of BSS between them.

3. Incubate the slides for 1–1½ hours in a humid 37°C environment.

4. Process the slides according to experimental plan, i.e., one by

direct methods for IgM PFC, the other by indirect methods for Ig of other classes. Include controls in which both layers are treated identically; it is necessary to establish in each experiment that the method is efficient in revealing on both slides plaques that are generated by one cell.

REFERENCES

Merchant, B., and Z. Brahmi. 1970. Duplicate plating of immune cell products: Analysis of globulin class secretion by single cells. *Science* **167**:69.

Nordin, A. A., H. Cosenza, and S. Sell. 1970. Immunoglobulin classes of antibody-forming cells in mice. II. Class restriction of plaque-forming cells demonstrated by replica plating. *J. Immunol.* **104**:495.

3.13 DETERMINATION OF IgM PLAQUE-FORMING CELLS DIRECTED AGAINST NUCLEATED CELL SURFACE ANTIGENS

Yvonne E. McHugh

The usefulness of the complement-dependent plaque assay (Jerne and Nordin 1963) has been extended through the utilization of nucleated target cells such as ascitic tumor cells (Fuji et al. 1971a; Nordin et al. 1971; Taylor and Bennett 1973) and a variety of normal lymphoid cells (Fuji et al. 1971b; McHugh and Bonavida 1977). Use of these target cells has facilitated the study of B cell populations producing cytolytic antibodies against H-2 (Malavé and Fuji 1975; Degovanni and Lejeune 1973) and Thy-1 (Fuji et al. 1971b; Lake 1976) alloantigens. In addition, this type of plaque assay has been employed to characterize B cell responses against both autoantigens (McHugh and Bonavida 1978) and tumor associated antigens (Fuji and Mihich 1975).

The major advantage of the assay described here is the simplicity with which it enables the kinetics and numbers of IgM antibody-secreting cells that react against nucleated cell surface antigens to be determined. It is also useful for assessing responses too low to be measured by analysis of the antibodies present in serum or culture supernatants.

One application of the plaque assay is the determination of the number of alloantibody-secreting cells following *in vivo* alloimmunization. In the prototype system described below, BALB/c mice (H-2^d) are immunized against mitomycin C-treated spleen cells from C57BL/6 mice (H-2^b). BALB/c spleen cells from immunized mice (or normal controls) are tested in the plaque assay at the peak of the alloantibody response (7–9 days after sensitization), using EL-4 tumor cells (H-2^b) as target indicator cells. To perform the assay, spleen cells from the allosensitized mice are mixed with target cells in medium containing agarose, and the mixture is plated onto microscope slides. When the mixture solidifies, the slides are flooded with medium. After an hour's incubation to allow for antibody secretion, the medium is drained off and the slides are flooded with target-absorbed rabbit complement. During the next hour of incubation, lysis of target cells occurs due to the activation of complement by target-bound IgM antibody. Because lysis of the nucleated target cells does not lead to rapid disintegration (as with red blood cells), the killed target cells are visualized by staining with trypan blue. The plaques surrounding alloantibody (anti-H-2^b)-secreting cells are then counted with 100× magnification. In the BALB/c anti–C57BL/6 system, a peak response of 6000–15 000 plaque-forming cells (PFC) per 10^8 spleen cells can be observed.

A. Alloimmunization

MATERIALS AND REAGENTS

Donor spleen cells from C57BL/6 mice, 8–12 weeks of age. Each donor spleen, after treatment with mitomycin C, will provide a sufficient number of cells to immunize approximately 3 recipients.

Recipient mice, BALB/c, 8–12 weeks of age

RPMI 1640 (Grand Island Biological, #320–1875)

Mitomycin C, lyophilized (Sigma Chemical, #M-0503), dissolved in RPMI 1640 to a concentration of 33 μg/ml just prior to use

Graduated centrifuge tubes, 12–15 ml

Needles, 25 gauge

Tuberculin syringes

Nitex monofilament nylon screen (TETKO, #HC3-110)

PROCEDURE

1. Prepare a suspension of dissociated spleen cells from donor mice as described in Section 1.2

2. Centrifuge the cells (200 × g, 10 min) and estimate the volume of the pellet.

3. Resuspend the cells in a volume of the mitomycin C solution that is 10× the volume of the pellet and incubate the suspension for 30 minutes at 37°C.

4. Wash the cells 4 times with RPMI and resuspend to 10^8 viable

cells/ml. Remove clumps by pouring the suspension through a nylon screen.

5. With a 25-gauge needle and tuberculin syringe, inject 0.2 ml/ mouse of this suspension intraperitoneally (2×10^7 viable cells/ mouse).

6. For assay, harvest spleens of immunized mice 7–9 days after sensitization.

COMMENTS

1. Prior treatment of donor cells with mitomycin C has resulted in the observation of an enhanced number of PFC, possibly because of the elimination of a graft-versus-host response.

2. The murine strain combination described above is only one of many that may be used.

B. Preparation of Target Cells

Depending on the antigen being studied, tumor, spleen, or thymus cells may be the preferred target (McHugh and Bonavida 1977; 1978).

1. Tumor Target Cells

MATERIALS AND REAGENTS

C57BL/6 mice, 8–15 weeks old
EL-4 (H-2^b) T lymphoma in ascitic form (Cell Distribution Center, Salk Institute)
RPMI 1640
Tuberculin syringes
Needles, 25 gauge
Pasteur pipettes and rubber bulb
Centrifuge tubes, 12–15 ml graduated, 50 ml
Nitex monofilament nylon screen (TETKO, #HC3-110)

PROCEDURE

1. Transfer the EL-4 lymphoma by peritoneal injection of 2×10^6 cells/mouse (0.2 ml of 10^7 washed cells/ml suspended in RPMI).

2. After 5–7 days, collect the ascitic tumor cells by opening the peritoneum and flushing it with RPMI repeatedly, using a Pasteur pipette and bulb; a total of 20 ml of RPMI should suffice. Deliver

each peritoneal wash into a 50-ml centrifuge tube through the nylon screen to eliminate clumps.

3. Wash cells two times and bring to a final concentration of 2×10^8 cells/ml in RPMI. Maintain the cell suspension on ice. Each mouse should yield $2-6 \times 10^8$ cells, and 93% or more of the cells should be viable. Red cell contamination should be minimal.

COMMENT

Each immune sample that will be assayed for plaque-forming cells requires 5×10^7 tumor target cells (to be divided between two slides). Each set of duplicate slides requires 2 ml of diluted complement previously absorbed with approximately 0.3 ml packed target cells ($\sim 1.5 \times 10^8$ EL-4 cells).

2. Thymocyte and Splenic Target Cells

MATERIALS AND REAGENTS

Spleen (Section 1.2) and thymus (Section 1.5) cell suspensions from C57BL/6 mice, each at 10^7 cells/ml in RPMI 1640
Fetal calf serum (FCS) or newborn calf serum (NCS): Either serum may be used; however, NCS is less expensive.
Hemolytic Gey's solution (Section 1.18)
Ficoll-Isopaque (Section 8.7)
RPMI 1640
RPMI 1640 containing 2% NCS (RPMI-2%NCS)
Polycarbonate tubes, 16×105 mm (Nalge, #3113)
Water bath adjusted to 20°C
Centrifuge, with rapid acceleration (adjusted to 20°C)

PROCEDURE

1. Treat spleen cell suspension with Gey's solution as described in Section 1.18 to remove red cells.

2. Layer spleen and thymus cell suspensions over Ficoll-Isopaque and centrifuge as described in Section 1.19 to remove dead cells and cell debris. After these manipulations, the cell yield will be approximately 7×10^7 thymocytes/thymus and 5×10^7 splenocytes/spleen.

3. Resuspend washed cells in RPMI-2%NCS to a concentration of 5×10^8 cells/ml and maintain the cell suspension on ice. At least 93% of the cells should be viable. Each immune sample (plated on

duplicate slides) will require 1.25×10^8 target cells in addition to those required for complement absorption (0.3 ml packed cells/sample; see Section 3.13C).

C. Preparation of Rabbit Complement

MATERIALS AND REAGENTS

> Lyophilized rabbit complement (Grand Island Biological, #640-9200)
> NCS
> RPMI 1640
> RPMI-2%NCS
> 0.15 M NaCl
> Graduated, conical centrifuge tubes, 15 ml and 50 ml
> Ice bucket with ice
> Target cells to be used in plaque assay
> Pipette, 10 ml

PROCEDURE

Note: See comments following plaque assay, Section 3.13E

1. Rehydrate the complement with ice cold 0.15 M NaCl (not the diluent provided with the complement). Leave on ice for 30–60 minutes to completely dissolve. Complement not needed should be aliquoted in 1-ml volumes and stored for future use at $-70°C$. Never thaw more than once.

2. Prepare target cells as for the plaque assay (Section 3.13B) but do not bother removing red or dead cells. In a 15-ml conical centrifuge tube, mix approximately 5 ml of undiluted rabbit complement with 0.5–1.0 ml packed target cells and resuspend the cells with a pipette. Leave on ice at least 45 minutes, swirling occasionally to maintain the cells in suspension.

3. Centrifuge the complement-target cell suspension at $400 \times g$ for 10 minutes in a refrigerated (4°C) centrifuge. Decant the complement and dilute 7-fold with RPMI-2%NCS.

D. Preparation of slide trays

MATERIALS AND REAGENTS

> Plexiglass trays, ($11 \times 11 \times \frac{1}{4}$ in.)
> 3 Pyrex tubes, about $\frac{3}{8}$-in. diameter, 24 in. long

Oxygen-acetylene or oxygen gas torch
Tinted protective goggles to use with torch
Water-insoluble glue

PROCEDURE

1. U-shaped glass tubes serve as a support for the microscope slides used in the plaque assay. Heat a glass tube at the midpoint region until it can be bent into a U-shape. The sides of the bent tube should be parallel to each other and about 2 in. apart, so that a microscope slide can rest securely across them.

2. Secure the bent tube to the plexiglass tray with glue. About three bent tubes can be placed side by side on a single tray. About 2 in. must be left in between these structures to allow for the safe manipulation of the slides. Six to eight slides can be placed adjacent to one another with $\frac{1}{4}$–$\frac{1}{2}$ in. between them.

E. Plaque Assay

MATERIALS AND REAGENTS

Target cells, prepared as described in Section 3.13B; adjust to the following concentrations in RPMI-2%NCS:

EL-4 tumor cells: 2×10^8 cells/ml

Spleen cells: 5×10^8 cells/ml

Thymocytes: 5×10^8 cells/ml

Effector spleen cells (Section 3.13A) and normal, unimmunized spleen cells, adjusted to 10^8 viable cells/ml in RPMI-2% NCS

NCS

RPMI-2%NCS

RPMI 1640, supplemented with 1.0 ml 200 mM glutamine and 1.0 ml 1 M HEPES buffer (Grand Island Biological, #380-5630) per 100 ml of medium

Agarose A37 (Indubois): Prepare a 2.5% solution of agarose in 0.15 M NaCl by heating over boiling water until dissolved. Distribute in 2-ml aliquots to 10×75-mm glass culture tubes. (These may be prepared beforehand and stored in the refrigerator.)

Rabbit complement, absorbed with target cells as described in Section 3.13D

Trypan blue: 0.1% (w/v) in 0.15 M saline

Formaldehyde: 0.2% (v/v) in 0.15 M saline

Culture tubes, 10×75 mm

2 racks for 10×75-mm tubes

Conical centrifuge tubes, 15 ml and 50 ml

Heating plate, with a 50-ml beaker of near-boiling water (1 in. deep)

Precoated microscope slides (1 × 3 in.); use unfrosted slides and coat one entire side of the slide with agarose by a method similar to that described in Section 3.2.

Slide trays (Section 3.13C)

Diamond tip pencil

Pasteur pipettes and rubber bulbs

Nitex monofilament nylon screens (TETKO, #HC3-110)

Glass pipettes, 1 ml, 5 ml, and 10 ml

Plastic pipettes, 1 ml

Water bath, adjusted to 42–43°C, (place one rack for the 10 × 75-mm culture tubes in waterbath)

Vortex mixer (fast setting)

Microscope, 100× magnification

Humidified CO_2 incubator, 5% CO_2 in air

Lint-free tissue paper

Staining dishes for microscope slides, rectangular with 200-ml volume

Hand counter

Capillary pipettes, 25 μl

PROCEDURE

1. Number the bottom side of each slide with a diamond tip pencil and place the slides on slide trays (agarose-coated side facing up). Place 10 × 75-mm tubes in the 42°C water bath.

2. Resolubilize agarose by placing in a boiling water bath.

3. With a Pasteur pipette and bulb, gently pass each cell suspension through a nylon screen to remove any clumps that may have formed.

4. Transfer 0.25 ml of target cells and 0.1 ml of effector cells or normal control cells into a series of 10 × 75-mm glass culture tubes. Place these in a rack at room temperature. Make all the cell mixtures to be used in the assay, at this time.

5. Add 0.4 ml of RPMI-2%NCS to one of the culture tubes in the 42°C water bath. Allow the temperature to equilibrate.

6. With a glass pipette, add 0.25 ml of the heated agarose solution to one of the tubes containing RPMI-2%NCS.

7. Place one of the tubes containing a cell mixture in the water bath for about 45 seconds. With a plastic 1-ml pipette, transfer the entire cell mixture to the agarose-medium mixture, vortex (2 seconds), and return the tube to the water bath.

8. With a new 1-ml plastic pipette, quickly transfer 0.35 ml of the agarose-cell mixture onto microscope slides (2 slides/sample tube). To do this, aspirate 0.4 ml of the cell mixture into the pipette, place the tip of the pipette at one end of the microscope slide, and allow the mixture to quickly drain onto the slide. While the mixture is draining out of the pipette, move the tip of the pipette *once* around the circumference of the slide. (Stay away from the edges; do not stir or clumps will form. Also, do not blow out the residual mixture in the pipette onto the slide.) Then quickly spread the mixture with the broadside of the pipette tip. The whole slide need not be covered. If the procedure is not performed quickly, clumps will form, making plaque enumeration impossible. The periphery of the agarose will be uneven because of the mode of application, but the thickness throughout should be relatively uniform. Before applying the second sample to a slide, blow out the residual mixture from the pipette.

9. Allow the agarose to solidify (1–3 minutes, depending on the room temperature). Prepare a new set of sample slides while waiting.

10. After the agarose has solidified deliver 1–2 ml of RPMI-2%NCS on top of the slides. Incubate the slides for 1 hour at 37°C in 5% CO_2 in air under humid conditions.

11. After this incubation, drain each slide by tipping it onto lint-free tissue and letting the liquid overlay flow off. Replace the overlay with 1–1.5 ml of diluted, absorbed rabbit complement. Control slides should receive only RPMI-2%NCS (see step 15). Again incubate at 37°C for 1 hour.

12. Following this incubation, drain off the complement and rinse the slides with 10 ml of RPMI-2%NCS per slide.

13. Overlay the slides with 2 ml trypan blue solution for 10 minutes at room temperature. Drain onto lint-free tissue. Overlay the slides with 3 ml RPMI without NCS. Allow the slides to destain for 3 minutes; then drain as above. Repeat 4 times. Further destaining and storage of the slides can be accomplished by maintaining the slides in 0.2% formaldehyde in staining dishes. Trypan blue-stained plaques will remain distinct for up to 12 hours.

14. Scan each entire slide under 100× magnification. Plaques appear as roundish areas of regularly spaced cells that have taken up trypan blue. The background of live cells are predominantly unstained.

15. Assay all samples in duplicate or triplicate. Controls should include target cells plated with normal splenocytes and sensitized

splenocyte-target cell slides overlayed with medium rather than complement.

16. The number of PFC per 10^8 viable spleen cells can be calculated by the following equations:

$$\text{PFC}/10^8 \text{ cells} = \frac{\text{number of PFC/slide}}{\text{number of cells/slide}} \times 10^8 \text{ cells};$$

Number of cells/slide $= (0.1 \text{ ml})(10^8/\text{ml})(0.35)$.

COMMENTS

1. It is advantageous to perform a pretest to make sure that the absorbed complement is active but not cytotoxic. Perform the assay as above but use 0.5 ml of RPMI-2%NCS (instead of 0.4 ml). Do not add effector splenocytes. On two slides spot heat-inactivated serum from "10-day" allosensitized mice in discrete areas on the agarose with a 25-μl capillary pipette. Do not overlay the slide with medium. Incubate for 1 hour at 37°C in a humid CO_2 incubator. Rinse each slide with 10 ml RPMI. On one of the slides add complement and on the other add RPMI-2%NCS. Incubate, rinse, and stain the slides (as above). If the complement is active and not cytotoxic, discrete areas of dead cells will appear where the antiserum was applied. Slides spotted with normal heat-inactivated serum serve as controls.

2. The strain combination presented above represents only one of many that may be used. However, because tumor cell lines vary greatly in size, their concentration must be adjusted accordingly when they are used as targets in the plaque assay. For instance, EL-4 (C57BL/6, H-2[b]) and D6 (C3H/HeJ, H-2[k]) are about the same size and are used at a concentration of 2×10^8 cells/ml. In contrast, the P815 (DBA/2, H-2[d]) mastocytoma is much larger and is used at 1.3×10^8 cells/ml. Too concentrated a target will make the plaques very small; too low a concentration will make them diffuse.

3. Antibodies other than IgM have not been measured successfully with this system.

REFERENCES

Degovanni, B. and G. Lejeune. 1973. Antibody response, measured by a plaque assay, compared to a cellular response after skin allograft in mice. *Transplant.* **20:**492.

Fuji, H., M. Zalenski, and F. Milgrom. 1971a. Plaque-forming-cell response to H-2 antigens of mice. *Proc. Soc. Exp. Biol. Med.* **136:**239.

Fuji, H., M. Zalenski, and F. Milgrom. 1971b. Immune response to alloantigens of thymus studied in mice with plaque assay. *J. Immunol.* **106:**56.

Fuji, H., and E. Mihich. 1975. Selection for high immunogenicity in drug-resistant sublines of murine lymphomas demonstrated by plaque assay. *Cancer Res.* **35:**946.

Jerne, N. K., and A. A. Nordin. 1963. Plaque formation in agar by single antibody-producing cells. *Science* **140:**405.

Lake, P. 1976. Antibody response induced *in vitro* to the cell-surface alloantigen, Thy-1. *Nature* **262:**297.

Malavé, I., and H. Fuji. 1975. Primary antibody response against K and D regions of the H-2[a] and H-2[d] haplotypes. *Transplant.* **20:**492.

McHugh, Y., and B. Bonavida. 1977. Antibody-forming cells with specificity for syngeneic and allogeneic (thymocyte) tissue antigens following lipopolysaccharide mitogenic stimulation. *Transplant. Proc.* **9:**1205.

McHugh, Y., and B. Bonavida. 1978. Autoreactive antibody-forming cells directed against thymocytes and thymus-derived lymphocytes. *J. Immunol.* **121:**1090.

Nordin, A. A., J.-C. Cerottini, and K. T. Brunner. 1971. The antibody response to allografts as determined by a plaque assay with allogeneic target cells. *Eur. J. Immunol.* **1:**55.

Taylor, G. M., and J. Bennett. 1973. A modified plaque test for the detection of cells forming alloantibody to alloantigens. *J. Immunol. Meth.* **2:**213.

4

Cell-Mediated
Cytolytic Responses

Kenneth Grabstein, with contributions from Yu-hua Una Chen

4.1 INTRODUCTION

The killing of target cells by sensitized T lymphocytes is an important type of cell-mediated immunity for which reliable quantitative assays have been developed. The reaction is antigen specific and requires contact between the specific effector T lymphocyte and a target cell carrying the appropriate cell surface antigen. Effector cells are generated in a manner analogous to the generation of antibody-forming cells. Antigens stimulate specific T lymphocyte precursors to proliferate and differentiate. The generation of cytolytic effectors has been extensively studied *in vitro* and appears to involve the cooperation of at least three types of cells: antigen-specific T effector precursors, antigen-specific T amplifiers (helpers), and nonspecific accessory cells.

Usually the responding lymphocytes and the immunizing target cells employed in these studies are from the same species. Cytolytic responses have been generated *in vitro* to sensitizing cells carrying major alloantigens* (Wunderlich and Canty 1970; Wagner and Feldmann 1972; Cerottini and Brunner 1974; Cerottini et al. 1974), minor alloantigens* (Bevan 1975; Miller and Mishell 1975), TNP-modified syngeneic surface structures (Shearer 1974), tumor-specific antigens (Gillis and Smith 1977), the male H-Y antigen (Simpson et al. 1975), and virus-specific antigens on tumor cells (Ting and Bonnard 1976).

Cell-mediated cytotoxicity is quantitated by using target cells that release a radioactive label ($^{51}CrO_4^=$) when killed by cytolytic effector cells. The amount of radioactivity released into the cell-free supernatant of mixtures of cytolytic lymphocytes and labeled target cells is directly proportional to the percentage of target cells killed. In this way, different populations of lymphocytes can be compared for their relative amount of cytolytic effector cells.

REFERENCES

Bevan, M. J. 1975. The major histocompatibility complex determines susceptibility to cytotoxic T cells directed against minor histocompatibility antigens. *J. Exp. Med.* **142**:1349.

Cerottini, J.-C., and K. T. Brunner. 1974. Cell-mediated cytotoxicity, allograft rejection, and tumor immunity. *Adv. Immunol.* **18**:67.

Cerrottini, J.-C., H. D. Engers, H. R. MacDonald, and K. T. Brunner. 1974. Generation of cytotoxic T lymphocytes *in vitro*. I. Response of normal and immune mouse spleen cells in mixed leukocyte cultures. *J. Exp. Med.* **140**:703.

Gillis, S., and K. A. Smith. 1977. *In vitro* generation of tumor-specific cytotoxic lymphocytes. Secondary allogeneic mixed tumor lymphocyte culture of normal murine spleen cells. *J. Exp. Med.* **146**:468.

Klein J. 1975. *Biology of the Mouse Histocompatibility-2 Complex: Principles of Immunogenetics Applied to a Single System.* Springer-Verlag, New York.

Miller, C. L., and R. I. Mishell. 1975. Differential regulatory effects of accessory cells on the generation of cell-mediated immune reactions. *J. Immunol.* **114**:692.

Shearer, G. M. 1974. Cell-mediated cytotoxicity to trinitrophenyl-modified syngeneic lymphocytes. *Eur. J. Immunol.* **4**:527.

Simpson, E., R. Gordon, M. Taylor, J. Mertin, and P. Chandler. 1975. Micromethods for induction and assay of mouse mixed lymphocyte reactions and cytotoxicity. *Eur. J. Immunol.* **5**:451.

Snell, G. D., J. Dausset, and S. Nathenson. 1976. *Histocompatibility.* Academic Press, New York.

---

* Two useful, comprehensive reviews of mouse histocompatibility genetics (Klein 1975; Snell et al. 1976) are listed in the references for this section.

Ting, C.-C., and G. D. Bonnard. 1976. Cell-mediated immunity to Friend virus-induced leukemia. IV. *In vitro* generation of primary and secondary cell-mediated cytotoxic responses. *J. Immunol.* **116**:1419.

Wagner, H., and M. Feldmann. 1972. Cell-mediated immune response *in vitro*. I. A new *in vitro* system for the generation of cell-mediated cytotoxic activity. *Cell. Immunol.* **3**:405.

Wunderlich, J. R., and T. G. Canty. 1970. Cell mediated immunity induced *in vitro*. *Nature* **228**:62.

4.2 *IN VITRO* GENERATION OF CYTOLYTIC T LYMPHOCYTES

The generation of cytolytic T lymphocytes was initially reported by Wunderlich and Canty (1970). Both the culture procedures developed by Mishell and Dutton (1966) and those developed by Marbrook (1967) have been used in generating cytolytic effector cells. The culture methods described in this chapter are essentially the same as those described for the generation of humoral responses (Section 2.2) except for the nature, preparation, and dose of the antigen.

MATERIALS AND REAGENTS

As described in Section 2.2 with the following exception:

SRBC are not used as antigen. The antigen may be cells from the spleen, lymph node, thymus, or a tumor cell line such as P815 mastocytoma (Cell Distribution Center, Salk Institute). The tumor cell line is most commonly used.

PROCEDURE

1. Harvest the cells that are the source of antigen and wash in a large volume of BSS. Resuspend to approximately 1×10^6 cells/ml in BSS and x-irradiate with 2000–3000 R. Wash again, count the cells, and adjust to 10^6 cells/ml in complete medium. Optimal immunizing doses may vary depending on the particular combination of responding cells and antigen being studied. For the responses by C57BL/6 spleen against DBA/2 antigens, a dose of 1 sensitizing cell (antigen) to 4 responding cells is satisfactory.

2. Precursors of cytolytic responder cells may be either spleen or lymph node cells. Culture these cells at a concentration of 4×10^6–2×10^7 cells/ml in 1-ml cultures.

3. The specific conditions desired at the assay stage (Section 4.3D, Section 4.3E) will dictate the number of cells initiated in culture at

this time. Determine what effector-to-target ratios will be used for the assay and calculate how many effector cells will be required. Cultures initiated with 2×10^7 cells at this time will provide enough effectors for titrations beginning at an effector-to-target ratio of 20 : 1 for the microwell assay (Section 4.3D) or 5 : 1 for the tube assay (Section 4.3E). Higher effector-to-target ratios may be used and will require the initiation of more effector cells at this stage. Cell recoveries in effector cell cultures usually approach 100%.

COMMENTS

1. The absolute frequency of precursors of cytolytic T cells can be estimated using limiting dilution analysis (Skinner and Marbrook 1976; Teh et al. 1977; and Lindahl and Wilson 1977). See Chapter 5.

2. Cytolytic T lymphocytes may also be generated in microcultures, as described by Simpson et al. (1975).

3. We have generally found that FCS that support primary humoral responses *in vitro* also support T-cell-mediated cytolytic responses *in vitro*. We at times test lots of FCS from various suppliers for use with primary humoral responses. Lots found satisfactory for use in that system are reserved by the companies for sale to those who specifically request them. The identification numbers of tested lots of FCS, if available, can be obtained from us by phone or mail.

REFERENCES

Lindahl, K. F., and D. B. Wilson. 1977. Histocompatibility antigen-activated cytotoxic T lymphocytes. II. Estimates of the frequency and specificity of precursors. *J. Exp. Med.* **145:**508.

Marbrook, J. 1967. Primary immune response in cultures of spleen cells. *Lancet* **ii:**1279.

Mishell, R. I., and R. W. Dutton. 1966. Immunization of normal mouse spleen cell suspensions *in vitro. Science* **153:**1004.

Simpson, E., R. Gordon, M. Taylor, J. Mertin, and P. Chandler. 1975. Micromethods for induction and assay of mouse mixed lymphocyte reactions and cytotoxicity. *Eur. J. Immunol.* **5:**451.

Skinner, M. A., and J. Marbrook. 1976. An estimation of the frequency of precursor cells which generate cytotoxic lymphocytes. *J. Exp. Med.* **143:**1562.

Teh, H.-S., E. Harley, R. A. Phillips, and R. G. Miller. 1977. Quantitative studies on the precursors of cytotoxic lymphocytes. I. Characterization of a clonal assay and determination of the size of clones derived from single precursors. *J. Immunol.* **118:**1049.

Wunderlich, J. R., and T. G. Canty. 1970. Cell mediated immunity induced *in vitro*. *Nature* **228**:62.

4.3 CHROMIUM RELEASE ASSAY

The quantitative assay of antigen-specific cytolytic T lymphocytes using ^{51}Cr released from labeled target cells was introduced by Brunner et al. (1968). First described for the assay of effector cell activity against major alloantigens, this assay has been adapted to measure activity against minor alloantigens (Bevan 1975; Miller and Mishell 1975), TNP-modified syngeneic cells (Shearer 1974), tumor-specific antigens (Gillis and Smith 1977), virus-specific antigens on infected macrophage monolayers (Zinkernagel and Doherty 1975), and the male H-Y antigen (Simpson et al. 1975). These adaptations will not be discussed here although most of them use the same basic procedure.

In the procedure described below, serial dilutions of cytolytic effector cell populations are incubated in the presence of a constant number of ^{51}Cr-labeled target cells at low effector-to-target ratios (10 : 1, 5 : 1, 2.5 : 1, and 1.25 : 1). At these low ratios, each effector cell is saturated with targets and kills at maximum efficiency. After 3 to 4 hours, the radioactivity released into the supernatants is measured and the percent specific cytotoxicity is calculated. Under these experimental conditions, the amount of lysis observed is usually linearly related to the number of effector cells; thus, titration of different effector populations will yield straight line graphs of cytotoxicity that may vary in slope (Henney 1971). Variations in the slopes reflect differences in both the frequency and the efficiency of cytolytic cells in the effector populations (Thorn and Henney 1976).

There are several variations of the chromium release assay, which differ in the number of cells and the assay volumes used. One of the techniques described below uses microwells and small volumes. The advantage of this method is that it makes it possible to run more complete titrations with fewer cells. Another technique described uses tubes and larger assay volumes. The procedure for the preparation and radiolabeling of the target cells is the same for both techniques.

A. Preparation of Target Cells

Various types of tumor cells, maintained *in vivo,* are good targets for cell-mediated cytotoxicity (CMC) assays. P815 (DBA/2) mastocytoma is the most widely used. Splenic blast cells induced by either concanavalin A (Con A) or lipopolysaccharide (LPS) may also be used as targets. However, mitogen-induced blasts give a relatively high spontaneous release of label. High spontaneous release also occurs with tumor cells maintained *in vitro*.

1. Tumor Cells

MATERIALS AND REAGENTS

DBA/2 mice

P815 tumor cells (Cell Distribution Center, Salk Institute)

Complete medium: Eagle's minimum essential medium (MEM) for suspension cultures (Microbiological Associates, #12-126) or RPMI 1640 (Grand Island Biological, #320-1875), which contains 1% sodium pyruvate (100 mM solution), 1% L-glutamine (200 mM solution), 1% Eagle's minimal medium nonessential amino acids (100× solution), and 5% fetal calf serum (FCS), pretested (Appendix A.1) and heat inactivated at 56°C for 30 minutes.

Balanced salt solution (BSS; Appendix A.3)

PROCEDURE

1. Obtain fresh P815 cells from the peritoneal cavities of DBA/2 mice (Section 1.3) that have been injected intraperitoneally 5 to 7 days previously with 10^7 viable tumor cells/mouse.

2. Wash cells in a large volume of BSS ($200 \times g$, 10 min, 4°C).

3. Resuspend to 2×10^7 cells/ml in complete medium for labeling.

2. Blast Cells

MATERIALS AND REAGENTS

Normal spleen cell suspension (Section 1.2)

Complete medium as described above for the preparation of tumor target cells, with the following exception and additions:

10% FCS, instead of 5%

5×10^{-5} M 2-mercaptoethanol (2-ME; Sigma Chemical, #M-6250); see Appendix A.6 for preparation.

1% penicillin-streptomycin (5000 units of penicillin, 5000 μg of streptomycin per ml of stock); optional

Concanavalin A (Con A), 2× crystallized in saturated NaCl (Miles Research Products) *or*

Bacto-lipopolysaccharide W (LPS), *S. typhosa* 0901 (Difco Laboratories)

BSS

Tissue culture dishes, 100 × 15 mm (Lux Scientific, #5211 and #5275)

Culture chamber (Bellco Glass, #7741-10005)

Gas mixture: 7% O_2, 10% CO_2, 83% N_2

PROCEDURE

1. Culture normal spleen cells (4 × 10^6/ml) in complete medium that contains 5 × 10^{-5} M 2-ME, 10% FCS, and either 2 μg/ml Con A or 10 μg/ml LPS. It is convenient to culture the cells in 10-ml volumes in 100-mm Petri dishes.

2. Culture cells in culture chambers containing the gas mixture. These cultures are not rocked.

3. Harvest the cells after 2–3 days and wash them twice in a large volume of BSS.

4. Resuspend cells to 2 × 10^7 cells/ml in complete medium for labeling; 100% cell recovery is not unusual.

B. Radioactive Labeling of Target Cells

Note: Established safety procedures must be followed in handling radioactive material.

MATERIALS AND REAGENTS

Complete medium as described for the preparation of tumor target cells (Section 4.3A)

BSS

$(Na)_2{}^{51}CrO_4$, 200–500 Ci/g, 1000 μCi/ml (New England Nuclear, #NEZ-030)

Centrifuge tube, 50 ml (Falcon, #2070 or similar)

PROCEDURE

1. Check age of $(Na)_2{}^{51}CrO_4$ and refer to the ^{51}Cr decay chart (Table 4.1) to determine current activity per ml.

2. Adjust the concentration of target cells to 10^7 cells/ml in complete

medium. Add an appropriate volume of $(Na)_2{}^{51}CrO_4$ so that there is 100 μCi ^{51}Cr/10^7 cells.

3. Incubate the mixture for 45 minutes to 1 hour at 37°C, swirling the tube periodically to maintain the cells in suspension. Wash the cells once in BSS (200 × g, 10 min). Then incubate the cells in 50 ml BSS for 30 minutes. (Incubating in a large volume of BSS for 30 minutes reduces nonspecific background radioactivity.) After each wash, discard the supernatant into a liquid radioactive waste container and shake the pellet gently in the residual liquid to resuspend the cells. Avoid pipetting since this may damage the cells and cause an increase in the nonspecific spontaneous release of ^{51}Cr.

4. Centrifuge the cells and wash once in complete medium. Adjust the cells in complete medium to 10^6 cells/ml for the microwell assay or 1.2 × 10^7 cells/ml for the tube assay.

C. Controls

Two controls must be included in the assay: for background (spontaneous) and for total ^{51}Cr release from the radiolabeled target cells.

MATERIALS AND REAGENTS

As described for sections 4.3D and 4.3E (see below), with the following additions:

Unsensitized spleen cells (optional), same strain as cytolytic effectors, 2 × 10^7/ml (microwell assay) or 1.2 × 10^7 cells/ml (tube assay) in complete medium
Nonidet P40 (NP40) (Particle Data Laboratories): 1% (w/v) in water

TABLE 4.1
^{51}Cr decay chart*

Days	μCi/ml	Days	μCi/ml	Days	μCi/ml	Days	μCi/ml
1	976	8	820	15	690	22	580
2	952	9	800	16	673	23	566
3	928	10	781	17	657	24	552
4	906	11	762	18	641	25	539
5	884	12	743	19	625	26	525
6	862	13	725	20	610	27	513
7	841	14	707	21	595	28	500

* To use the chart, determine the number of days that have elapsed since the ^{51}Cr sample was 1000 μCi/ml (as ascertained by supplier).

PROCEDURE

1. *Background release*: Background release is the amount of label released by the target cells in the absence of cytolytic effector cells. To provide for the measurement of background release, either incubate the labeled target cells alone or incubate them together with unsensitized spleen cells of the same strain as the cytolytic effectors. However, because ^{51}Cr spontaneously released by the target cells can be taken up by the normal spleen cells, the latter procedure often gives lower values of apparent spontaneous release.

2. *Total release*: To measure total release, all target cells must be lysed. The usual method used to lyse the cells is to suspend the labeled target cells in water and freeze-thaw 3 times. An alternate method is to add 1.0% NP40 to microwells (0.1 ml/well) or tubes (0.5 ml/tube) containing the target cells. The total release control lines are then treated the same as all the other lines. Although the use of NP40 is convenient, it does give a higher total release value than the freeze-thaw method; this results in lower values for specific release.

D. Microwell Assay

To have sufficient numbers of effector cells for a quantitative assay, initiate effector cell cultures with a total of 2×10^7 cells for each experimental line (Section 4.2). This will provide enough cells for effector-to-target ratios beginning at 20:1. Cell recoveries in effector cell cultures usually approach 100% and need not be calculated at this time. Titrations of effector cells are based on the number of cells initiated in culture for the generation of effector cells (Section 4.2).

MATERIALS AND REAGENTS

^{51}Cr-labeled target cells (Section 4.3B)
Complete medium as described for preparation of tumor target cells (Section 4.3A)
BSS
NP40: 1% (w/v) in water
Gas mixture: 7% O_2, 10% CO_2, 83% N_2
Disposable glass culture tubes, 12 × 75 mm
Culture chamber (Bellco Glass, #7741-10005)

Linbro Disposo multiwell tray, 96 wells (Flow Laboratories #76-362-05) and cover for Disposo multiwell tray (Flow Laboratories #76-406-05)

Centrifuge carriers, holding 5 microwell plates each (Cooke Laboratory Products, #18-082)

Horizontal centrifuge rotor, 4-place pin-type (Damon/IEC Division, #IEC 276)

Pipetman, 20–200 μl (West Coast Scientific, #P-200D)

Pipette tips (E & K Scientific Products, #7505)

PROCEDURE

1. Prepare ^{51}Cr-labeled target cells (Section 4.3B). Adjust to 10^6 cells/ml in complete medium.

2. Harvest cytolytic effector cell cultures and pool replicates. Pellet the cells (200 $\times$ g, 10 min, 4°C) and wash once in BSS. Resuspend each line to 1.0 ml (2 $\times$ 10^7 cells/ml assuming 100% recovery) in complete medium.

3. Make serial 2-fold dilutions in complete medium. At least three dilutions of each effector population should be run. The dilutions chosen may vary depending on the expected activity.

4. To each well add 0.1 ml of effector cell suspension (ranging from undiluted to a dilution of 1 : 16). These dilutions result in effector: target ratios ranging from 20 : 1 to 1.25 : 1. Run each experimental point in triplicate.

5. To each well add 0.1 ml of labeled target cell suspension (10^5 cells/well).

6. Control wells for background ^{51}Cr release receive labeled target cells and either 0.1 ml of unsensitized effector cells or 0.1 ml of complete medium. Control wells for total ^{51}Cr release receive labeled target cells and 0.1 ml of 1% NP40 (see Section 4.3C).

7. Cover plates with lids. Place plates in a humidified culture chamber and exchange the air with the gas mixture. Incubate the cultures at 37°C for 3–4 hours.

8. After 3–4 hours of incubation, place the plates in centrifuge carriers for centrifugation. Centrifuge at 250 $\times$ g for 10 to 20 minutes.

9. Remove 80 or 100 μl of supernatant from each well, taking care not to disturb the pellet. Tilt plate to facilitate the harvesting of supernatant. Place supernatants in disposable 12 $\times$ 75-mm glass tubes and count samples in a gamma counter adjusted for ^{51}Cr.

E. Tube Assay

Effector cell cultures initiated with 4×10^7 cells for each experimental line (Section 4.2) will provide enough cells for effector-to-target ratios beginning at 10 : 1. Cell recoveries in effector cell cultures usually closely approach 100% and need not be calculated at this time. Titrations of effector cells are based on the number of cells initiated in culture for the generation of effector cells (Section 4.2).

MATERIALS AND REAGENTS

^{51}Cr-labeled target cells
Complete medium as described for preparation of tumor target cells (Section 4.3A)
BSS
NP40: 1% (w/v) in water
Gas mixture: 7% O_2, 10% CO_2, 83% N_2
Disposable glass culture tubes, 12 × 75 mm
Culture chamber (Bellco Glass, #7741-10005)
Disposable clear plastic tubes with caps, 12 × 75 mm (Falcon, #2054)
Carrier, $\frac{3}{4}$ in. trunnion, 28 places (Damon/IEC Division, #IEC 1021)
Biopette with Biotips (Schwarz/Mann, #0010-29 and #0010-30)
Slant tube rack to hold tubes in culture chamber (Bellco Glass, #2028-50008)

PROCEDURE

1. Prepare ^{51}Cr-labeled target cells as described above (Section 4.3B). Resuspend to 1.2×10^7 cells/ml in complete medium.

2. Harvest, pool and wash cytolytic effector cell cultures. Resuspend cells to 3.3 ml, containing approximately 1.2×10^7 recovered cells/ml (assuming 100% recovery).

3. Make serial 2-fold dilutions in complete medium. At least three dilutions of each effector population should be tested. The three dilutions chosen may vary depending on the expected activity.

4. Place tubes in slanted rack.

5. To each tube add 0.5 ml of effector cell suspension (ranging from undiluted to a dilution of 1 : 8). These dilutions result in effector: target ratios ranging from 10 : 1 to 1.25 : 1.

6. To each tube add 0.05 ml of labeled target cell suspension (6×10^5 cells/tube).

7. Control tubes for background (spontaneous) ^{51}Cr release receive

0.05 ml of labeled target cells and either 0.5 ml of unsensitized effector cells (Section 4.3C) or 0.5 ml of complete medium. Control tubes for total ^{51}Cr release receive 0.05 ml of labeled target cells and 0.5 ml of water (or other lysing agent—see Section 4.3C). If water is used, freeze and thaw the tubes 3 times.

8. Cap the tubes loosely to allow gas exchange. Place rack into culture chamber and exchange the air with the gas mixutre. Incubate the cultures at 37°C for 3–4 hours.

9. After 3–4 hours incubation, place tubes in 28-place trunnions and centrifuge at 250 × g for 10 minutes.

10. Remove 0.2 or 0.3 ml of supernatant from each tube with the Biopette. Place supernatants in disposable glass tubes and count samples in a gamma counter adjusted for ^{51}Cr. Take care not to disturb the pellet when removing the supernatants.

F. Calculations

Assay serial dilutions of each effector cell culture for cytotoxic activity. Run each experimental point in triplicate. Average the counts per minute (cpm) for the triplicates and calculate the percent specific cytotoxicity using the formula:

% specific cytotoxicity =

$$\frac{\text{experimental cpm} - \text{background release cpm}}{\text{total release cpm} - \text{background release cpm}} \times 100$$

Represent the percent specific cytotoxicity graphically as a function of culture dilution or effector cell number. Under the conditions of this assay, the percent specific cytotoxicity is linearly related to the number of effector cells. The slope of the line will vary depending on the proportion of cytolytic cells and the efficiency of cytolysis in the effector population (Thorn and Henney 1976). Compare different effector cell cultures by determining what dilution of each culture produces a particular amount of killing (e.g., 10% specific cytotoxicity).

The results can also be expressed in lytic units (Cerottini et al. 1974). One lytic unit is defined as the fraction of one culture required to achieve a particular amount of killing (e.g., 10% specific release). If ¼ of one culture is required to give 10% specific release, that culture has a total of 4 lytic units. Compare different effector cell cultures by determining how many lytic units each culture contains.

The two methods of expressing specific cytotoxicity (percent specific cytotoxicity and lytic units) are basically the same, differing only by the magnitude of the number reported.

COMMENTS for 4.3

The method described above cannot distinguish between differences in cytolytic cell frequency and cytolytic cell efficiency. Several approaches have been used to make such distinctions:

1. The absolute frequency of cytolytic effector cells can be estimated as described by Henney (1977). By manipulating the presence of Mg^{2+}, Ca^{2+}, and cytochalasin B in the mixture of effector cells and target cells, it is possible to obtain conditions such that each effector cell can kill only a single target cell.

2. Alternatively, the absolute frequency of cytolytic cells can be estimated by limiting dilution analysis (Lindahl and Wilson 1977). Effector cells are titrated against an optimal number of labeled targets in order to find a dose that produces one effector cell for each culture in which cytolysis is detected. This method requires very sensitive assay techniques that produce low values of spontaneous background release.

3. The relative frequency and efficiency of cytolytic effector cells can be estimated by titrating labeled target cells against a constant number of effector cells and analyzing the kinetics of target cell destruction (Thorn and Henney 1976).

REFERENCES

Bevan, M. J. 1975. The major histocompatibility complex determines susceptibility to cytotoxic T cells directed against minor histocompatibility antigens. *J. Exp. Med.* **142**:1349.

Brunner, K. T., J. Mauel, J.-C. Cerottini, and B. Chapuis. 1968. Quantitative assay of the lytic action of immune lymphoid cells on ^{51}Cr-labelled allogeneic target cells *in vitro*; inhibition by isoantibody and by drugs. *Immunology* **14**:181.

Cerottini, J.-C., H. D. Engers, H. R. MacDonald, and K. T. Brunner. 1974. Generation of cytotoxic T lymphocytes *in vitro*. I. Response of normal and immune mouse spleen cells in mixed leukocyte cultures. *J. Exp. Med.* **140**:703.

Gillis, S., and K. A. Smith. 1977. *In vitro* generation of tumor-specific cytotoxic lymphocytes. Secondary allogeneic mixed tumor lymphocyte culture of normal murine spleen cells. *J. Exp. Med.* **146**:468.

Henney, C. S. 1971. Quantitation of the cell-mediated immune response. I. The number of cytolytically active mouse lymphoid cells induced by immunization with allogeneic mastocytoma cells. *J. Immunol.* **107**: 1558.

Henney, C. S. 1977. T-cell-mediated cytolysis: An overview of some current issues. *Contemporary Topics in Immunobiology* **7**:245.

Lindahl, K. F., and D. B. Wilson. 1977. Histocompatibility antigen-activated cytotoxic T lymphocytes. I. Estimates of the absolute frequency of killer cells generated *in vitro. J. Exp. Med.* **145**:500.

Miller, C. L., and R. I. Mishell. 1975. Differential regulatory effects of accessory cells on the generation of cell-mediated immune reactions. *J. Immunol.* **114**:692.

Shearer, G. M. 1974. Cell-mediated cytotoxicity to trinitrophenyl-modified syngeneic lymphocytes. *Eur. J. Immunol.* **4**:527.

Simpson, E., R. Gordon, M. Taylor, J. Mertin, and P. Chandler. 1975. Micromethods for induction and assay of mouse mixed lymphocyte reactions and cytotoxicity. *Eur. J. Immunol.* **5**:451.

Thorn, R. M., and C. S. Henney. 1976. Kinetic analysis of target cell destruction by effector T cells. I. Delineation of parameters related to the frequency and lytic efficiency of killer cells. *J. Immunol.* **117**:2213.

Thorn, R. M., and C. S. Henney. 1977. Kinetic analysis of target cell destruction by effector T cells. II. Changes in killer cell avidity as a function of time and antigen dose. *J. Immunol.* **119**:1973.

Zinkernagel, R. M., and P. C. Doherty. 1975. Peritoneal macrophages as target cells for measuring virus-specific T cell-mediated cytotoxicity *in vitro. J. Immunol. Meth.* **8**:263.

5

Limiting Dilution Analysis

Claudia Henry, John Marbrook, Douglas C. Vann,
Dankward Kodlin, and Carla Wofsy

5.1 INTRODUCTION

This section discusses the determination of frequencies of specific B cells and T cells in lymphocyte suspensions and the average clonal yield of a stimulated B precursor. Methods based on the reasoning summarized below can also be used to answer other questions.

B cells and T cells of a single specificity occur in very low frequency in lymphocyte populations (10^{-4} to 10^{-7} in suspensions from unprimed animals and frequencies 10- to 100-fold higher in suspensions from primed animals). The distribution of interest for estimating these frequencies is the Poisson distribution. It is essential to understand the fundamental assumptions of this distribution.

The frequency distribution of cells in a hemacytometer counting chamber is a good example of the realization of the Poisson distribution. Here N cells can be thought to make trials, each independently, with probability p of success of falling into a given small square. The Poisson distribution then gives the relative frequency of squares containing 0, 1, 2, 3, . . . r cells.

The general term of the Poisson formula

$$F_r = \frac{(m^r)(e^{-m})}{r!}$$ (1)

gives the probability of precisely r cells in a square where $m = Np$ is the mean number of cells per square.

It follows from (1) that the frequency of squares containing no cells is

$$F_0 = \frac{(m^0)(e^{-m})}{0!} = e^{-m}. \tag{2}$$

Furthermore, the frequency of squares containing *precisely* 1 cell is

$$F_1 = \frac{(m)(e^{-m})}{1!}, \text{ and so on.}$$

Table 5.1 works the Poisson formula for $r = 0, 1, 2, \ldots 5,$ and >5 for two special cases of a *mean number of cells per square* of $m = 1$ and $m = 2$. Note that the sum of the relative frequencies is 1.0. The agreement between such theoretical frequencies and observations is well established (Fisher 1938). One would also expect a distribution of this kind when dealing with lymphocytes that fall randomly into cultures; the cultures correspond to the squares of the counting chamber. It is worthwhile to stress that the distribution holds only if the trials in question are truly independent, that is, only if there is no crowding or clustering. Futhermore, N must be large and p very small. These assumptions seem reasonable for dilution assays of antigen-specific lymphocytes.

We will now use the notions discussed above to estimate the concentrations of specific B and T cells in a given suspension of lymphocytes. The so-called "dilution assay" simply determines the fraction of cultures that is negative at given steps in the dilution and does not attempt to determine which cultures contain precisely 1, 2, 3, . . . specific cells. Equating the

TABLE 5.1
Poisson distribution of cells in small squares

No. of cells per square (r)	Relative frequency (F_r) of r	
	for $m = 1$	for $m = 2$
0	.368	.135
1	.368	.270
2	.184	.270
3	.061	.180
4	.014	.090
5	.003	.036
>5	.002	.019
	1.000	1.000

zero term of the Poisson distribution with the observed fraction of negative cultures, say s, we get

$$e^{-m} = s$$

or $$-\ln s = m \tag{3}$$

For instance, if a given dilution gave no response in 3 out of 10 cultures,

$$m = -\ln .3 = 1.2$$

If a dilution series is properly designed, a fraction of negative cultures can be observed at various dilution levels. In practice, decreasing numbers of cells of the sample under consideration are cultured to cover a range of dilutions in which only a fraction of cultures respond. When the negative of the logarithm of the fraction of nonresponding cultures is plotted on the y axis against the total cell dose (D) on the x axis (on a linear scale), the points should fit a straight line. This follows from Equation (3) because m is a constant fraction of the total cell dose, D. Since $m = 1$ when $F_0 = .37$, one can conveniently find the cell dose containing 1 antigen-specific cell from the graph by locating on the x axis the dose corresponding to 0.37 nonresponding cultures. This is the cell dose that contains a mean of 1 specific cell. The frequency of specific cells is thus $1/D_{.37}$. See Figure 5.1, plot a, where there is a mean of 1 specific cell in 10^5 total cells: a relative frequency of 10^{-5}.

Unlike the hemacytometer example where it is possible to observe directly the presence of a cell, a dilution assay makes it possible to observe only whether a specific cell is responding under the culture conditions.

A dish or well is considered to have received at least one responsive cell if after culture it contains specific antibody-secreting cells or specific antibody released by them. In calculating T or B cell frequencies from the zero term of the Poisson distribution, we are not concerned with the *magnitude* of the response of each culture but merely whether the culture *responds* or *not*. It is sufficient to do a "spot" test with the culture fluids on the appropriate indicator cells (Section 2.9) or to do a plaque assay *in situ* (Section 3.6). There is no ambivalence in distinguishing positive and negative responses in the "spot" test or in plaque-forming cell assays where the clonal yield is large. If the clonal yield is small (e.g., in responses to T "independent" antigens and in some microculture assays), it may be necessary to examine histograms of responses in the limiting dilution region for evidence of bimodality. The lower modal group should correspond to that given by known negative cultures. The saddle between

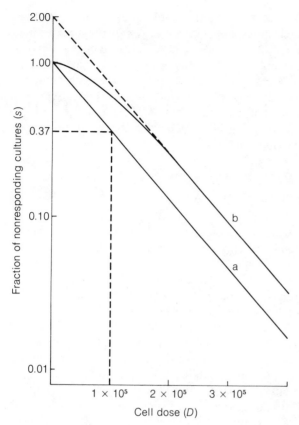

FIGURE 5.1
Dilution analysis.

the two modes is then taken as the breakpoint between positivity and negativity (Groves et al. 1970; Hunter and Kettman 1974).

For the dilution assay discussed above, we have made the further important assumptions that one specific responsive cell is sufficient to give a positive culture and that only one cell type is being diluted even if more than one cell type participates in generating a response. *Linearity of the semilogarithmic plot is obtained only if both of these assumptions are true.* Since most immune responses depend on the fruitful interaction of at least three cell types (B cells, T cells, and macrophages), a straight line would not be obtained if a spleen cell suspension were titrated as above. In practice, this problem is surmounted for a B cell titration by diluting out a source of B cells and providing each culture with a plentiful supply of helper T cells and macrophages. Similarly, for a T cell titration, a source of T cells is diluted into cultures containing nonlimiting numbers of B cells and macrophages. Straight-line plots such as plot a in Figure 5.1 should then be obtained, if one B cell or one T cell is sufficient to give a response.

If a response depends on the interaction of two different cell types, $F_0 = 1 - (1 - e^{-m_1})(1 - e^{-m_2})$ where m_1 and m_2 are the mean number of cells of each cell type present. The product term in this expression represents the probability that a given culture will contain 1 or >1 cells of each cell type. If $m_1 = m_2$, that is, if each cell type is present in equal amounts in the sample being diluted,

$$F_0 = 1 - (1 - e^{-m_1})^2 \doteq 2e^{-m_1}$$

or $$-\ln F_0 \doteq -\ln 2 + m_1$$

so that a plot of $-\ln F_0$ against m_1 would extrapolate to 2 on the y axis. Plot b in Figure 5.1 was obtained on this assumption. Such a curve exhibits an initial shoulder and then becomes linear. Dilution assays involving more than one cell type generally yield nonlinear curves that are more difficult to analyze, since different cell types are never present in equal amounts. Other dose response models give other types of curves. We do not pursue the question further here but refer the reader to the literature (Timoféeff-Ressovky and Zimmer 1947; Mosier and Coppleson 1968; Groves et al. 1970; Henry and Kodlin 1971). Nor do we discuss other variants of dose response models, such as target variability (Henry et al. 1977).

We restate that the analysis based on (3) is only valid for single-hit events: Equation (3) is not applicable if the experimental points do not fall on a straight line through the origin. Such results probably indicate that more than one essential cell type is being diluted or that more than one cell is required to give a response. Although results giving a nonlinear plot might well indicate something of fundamental importance, they do not lend themselves to the estimation procedures discussed above.

5.2 FREQUENCY OF B CELL PRECURSORS

MATERIALS AND REAGENTS

A source of B lymphocytes: Use spleen suspensions from normal or primed mice that have been depleted of T cells by rabbit anti–mouse brain (RAMB) and complement (Section 9.2), or spleen cells from nude mice.

A good source of T helper cells and macrophages: If studying responses to hapten-protein conjugates, use spleen suspensions from mice primed to the protein. If one is estimating B precursor frequencies in unprimed B cell suspensions, it is necessary to remove B cell activity in the T-macrophage source by either irradiation (Section 10.4) or depletion of B cells (Section 9.4 or 9.7). For responses to some antigens (e.g., SRBC), irradiated allogeneic lymphocytes are often satisfactory. Cell preparations should be titrated beforehand to obtain a cell dose that gives optimal responses with the B cells under study.

A source of "filler" cells that does not contribute to the response. Frequently required, such cells are used to maintain a constant and optimal cell density in all cultures. Irradiated B cells or thymocytes depleted of B cells can be used for this purpose.

Materials and media required for cultures: either 10-μl microcultures (Section 2.9), 100-μl minicultures (Sections 2.7 and 2.8), or conventional 1-ml culture (Section 2.2). Since the confidence in determinations of precursor frequency increases with an increasing number of replicate cultures for each dilution, 10-μl microcultures have an obvious advantage. In this system, estimates are usually based on results of 60–180 microcultures for each B cell dilution.

PROCEDURE

1. Dilute the B cell source in culture medium, preferably in 2-fold steps to cover the range of expected responding and nonresponding cultures. (The range depends on the antigen being used and whether the B cells are from normal or primed animals.)

2. Prepare mixtures of each B cell dilution with a constant, optimal number of T helper cells and macrophages and a variable number of "filler" cells so that the cell density is 1–2 $\times$ 10^7 cells/ml. Add antigen at the optimal concentration.

3. Distribute each mixture into the allocated number of cultures. For 10-μl microcultures use 60–180 replicas; for 1-ml cultures it is usually practical to have only 10–20 replicas. For other sizes of culture dishes use an intermediate number.

4. Culture for the optimal period (4–5 days depending on antigen).

5. Assay culture fluid by "spot" test (Section 2.9) or wash cells and assay for plaque-forming cells (Chapter 3).

6. Plot the fraction of nonresponders, s, against the dose of B cells on semilogarithmic paper. Verify linearity and determine the B cell dose that gives 0.37 negative culture. This cell dose contains an average of 1 specific B cell precursor.

5.3 AVERAGE CLONE SIZE OF RESPONDING B CELL PRECURSORS

MATERIALS AND REAGENTS

The materials and reagents required are the same as those in Section 5.2.

We find that cultures in conventional 1-ml dishes engender clone sizes that are larger and vary less from dish to dish, possibly because of better culture conditions and less chance for procedural error in recovering cells and in plating for plaque-forming cells (PFC). However, one usually compares clone sizes under different conditions of stimulation. Microcultures are satisfactory when clone sizes under different conditions are quite different. They have the advantage of giving information from large numbers of cultures and thus allowing better determinations of B cell frequency.

PROCEDURE

Steps 1 to 4 are as described in Section 5.2.

5. Harvest cells from individual dishes, wash, and plate the entire contents of each culture for PFC. Cultures containing B cell dilutions that give only a fraction of positive cultures are of greatest value, because many such positive cultures will contain only a single precursor. Note that some may contain 2 precursors, and a few 3: When 37% of the cultures are negative, 37% contain 1 precursor, 18% have 2 precursors, 6% have 3 (see Table 5.1). With larger numbers of B cells per culture, a marked quantal distribution of PFC in the individual dishes is observed, as one would predict from the Poisson formula (see also Table 5.1), with "jumps" corresponding to the clonal yield of a B cell. Such jumps are easily recognized if the clone size is large (100 or greater).

6. The clone size is determined by using the estimations of precursor concentration and the average number of precursors per culture (m) for the dilution of B cells under consideration (Section 5.2). If the number of cultures assayed is C, the average clone size (c) is

$$c = \frac{\Sigma\text{PFC}}{C \times m}$$

where ΣPFC is the total number of PFC found in C wells.

Alternatively, a reasonably good estimation of the clone size can be obtained by analyzing the response distribution by Poisson expectation and finding the arithmetic mean of PFC per B precursor.

5.4 FREQUENCY OF HELPER T CELLS

MATERIALS AND REAGENTS

The source of T cells to be assayed: When one is studying anti-hapten responses, spleen suspensions from mice primed with the protein carrier are used (e.g., see Sections 2.5, 2.6). In some circumstances, it may be necessary to deplete the suspensions of B cells by anti-Ig rosetting (Section 9.4), nylon wool filtration (Section 7.4), or panning (Section 9.7). Irradiated allogeneic cells can be used for anti–red cell responses.

A source of B cells and macrophages: Each culture should contain a nonlimiting number of B cells and macrophages. For anti-hapten responses, it is usually most convenient to use anti–mouse brain and complement-treated spleen suspensions (Section 9.2) obtained from mice primed against the hapten.

A source of noncontributing "filler" cells (e.g., irradiated B cells)

Materials and media as in Section 5.2

PROCEDURE

1. Dilute the T cell source in culture media preferably in 2-fold steps to cover a range that will give positive and negative cultures.

2. Prepare mixtures of each T cell dilution, a constant nonlimiting number of B cells and macrophages, and a variable number of "filler" cells to maintain a constant density of $1-2 \times 10^7$/ml. Add antigen to the optimal concentration.

3. Distribute each mixture into the allocated number of cultures.

4. Culture for the optimal period (4–5 days).

5. Assay fluid by "spot" test (Section 2.9) or wash cells and assay for PFC (Chapter 3).

6. Plot the fraction of nonresponding cultures, s, against the dose of T cells on semilogarithmic paper. Verify that the experimental points fit a straight line through the origin. Determine the T cell dose that yields 0.37 negative culture. This cell dose contains on the average of 1 specific helper T cell.

5.5 FREQUENCY OF CYTOLYTIC T CELL PRECURSORS

The limiting dilution assays described above use nonporous plastic culture dishes or microwell plates. An alternative technique uses the polyacrylamide raft (Skinner and Marbrook 1976). Briefly, it is a vessel constructed of polyacrylamide that has an array of 64 depressions or "dimples" in the bottom. The vessel is filled with a suspension of cells which settle down into the 64 dimples. The culture can be harvested at the appropriate time. Adjustments in the cell concentration enable the number of dimples containing effector cells to indicate the number of clones. Polyacrylamide was selected because it is a nontoxic, transparent polymer to which cells do not adhere. As it is a porous material, the settled cells are effectively surrounded by nutrient medium. The particular procedure we have selected to illustrate the technique measures the number of precursors of cytolytic lymphocytes in a murine spleen. This procedure can also be used to determine the frequency of B cells or clone size, if 1.4×10^7 thymus cells are used as "filler" cells.

MATERIALS AND REAGENTS

Polyacrylamide Rafts

Eagle's minimum essential medium (MEM) (with and without bicarbonate)
RPMI 1640 (with bicarbonate)
Phosphate-buffered saline (PBS; Appendix A.8)
Acrylamide. Caution: Acrylamide is a neurotoxin. Wear a mask when weighing and use gloves when handling solutions.
Bis-acrylamide
Ammonium persulphate
TEMED (N,N,N′,N′-Tetramethyl-1,2-diaminoethane)
Distilled water
CO_2
Mold for the polyacrylamide vessel
Wide-mouthed polycarbonate jar
Sealed container

Generation and Assay of Cytolytic T Cell Precursors

CBA and CBA/DBA mice (or similar combinations)
^{51}Cr-labeled mastocytoma cells for cytotoxic assay (Section 4.3)
Fetal calf serum (FCS), heat inactivated (56°C, 30 min)
Culture medium (as described in Section 2.3)
Materials to prepare spleen cell suspensions (as described in Section 1.2)

95% ethanol
CO_2
Vortex mixer

PROCEDURE

Construction of the Mold

A scale diagram of the mold for the polyacrylamide vessel is presented in Figure 5.2. The mold is constructed from Perspex (methacrylate) and can be made by any competent workshop technician. It is designed to make four rafts at a time. Since the mold is symmetrical, only one section is drawn in detail. The mold is made in two pieces: a base piece (unshaded) and a frame piece (shaded). The two pieces are glued together after the dimpled surface on the base piece has been fabricated. The dimpled surface is made by cutting V-shaped grooves at right angles to each other with a 60° milling tool (Figure 5.3 a,b). This results in pyramid-shaped projections. The pointed tops of the projections are subsequently removed (Fig. 5.3 c) so that rafts made from the mold have a dimpled surface in which the depressions (or wells) have a flat bottom of approximately 1 mm square.

Preparation of the Polyacrylamide Raft

1. Make up three solutions of acrylamide mixture in the following proportions:

    Solution A: 8.4 g acrylamide, 0.2 g bis-acrylamide in 50 ml distilled water.
    Solution B: 70 mg ammonium persulphate in 10 ml distilled water.
    Solution C: 0.05 ml TEMED in 40 ml distilled water.

2. Mix the three solutions and pour into the mold until the mold is completely full. Place a sheet of plate glass over the mold (excluding all air bubbles) and allow the polymerization to continue for about 15–20 minutes. Remove the polyacrylamide raft from the mold with a spatula that has no sharp edges. Wash in several changes of distilled water including an overnight soak. Place in a polycarbonate wide-mouthed bottle with a screw cap and soak in phosphate-buffered saline. Autoclave the contents of the bottle and store at 4°C.

3. Before use, wash in Eagle's MEM (without bicarbonate) and soak in MEM plus bicarbonate overnight. Change the medium and soak in RPMI 1640 with bicarbonate overnight. This procedure, which is carried out using standard sterile techniques, washes all the

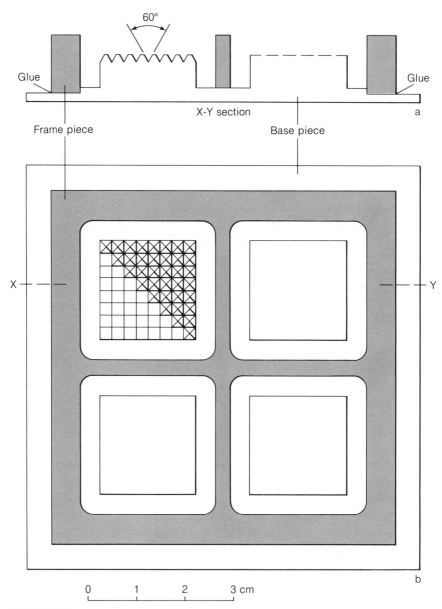

FIGURE 5.2
Scale diagram of the mold used in constructing polyacrylamide rafts: (a) side view through section X-Y; (b) surface view. The 60° angle in (a) indicates the groove cut by the milling tool. The bottom of the groove must be V-shaped; otherwise the raft will have a slight shelf that will prevent some of the cells from settling into the bottom of the depressions. The base piece (unshaded area) and frame piece (shaded area) are glued together after the milling process. (From Marbrook and Haskill 1974.)

unpolymerized reagents from the gel and replaces the buffered saline with the medium to be used in the culture. It has been found unnecessary to include fetal calf serum in the medium used to wash the rafts. The medium that contains bicarbonate should be gassed with sterile 10% CO_2 in air so that it is slightly orange. With a sealed container the washing procedure can be carried out under slightly acid conditions.

Generation of Cytolytic Lymphocytes

A one-way, mixed lymphocyte reaction, using mixtures of F_1 and parental strain spleen cells, is used for the generation of cytolytic lymphocytes.

1. Warm the bottle of rafts to 37°C. If cultures are set up cold and subsequently warmed, the change of dimensions of the raft causes a slight meniscus to form, which prevents the random settling of the cells over the whole raft. Decant off the excess medium and remove a raft from the bottle and place in a 60-mm glass Petri dish. The best instrument for this is a long-handled, stainless steel dessert spoon. (If the spoon is held in a beaker of 95% ethanol, it can be drained and flamed to maintain sterile conditions while handling the raft.)

2. Make up a suspension of cells in culture medium containing 1.3×10^7 (CBA × DBA)F_1 spleen cells and 8×10^4 CBA spleen cells in each 3.5 ml. With a 5-ml pipette, place 3.5 ml of cell suspension in each raft. Adjust the volume for the particular raft

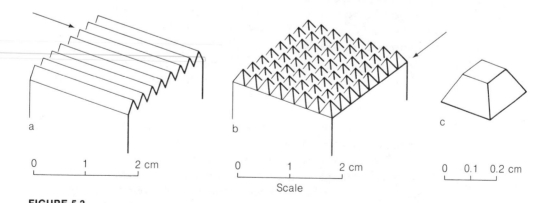

FIGURE 5.3
Diagram of milling procedure to produce dimpled surface for mold. (a) Using a 60° milling tool, start from one edge of the square plastic block and cut grooves 0.2 cm deep at 0.2-cm intervals. (b) Cut similar grooves at 90° angle to (a), thereby creating 100 pyramid-shaped projections. (c) Mill down tip of each pyramid to produce a flat, 1-mm square for each projection.

so that no meniscus forms. Place 10 ml of medium in the dish outside the raft. Place the lid on the Petri dish and incubate in 5% CO_2 in air in the incubator.

Assay for Cytolytic Lymphocytes

The procedure described uses plastic centrifuge tubes, although it can be modified to use microwell plates.

1. Prepare ^{51}Cr-labeled mastocytes as described in Section 4.3. Dilute the radioactive cells to a concentration of 5×10^4/ml using medium containing heat-inactivated fetal calf serum, and hold at room temperature.

2. Pipet 0.3 ml of culture medium into each tube.

3. Carefully remove the medium from the Petri dish and the 3.5 ml from the raft. Remove the cells from each dimple with a fine Pasteur pipette and place them in the tubes. Perform this operation under a low power dissecting microscope. With a little practice, it is possible to harvest 64 dimples in 10–15 minutes.

4. Add 0.2 ml of radioactive mastocytes to each tube. Shake to mix the cell suspensions, and centrifuge the tubes at $200 \times g$ for 3 minutes. Place tubes in a 5% CO_2 incubator at 37°C for 4 hours.

5. Mix the contents of each tube on a Vortex mixer and centrifuge at $200 \times g$ for 7 minutes. Carefully remove 0.2 ml without disturbing the pellets of cells, and count the radioactivity. Include a number of tubes without cytotoxic cells to make it possible to estimate the spontaneous and maximum release of chromate. The percent specific release can be calculated for each dimple.

Expression of Results

Cells from a single dimple that yield more than 10% specific lysis are usually scored as positive. The arbitrary percentage is a figure well above any lysis due to errors in isotope counting or manipulations, so that the calculation of the total number of positive foci or clones is a conservative estimate. The reference of Skinner and Marbrook (1976) contains data expressed in two ways. As discussed above, there should be a linear relationship between the logarithm of the fraction of negative dimples and the number of CBA cells cultured. There will be 37% negative dimples when there is an average of 1 precursor cell per dimple.

The linear relationship between the number of clones and the number of cells cultured can be plotted directly if the number of positive dimples is corrected for the coincidence of more than one clone in the same dimple. The correction factor can be derived from the formula:

$$s = \left(1 - \frac{1}{C}\right)^r$$

where s is the fraction of negative dimples, C is the number of dimples, and r is the *corrected* number of precursors—clones (see Marbrook and Haskill 1974).

REFERENCES

Booth, R. J., J. M. Booth, and J. Marbrook. 1976. Immune conservation: A possible consequence of the mechanism of interferon-induced antibody suppression. *Eur. J. Immunol.* **6**:769.

Fisher, R. A. 1938. *Statistical Methods for Research Workers.* Oliver and Boyd, Edinburgh.

Groves, D. L., W. E. Lever, and T. Makinodan. 1970. A model for the interaction of cell types in the generation of hemolytic plaque forming cells. *J. Immunol.* **104**:148.

Henry, C., E. L. Chan, and D. Kodlin. 1977. Expression and function of I region products on immunocompetent cells. II. I region products in T-B interaction. *J. Immunol.* **119**:744.

Henry, C., and D. Kodlin. 1971. Cell interaction in the secondary immune response. *Cell. Immunol.* **2**:521.

Hunter, P., and J. R. Kettman. 1974. Mode of action of a supernatant activity from T cell cultures that nonspecifically stimulates the humoral immune response. *Proc. Natl. Acad. Sci.* (USA) **71**:512.

Marbrook, J., and J. S. Haskill. 1974. The *in vitro* response to sheep erythrocytes by mouse spleen cells: Segregation of distinct events leading to antibody formation. *Cell. Immunol.* **13**:12.

Marrack, P., J. W. Kappler, and J. R. Kettman. 1974. The frequency and activity of single helper T cells. *J. Immunol.* **113**:830.

Mosier, D. E., and L. W. Coppleson. 1968. A three-cell interaction required for the induction of the primary immune response *in vitro.* *Proc. Natl. Acad. Sci.* (USA) **61**:542.

Quintans, J., and I. Lefkovits. 1973. I. Precursor cells specific to sheep red cells in nude mice. Estimation of frequency in the microculture system. *Eur. J. Immunol.* **3**:392.

Skinner, M. A., and J. Marbrook. 1976. An estimation of the frequency of precursor cells which generate cytotoxic lymphocytes. *J. Exp. Med.* **143**:1562.

Timoféeff-Ressovsky, N. W., and Z. G. Zimmer. 1947. *Das Trefferprinzip in der Biologie (Hit Theory in Biology)*. S. Hirzel, Leipzig.

Vann, D. C., and C. R. Dotson. 1974. Cellular cooperation and stimulatory factors in antibody responses: Limiting dilution analysis *in vitro*. *J. Immunol.* **112:**1149.

Waldman, H., I. Lefkovits, and J. Quintans. 1975. Limiting dilution analysis of helper cell function. *Immunology* **28:**1135.

6

Cell Proliferation

6.1 INTRODUCTION

Linda M. Bradley

Lymphocytes proliferate when stimulated by a variety of agents, including several plant lectins and the constitutive elements of bacterial cell membranes. Substances that evoke significant proliferation on a nonimmune basis are known collectively as mitogens. The specific recognition of antigens also induces lymphocyte division. This chapter describes procedures for inducing and measuring proliferation in response to mitogens and antigens *in vitro*.

Several mitogens selectively stimulate different lymphocyte subpopulations. For example, concanavalin A (Con A) stimulates both immature and mature murine thymocytes, whereas phytohemagglutinin (PHA) stimulates only the mature subpopulation. These mitogens also activate peripheral T lymphocytes. Other mitogens (for example, bacterial lipopolysaccharide and bacterial lipoprotein) are specific for B lymphocytes and probably stimulate different B cell subpopulations. Because of their selectivity, mitogens are frequently used to characterize lymphocyte subpopulations obtained from different tissue sources or prepared by various cell purification procedures. Mitogens are also employed to study the surface membrane alterations and intracellular metabolic events involved in cellular activation.

In vitro assays of antigen-specific proliferation primarily detect T cell responses. In order to elicit significant proliferation in response to soluble antigens, prior immunization of the lymphocyte donors is necessary. However, surface antigens of allogeneic cells (e.g., Ia and H-2 antigens) induce strong T cell responses *in vitro* without previous exposure *in vivo*. These allogeneic reactions are termed mixed lymphocyte responses (MLR). Both types of antigen-induced proliferative responses are used to study the genetic and cellular requirements for immune induction. MLR are also employed in clinical tests of T cell function.

A convenient method for quantitating cellular proliferation is to assay DNA synthesis. Incorporation of exogenous radiolabeled (^{3}H or ^{14}C) thymidine into material precipitable by trichloracetic acid over a specified period of time is measured by scintillation counting. For this purpose it is necessary to use low-specific-activity radiolabeled thymidine both to prevent radiation damage and to insure that sufficient exogenous thymidine is available to maintain the incorporation throughout the pulse period. Although labeling periods of 4 to 6 hours are sufficient to demonstrate significant incorporation, longer labeling (18 to 24 hours) is usually used for convenience as well as to minimize the effects of asynchronous DNA synthesis by lymphocytes. The magnitude of the response of cells to a particular stimulus varies with the culture conditions, the cell density, the concentration of the activating agent, as well as with the tissue source of responding cells and the mouse strain employed. The time and duration of the peak response varies with the cell type activated, the particular activator used, and the concentration of the activating agent. For example, optimal incorporation in response to many mitogens occurs within 2 to 4 days, whereas peak responsiveness to antigens usually occurs between days 4 and 7 of culture. The optimal conditions for a particular assay must be empirically derived from the analysis of the variables described above.

Careful technique is required in the execution of the methods for quantitating cellular proliferation. The experimental results are particularly sensitive to technical inaccuracies (e.g., errors in pipetting and in dilutions). The maintenance of sterile conditions is essential. Bacterial contamination can distort the results either by causing excess label to be incorporated into the DNA of replicating bacteria or by interfering with the response of the lymphoid cells. Contamination will usually be detected by high backgrounds, poor correspondence of triplicate cultures, or both.

Another method sometimes used for studying proliferative phenomena is autoradiography. While the procedure examines relatively few cells and is considerably more complex than scintillation counting, it is useful for determining the actual proportion of cells that incorporate radiolabel.

When interpreting incorporation data obtained by the methods described in this section, one should consider several points. Because some of the cells that synthesize DNA do not necessarily divide, the data provide only an estimate of cell proliferation. Moreover, experimental manipulations can influence incorporation levels indirectly by affecting cooperating cells that are not themselves dividing. Finally, some of the incorporation may be indirect, caused by cells responding to products of other cells which are in turn directly stimulated by the activating agents.

REFERENCES

Bach, F., and K. Hirschhorn. 1964. Lymphocyte interaction: A potential histocompatibility test *in vitro*. *Science*. **143**:813.

Bain, B., M. R. Vas, and L. Lowenstein. 1964. The development of large immature mononuclear cells in mixed leukocyte cultures. *Blood* **23**:108.

Corradin, G., H. M. Etlinger, and J. M. Chiller. 1977. Lymphocyte specificity to protein antigens. I. Characterization of the antigen-induced *in vitro* T cell-dependent proliferative response with lymph node cells from primed mice. *J. Immunol.* **119**:1048.

Dutton, R. W., and J. D. Eady. 1964. An *in vitro* system for the study of the mechanism of antigenic stimulation in the secondary response. *Immunology* **7**:40.

Klein, J. 1975. *Biology of the Mouse Histocompatibility-2 Complex: Principles of Immunogenetics Applied to a Single System*. Springer-Verlag, New York.

Nowell, P. C. 1960. PHA: An initiator of mitosis in cultures of normal human leukocytes. *Cancer Res.* **20**:562.

Oppenheim, J. J., and D. L. Rosenstreich. 1976. *Mitogens in Immunobiology*. Academic Press, N.Y.

Oppenheim, J. J., and B. Schecter. 1976. Lymphocyte transformation. In N. R. Rose and H. Friedman (Eds.), *Manual of Clinical Immunology*. American Society of Microbiology, Washington.

Rosenwasser, L. J., and A. S. Rosenthal. 1978. Adherent cell function in murine T lymphocyte antigen recognition. I. A macrophage-dependent T cell proliferation assay in the mouse. *J. Immunol.* **120**:1991.

Schwartz, R. H., L. Jackson, and W. E. Paul. 1975. T lymphocyte-enriched murine peritoneal exudate cells. I. A reliable assay for antigen-induced T lymphocyte proliferation. *J. Immunol.* **115**:1330.

Snell, G. D., J. Dausset, and S. Nathenson. 1976. *Histocompatibility*. Academic Press, New York.

Waithe, W. I., and K. Hirschhorn. 1978. The lymphocyte response to activation. In D. M. Weir (Ed.), *Handbook of Experimental Immunology*, 3rd edition. Blackwell Scientific Publications, Oxford.

6.2 MITOGEN-INDUCED RESPONSES

Linda M. Bradley

Methods for generating and assaying proliferative responses to mitogens with macrocultures and microcultures are described in this section. The T cell mitogens phytohemagglutinin and concanavalin A, and the B cell mitogen lipopolysaccharide are used as examples. Each commercial batch of these mitogens may differ in the dose required to induce optimal proliferation; thus, individual lots must be titrated. Variations from the experimental conditions outlined below can alter both the magnitude and the kinetics of these responses. Moreover, if different mitogens are used, it may be necessary to modify the procedures. As described in Section 6.1, the optimal conditions for each experimental system must be derived empirically.

A. Macrocultures

MATERIALS AND REAGENTS

Cell Culture

Spleen cells (Section 1.2), thymus cells (Section 1.5), or lymph node cells (Section 1.9)

RPMI 1640, supplemented with L-glutamine, sodium pyruvate, nonessential amino acids, penicillin/streptomycin (optional) as described in Section 2.2, and 5% fetal calf serum (FCS; a lot screened for low background in proliferative cultures)*

^{3}H-methyl-thymidine, specific activity 2 Ci/mmol (New England Nuclear) *or*

^{14}C-thymidine, specific activity 50 mCi/mmol (Schwarz/Mann)

Mitogens

    Phytohemagglutinin (PHA), purified (Wellcome Reagents Division)

    Concanavalin A (Con A), 2× crystallized in saturated NaCl (Miles Research Products)

    Bacto-lipopolysaccharide W (LPS), *S. typhosa* 0901 (Difco Laboratories)

---

* We at times test lots of FCS from various suppliers. Lots of FCS found satisfactory for use in this system are reserved by the companies for sale to those who specifically request them. The identification numbers of tested lots of FCS, if available, can be obtained from us by phone or mail.

Tissue culture tubes with caps, 12 × 75 mm (Falcon, #2054)

Slant tube rack to hold tubes in culture chamber (Bellco Glass, #2028-50008)

Culture chamber (Bellco Glass, #7741-10005) and gas mixture of 7% O_2, 10% CO_2, 83% N_2, *or*

Humidified incubator with an atmosphere of 5% CO_2 in air

Cell Harvest

Balanced salt solution (BSS; Appendix A.3)

10% trichloroacetic acid (TCA)

95% ethanol or absolute methanol

Scintillation fluid: 1 gallon scintillation-grade toluene plus 1 galpack Omnifluor (New England Nuclear) *or* 5 g PPO (2,5-diphenyloxazole) and 100 mg POPOP (*p-bis*-[2-(5-phenyloxazolyl)]benzene) per liter of toluene (Amersham is the supplier of both PPO and POPOP)

Scintillation vials

Millipore filter assembly or similar device (Millipore)

Whatman glass fiber filter paper GF/A *or* 0.45-μm Millipore filters

Beta scintillation counter

PROCEDURE

Note: Established safety procedures must be followed when handling radioactive materials.

Cell Culture

1. Prepare sterile suspensions of cells from spleen (Section 1.2), thymus (Section 1.5), or lymph node (Section 1.9).

2. Suspend the cells in sterile, supplemented medium to a concentration of 1×10^6 cells/ml for spleen or lymph node cells; 5×10^6 cells/ml for thymocytes. Add 1 ml of suspension/tube. Control and experimental cultures should be run in triplicate.

3. Dilute PHA, Con A, or LPS in sterile BSS or supplemented medium. Optimal mitogenic responses have been obtained with 1–2 μg/ml PHA, 1–4 μg/ml Con A, and 2–25 μg/ml LPS (final concentrations in culture). As noted above, each lot of mitogen may differ and should be titrated. Make up mitogens at 10× final desired concentration. Add 0.1 ml/culture. Control cultures receive 0.1 ml of BSS or medium.

4. Place the tubes in the slant tube rack. Incubate the cultures in a 37°C humidified incubator in an atmosphere of 5% CO_2 in air or, alternatively, incubate the cultures in a culture chamber filled with

a gas mixture of 7% O_2, 10% CO_2, 83% N_2 and incubate at 37°C without rocking or feeding.

5. Radiolabeled thymidine (1–2 μCi) is added to each culture in a volume of 0.1 ml. As previously indicated, the optimal pulse period for a particular experimental system must be derived empirically. We have found that a pulse period from 24 to 48 hours is optimal for PHA, whereas a pulse period from 48 to 72 hours is optimal for Con A or LPS.

Cell Harvest

1. Place filter disk(s) on Millipore filter assembly or other similar device; turn on suction.
2. Vortex the culture tube and decant the culture onto filter.
3. Add 2 ml of cold BSS to the culture tube, vortex, and decant onto filter.
4. Repeat step 3.
5. Extract and discard the TCA soluble material by washing the cells on the filter with 10 ml of cold 10% TCA (2 sequential washes).
6. Wash the precipitate with 2 ml 95% ethyl alcohol or absolute methanol (3 washes).
7. Remove the filter; place in a scintillation vial.
8. When all cultures have been processed, place the scintillation vials in a 37°C incubator or drying oven for 60 minutes, or leave to dry overnight at room temperature.
9. Add 5 ml of scintillation fluid to each vial; if completely dried, the filters will become transparent upon addition of scintillation fluid.
10. Chill the vials at 4°C for 45 minutes in a dark place.
11. Count in a beta scintillation counter at appropriate settings to determine counts/minute.

B. Microcultures

MATERIALS AND REAGENTS

Cell Culture

Spleen cells (Section 1.2), thymus cells (Section 1.5), or lymph node cells (Section 1.9)

RPMI 1640, supplemented as described for macrocultures (Section 6.2A)

^{3}H-methyl-thymidine *or* ^{14}C-thymidine, as described for macrocultures (Section 6.2A)

Mitogens: PHA, Con A, LPS, as described for macrocultures (Section 6.2A)

Microwell plates, flat-bottom wells (Falcon, #3040) with lids (Falcon, #3041)

Hamilton gas-tight syringes with repeating dispenser (Hamilton, #PB 600-1 and #PB 600-10):

   10-ml syringe delivers 0.2 ml (Hamilton, #1010LT)
   5-ml syringe delivers 0.1 ml (#1005LT)
   2.5-ml syringe delivers 0.05 ml (#1002LT)
   1-ml syringe delivers 0.02 ml (#1001LT)

Sterile needles, 18 or 22 gauge

Culture chamber (Bellco Glass, #7741-10005) and gas mixture of 7% O_2, 10% CO_2, 83% N_2, *or*

Humidified incubator with an atmosphere of 5% CO_2 in air

Cell Harvest

Saline: 0.85% NaCl (w/v)

5% trichloroacetic acid (TCA)

Absolute methanol

Glass fiber filter paper, type A-E, cut into strips $\frac{3}{4}$ in. $\times$ 8 in. (Gelman Sciences)

Scintillation fluid as described for macrocultures (Section 6.2A)

Scintillation vials

Automated sample harvester (Otto Hiller)

Beta scintillation counter

PROCEDURE

Cell Culture

1. Prepare sterile suspensions of cells from spleen (Section 1.2), thymus (Section 1.5), or lymph node (Section 1.9).

2. Suspend the cells in sterile, supplemented medium. The final number of cells/well should be 5–6 $\times$ 10^5 for spleen or lymph node cells, 1–1.2 $\times$ 10^6 for thymocytes. Depending on the protocol, the cells may be added to the wells in 0.2-ml, 0.1-ml, or 0.05-ml volumes; the cell concentration is adjusted accordingly. Control and experimental cultures should be run in triplicate.

3. Dilute the mitogens in sterile, supplemented medium. The mitogens can be added to the wells in any desired volume (see above), but the total culture volume should not exceed 0.25 ml. It is usually most convenient to add cells and mitogens separately in 0.1-ml

volumes. As with macrocultures, optimal mitogenic responses have been obtained with 1–2 μg/ml PHA, 1–4 μg/ml Con A, and 2–25 μg/ml LPS (final concentration in culture). As previously indicated, each lot of mitogen should be titrated. Control cultures receive supplemented medium instead of mitogen.

4. The cells, mitogens, and medium can be conveniently and accurately dispensed with Hamilton syringes and repeating dispenser. The syringes can be stored filled with 70% ethanol and used for sterile work.

   a. Empty the ethanol from the syringe, and replace needle with a sterile 18- or 22-gauge needle.

   b. Rinse the syringe 3 to 5 times with sterile BSS to thoroughly remove the ethanol. On the last rinse, fill the syringe partially, and with needle up, let air in. With syringe in same position, push out all air so that no bubbles are present (bubbles distort the volume when dispensing).

   c. Fill the syringe with cell suspension or mitogen solution slowly so as not to let air in. Discard the first volume delivered (which may be inaccurate) and dispense to wells.

   d. If the same syringe is to be used for additional mitogens or cell suspensions, rinse the syringe 3 to 5 times with sterile BSS before refilling.

5. Incubate the cultures in a humidified 37°C incubator in an atmosphere of 5% CO_2 in air or in a culture chamber filled with a gas mixture of 7% O_2, 10% CO_2, and 83% N_2; incubate at 37°C without rocking or feeding.

6. Add 1 μCi radiolabeled thymidine per well in a volume of 0.02 ml, with a 1-ml Hamilton syringe. For further information on pulse periods, see description for macrocultures.

Cell Harvest

1. Depending on the model, automated sample harvester units harvest 12 or 24 culture wells at a time (1 or 2 rows of a microwell plate) by aspiration onto filter strips. Wash the wells sequentially with saline, 5% TCA, and absolute methanol, according to the instructions for use of the harvester.

2. Place individual filter disks in scintillation vials and dry in a 37°C incubator or drying oven for 60 minutes, or leave to dry overnight at room temperature.

3. Add 5 ml of scintillation fluid to each vial.

4. Chill the vials at 4°C for 45 minutes in a dark place.

5. Count in a beta scintillation counter at appropriate settings to determine counts/minute.

C. Representation of Data

Control and experimental cultures should be performed in triplicate. Data can be expressed in one of three ways:

1. Average counts per minute (cpm): The arithmetic mean of cpm from triplicate cultures and the standard error.

2. Δcpm: The arithmetic mean of cpm from triplicate experimental cultures (stimulated cultures) minus the mean of control cultures.

3. Stimulation index (S.I.): The ratio of the mean cpm of experimental cultures to the mean cpm of control cultures (i.e., experimental/control).

Both 2 and 3 are based on the assumption that the amounts of proliferation in control and experimental cultures are affected similarly by external variables and are proportional. However, depending on the treatment under study, this assumption is not necessarily valid. Thus, the average cpm (1) should always be indicated as well for valid interpretation of data. Variations in the cpm of individual cultures in excess of 15–20% of the mean of replicate cultures indicate technical errors or contamination.

REFERENCES

Macrocultures

Andersson, J., G. Möller, and O. Sjöberg. 1972. Selective induction of DNA synthesis in T and B lymphocytes. *Cell. Immunol.* **4:**381.

Microcultures

Hartman, R. J., M. L. Bach, F. H. Bach, G. B. Thurman, and K. W. Sell. 1972. Precipitation of radioactively labeled samples: A semi-automatic multiple-sample processor. *Cell. Immunol.* **4:**182.

Janossy, G., M. F. Greaves, M. J. Doenhoff, and J. Snajder. 1973. Lymphocyte activation. V. Quantitation of the proliferative response to mitogens using defined T and B cell populations. *Clin. Exp. Immunol.* **14:**581.

Pick, A. B., and F. H. Bach. 1973. A miniaturized mouse mixed lymphocyte culture in serum-free and mouse serum supplemented media. *J. Immunol. Meth.* **3:**147.

Strong, D. M., A. A. Ahmed, G. B. Thurman, and K. W. Sell. 1973. *In vitro* stimulation of murine spleen cells using a microculture system and a multiple automated sample harvester. *J. Immunol. Meth.* **2:**279.

6.3 MIXED LYMPHOCYTE RESPONSES

Linda M. Bradley

The mixing of two populations of allogeneic lymphoid cells results in T cell proliferation, which is termed a mixed lymphocyte response (MLR). Cell surface antigens encoded by genes of the major histocompatibility complex and/or the M locus are the major stimuli of this response. MLRs may be induced in either macro- or microcultures. The methods for cell culture and harvest are similar to those described for mitogen responses (Section 6.2). MLRs may be either unidirectional or bidirectional. For unidirectional responses, one population of allogeneic cells serves as antigen (the stimulator cells) and is inhibited from proliferating by procedures that arrest cell division. Thus, only proliferation by the second cell population (the responder cells) is measured. In bidirectional MLRs, neither population is inhibited from dividing and the combined response of both cell populations is measured. Procedures for unidirectional reactions are described in this section.

A. Macrocultures

MATERIALS AND REAGENTS

Cell Culture

As described in Section 6.2A, with the deletion of mitogens, and the addition of:

> Mice which differ at the H-2 and/or M loci
> Mitomycin C, lyophilized (Sigma Chemical, #M-0503)

Cell Harvest

As described in Section 6.2A

PROCEDURE

Cell Culture

1. Prepare the responder and stimulator cell populations. For the responder population, spleen cells (Section 1.2), lymph node cells (Section 1.9), or the functionally mature subpopulation of thymocytes (Sections 1.7 or 9.6A) may be used. For the stimulator population, spleen or lymph node cells are usually used.

2. Treat the stimulator cells and an aliquot of the responder cells (for use in the control) with mitomycin C (Section 10.3) or with 2000 R x-irradiation (Section 10.4) to inhibit proliferation.

3. Suspend the untreated responder cells and the treated stimulator and responder cells to 2×10^6 cells/ml in supplemented medium.

4. For the control cultures, mix 0.5 ml of the untreated responder cells with 0.5 ml of the treated responder cells in a 12×75-mm culture tube. For the experimental cultures, mix 0.5 ml of the untreated responder cells with 0.5 ml of the treated stimulator cells. Run both control and experimental lines in triplicate.

5. Culture cells as described in Section 6.2A.

6. Pulse the cultures with ^{3}H-thymidine as described in Section 6.2A. Optimal pulse periods for MLRs in macrocultures are 72–96 hours or 96–120 hours.

Cell Harvest

Follow the procedure outlined in Section 6.2A.

B. Microcultures

MATERIALS AND REAGENTS

Cell Culture

As described in Section 6.2B, with the deletion of mitogens, and the addition of:

Mice which differ at the H-2 and/or M loci
Mitomycin C, lyophilized (Sigma Chemical, #M-0503)

Cell Harvest

As described in Section 6.2B

PROCEDURE

Cell Culture

1. Prepare responder and stimulator cell populations for culture as described for macrocultures above (Section 6.3A).

2. Treat the stimulator cells and an aliquot of the responder cells (for use in the control) with mitomycin C (Section 10.3) or with 2000 R x-irradiation (Section 10.4) to inhibit proliferation.

3. Suspend the untreated responder cells and the treated stimulator and responder cells to 5×10^6 cells/ml in supplemented medium.

4. For the control cultures, mix 0.1 ml of untreated responder cells with 0.1 ml of treated responder cells in the wells of a microwell plate. For the experimental cultures, mix 0.1 ml of untreated re-

sponder cells with 0.1 ml of treated stimulator cells. Run both control and experimental cultures in triplicate.

5. Culture the cells as described in Section 6.2B.

6. Pulse the cultures with ^{3}H-thymidine as described in Section 6.2B. Optimal pulse periods for MLRs in microculture are 72–96 hours or 96–120 hours.

Cell Harvest

Follow the procedure outlined in Section 6.2B.

6.4 ANTIGEN-INDUCED T CELL PROLIFERATIVE RESPONSES

Linda M. Bradley, with contributions from
Jessica Clarke and Alexander Miller

Parameters for inducing antigen-specific proliferation by primed lymph node T cells *in vitro* have been described by Corradin et al. (1977). Secondary responses are generated with inguinal and periaortic lymph node cells, usually from mice primed 5 to 8 days before the experiment by subcutaneous immunization at the base of the tail. (Substantial *in vitro* responses can be observed as early as 4 days after the initial priming and as late as 30 days.) The *in vitro* proliferative response is maximal 5 days after the initiation of culture. The antigen may be emulsified in either complete or incomplete Freund's adjuvant for *in vivo* immunization. The optimal dose of soluble antigen *in vitro* and the kinetics of the response must be empirically determined for each antigen.

MATERIALS AND REAGENTS

Immunization

Protein antigen, 5 mg/ml in balanced salt solution (BSS; Appendix A.3) or phosphate-buffered saline (PBS; Appendix A.8)

Complete or incomplete Freund's adjuvant (Difco Laboratories). Note: Freund's adjuvant is a potentially hazardous agent (see Appendix F).

Syringes, 1 ml

Needles, 25 gauge

Cell Culture

Lymph node cells (Section 1.9)

Antigen, 200–500 µg/ml in medium, sterilized by membrane filtration (Appendix C.2)

BSS
Modified Click's medium (Appendix A.15)
Gas mixture: 98% air, 2% CO_2
Syringes, 5 ml with 18-gauge needles
Fine-mesh stainless steel screen
Microwell plates, flat bottom with lids (Falcon, Microtest II, #3042)
Syringe, 5 ml with repeating dispenser delivering 0.1 ml (Hamilton, #1005LT and #PB600-10, respectively)
Needles, 18 gauge

Cell Harvest

As described in Section 6.2B.

PROCEDURE

Immunization

1. Emulsify the antigen in an equal volume of either complete or incomplete Freund's adjuvant as described in Appendix F.
2. Inject 0.04 ml of the emulsion (100 μg of antigen) subcutaneously at the base of the tail.

Cell Culture

1. Aseptically remove inguinal and periaortic lymph nodes 5–8 days after *in vivo* immunization.
2. Trim nodes free of fat, and tease. Further dissociate cells by gently forcing through a 5-ml syringe with an 18-gauge needle, 3–5 times.
3. To obtain a single cell suspension free of debris, pass the cells through a fine-mesh stainless steel screen.
4. Wash the cells twice with BSS. Resuspend the cells to a concentration of 4 × 10^6 cells/ml in medium.
5. Dispense 0.1 ml of cell suspension (4 × 10^5 cells) and 0.1 ml of antigen (20–50 μg, final concentration of 100–250 μg/ml) to individual microtiter wells using a Hamilton syringe. (The use of Hamilton syringes for culture is described in Section 6.2B.)
6. Culture the cells for 5 days at 37°C in a humidified atmosphere of 98% air, 2% CO_2 (without rocking).

Cell Harvest

On day 4 of culture, pulse each well with 1 μCi ^{3}H-thymidine and harvest 18–24 hours later. The procedure for pulsing cultures with ^{3}H-thymidine, harvesting the cells, and preparing the filter discs for scintillation counting is described in Section 6.2B.

Editors' note

Rosenwasser and Rosenthal (1978) have suggested that this method for generating antigen-induced proliferation by primed lymph node T cells (based on that originally described by Corradin et al. 1977) may measure the proliferation of recruited B cells as well as that of the antigen-specific T cells. They have described an alternative procedure employing nylon-wool-purified primed T cell populations. This method is described in detail in the 1978 reference cited below. The presence of contaminating B cells can be assessed by measuring the proliferative response to LPS. An alternative method for detecting antigen-specific T cell proliferation, using peritoneal exudate, T lymphocyte enriched cells (PETLES), is described in the references by Schwartz et al. (1975) and Yano et al. (1977).

REFERENCES

Corradin, G., H. M. Etlinger, and J. M. Chiller. 1977. Lymphocyte specificity to protein antigens. I. Characterization of the antigen-induced *in vitro* T cell-dependent proliferative response with lymph node cells from primed mice. *J. Immunol.* **119**:1048.

Rosenwasser, L. J., and A. S. Rosenthal. 1978. Adherent cell function in murine T lymphocyte antigen recognition. I. A macrophage-dependent T cell proliferation assay in the mouse. *J. Immunol.* **120**:1991.

Schwartz, R. H., L. Jackson, and W. E. Paul. 1975. T-lymphocyte-enriched murine peritoneal exudate cells. I. A reliable assay for antigen-induced T-lymphocyte proliferation. *J. Immunol.* **115**:1330.

Yano, A., R. H. Schwartz, and W. E. Paul. 1977. Antigen presentation in the murine T-lymphocyte proliferative response. I. Requirement for genetic identity at the major histocompatibility complex. *J. Exp. Med.* **146**:828.

6.5 AUTORADIOGRAPHY OF SPLEEN CELL CULTURES

James Watson

Autoradiography allows the visual localization of a radioactive precursor incorporated into cellular macromolecules. Cells that have been exposed to radiolabels are mounted and fixed on microscope slides. The slides are coated with a photographic emulsion that undergoes photochemical changes wherever radioemissions occur. After a suitable exposure time, the emulsion-coated slides are developed, fixed, and stained. They are then ready for examination under a light microscope. Cells that have incorporated radiolabel are recognizable by the black reduced silver grains in the overlying emulsion.

The procedure outlined below works well for counting the number of spleen cells that have incorporated radioactive thymidine during culture. There are many variations to the techniques given. For example, there are a variety of films and emulsions for detecting radioactive emissions, each with its own purpose and specifications. The reference cited for this section or a similar comprehensive text should be consulted for specific details. The necessity for immaculately clean working conditions is a theme throughout almost every procedure given. Consistently clean conditions are essential to reduce the nonspecific background that can so easily become a problem.

A. Preparation of Coated Slides

Agarose provides a uniform, adhesive layer for cell smears on glass slides.

MATERIALS AND REAGENTS

Coating solution made by dissolving 250 mg of agarose in 50 ml of balanced salt solution (BSS; Appendix A.3). After heating, filter the solution through a 0.45-μm membrane filter and keep at 45°C.

Acid bath consisting of a mixture of 5% nitric acid and 5% hydrochloric acid. This bath will last for several weeks. Any corrosive material can be skimmed off the top.

Slides, frosted on one end

Detergent for glassware (7X; Linbro Scientific)

PROCEDURE

1. Wash the slides with detergent and rinse them thoroughly in distilled water.
2. Wash overnight in acid bath. (Glass slide holders designed to keep slides separated are best; most metal or plastic slide holders are unsuitable).
3. Wash several hours in running distilled (or deionized) water.
4. Wash in two, separate changes of double-distilled water (30 minutes each).
5. Paint the slides with the agarose solution, using a cleaned paint brush. Allow to dry in a dust-free environment.
6. Coated slides may be stored for several weeks in a dust-free slide box.

B. Preparation of Labeled Cell Sample

MATERIALS AND REAGENTS

Labeling Cell Cultures

^{3}H-thymidine, 40–60 Ci/mmol, 1000 μCi/ml (New England Nuclear, #NET-027Z)
Thymidine (unlabeled), 10^{-3} M in BSS

Fixing Labeled Cells on Slides

2% acetic acid
Agarose-coated slides for autoradiography
Diamond-tipped pen

PROCEDURE

1. Add 10 μCi (10 μl) of diluted ^{3}H-thymidine per ml of cultured spleen cells. Incubate, with rocking, for approximately 6 hours.
2. Remove the labeled cells from the culture dish to a test tube. Wash twice in 10^{-3} M unlabeled thymidine.
3. Resuspend in BSS at 1–2 × 10^6 cells/ml.
4. Label slides on the frosted end by etching with a diamond-tipped pen. Do not mark with anything that contains a metal (e.g., lead) or that is soluble in organic reagents.
5. Place 0.1 ml of the spleen cell suspension in the middle of an agarose-coated slide. Drop 0.1 ml of 2% acetic acid onto the same area of the slide. Spread the liquid evenly by rolling the thin end of a clean Pasteur pipette over the unfrosted portion of the slide.
6. Dry the slide by repeated, rapid passages over a low flame. Do not allow the slide to get hotter than is comfortable to touch with your bare hand. Do not allow the slide to air dry.
7. After the slides have dried and cooled, dip them 15 to 20 times in a distilled water bath to remove salt crystals.
8. Store in a dust-free slide box.

C. "Defatting Slides"

This procedure is not absolutely required, but it will improve the staining of the cells and increase the number of visible silver chloride grains by removing lipid from both the agarose layer and the cellular surface. Defatting thereby reduces the length of the path a radioactive emission must travel before reaching the emulsion layer.

MATERIALS AND REAGENTS/PROCEDURE

Dip the slides in the following solutions for the specified amount of time. This is most conveniently done using a multiple slide holder. Each listing represents a separate solution.

Solution	Time of incubation
1. Distilled water	5 min
2. 50% ethanol	5 min
3. 70% ethanol	5 min
4. 100% ethanol	5 min
5. 100% ethanol	5 min
6. 100% N-butanol	5 min
7. Xylene	45 min
8. Xylene	45 min
9. 100% N-butanol	2 min
10. 100% ethanol	2 min
11. 95% ethanol	2 min
12. 70% ethanol	2 min
13. 50% ethanol	2 min
14. Distilled water	15 min
15. Distilled water	15 min

After the slides have dried, they are ready to be dipped in emulsion.

D. Coating Slides with Emulsion

Because it is difficult to maintain an emulsion layer at constant thickness, the use of liquid emulsion is generally reserved for qualitative work, although quantitative work using liquid emulsion can be done under special conditions (see Rogers 1973). The minimum usable thickness for the emulsion layer is 1.5 μm. Parameters that influence the thickness are the temperature of the emulsion, the dilution of the emulsion, and the temperature and wetness of the slides. The following precautions should be observed:

1. Use only glassware that has been thoroughly washed with soap and water, rinsed in an acid bath, and then extensively rinsed with distilled water. Keep all clean glassware dust free.
2. Treat the emulsion as one would any film; expose only to an appropriate safelight, and protect from radioactivity during storage.

3. Do not allow the emulsion to come in contact with any type of metal.

4. Work as gently as possible to avoid friction that will expose the emulsion.

MATERIALS AND REAGENTS

NTB-2 nuclear track emulsion (Eastman Kodak)
Beaker, 100 ml
Graduated cylinder, 100 ml, filled with distilled water
Cylinder for holding emulsion and dipping slides. (This should be a vessel that closely approximates the dimensions of a slide. A 100-ml graduated cylinder cut off at approximately the 45-ml mark works well.)
Plastic spoon
Kimwipes
Test tube rack (for holding slides upright)
Parafilm
Pads to cover bench
Water bath at 39°C
Light-tight slide box containing small amount of Drierite
Slides to be coated

PROCEDURE

1. Take the materials and reagent into a darkroom.

2. Cover a bench area in the darkroom with bench pads and organize equipment. The following steps must be done in the dark with the appropriate safelight as the only source of light.

3. Melt the emulsion in a covered beaker at 39°C. The background steadily increases with the amount of time the emulsion is at a high temperature.

4. Dilute the emulsion with an equal volume of distilled water in the "dipping cylinder." Mix slowly as friction will expose grains in the emulsion. Remove any bubbles from the top of the diluted emulsion. A total volume of 40 ml is sufficient to coat approximately 50 slides. Any concentrated, unused emulsion may be poured back into the stock emulsion.

5. Dip a few blank slides into the emulsion by slowly lowering each slide into the emulsion and then withdrawing it in one even movement. Repeat until there are no bubbles on the slide. Continue as above with the experimental slides.

6. Wipe the backs of the slides and place them upright in a test tube rack. The slides should not be allowed to completely dry at room temperature since this leads to cracking of the emulsion.

7. When all of the slides are coated, place them in a light-tight slide box containing Drierite. Immediately place the slides at 4°C.

E. Developing and Fixing Autoradiograms

Expose autoradiograms for approximately 7 days when using ^{3}H-thymidine with a specific activity of 40–60 Ci/mmol. Lower specific activity requires a longer exposure time. In any case, develop a few test slides on successive days, bracketing the estimated exposure time. Autoradiograms should not be exposed to any light except the appropriate safelight until after they have been developed and fixed.

MATERIALS AND REAGENTS

D-19 developer (Eastman Kodak) at 16°C
Rapid Fix (Eastman Kodak)
Glass or plastic multiple slide holder

PROCEDURE

1. Remove the slides from the slide box and place in a plastic or glass slide holder (do not use metal).

2. Develop 3–5 minutes in the D-19 at 16°C. Determine exact development times by analyzing the test slides developed for different time intervals.

3. Wash gently in distilled water for 3–5 minutes.

4. Place in Rapid Fix for 8–10 minutes.

5. Wash thoroughly with running water.

6. Proceed to staining procedures. Do not allow the slides to dry.

F. Staining Cells

MATERIALS AND REAGENTS

In addition to reagents listed in procedure:

Cresyl violet stain
Stock dye: 1.2 g cresyl violet (Matheson Coleman and Bell) in 500 ml water

Acetate buffer: 6 ml 1 M acetic acid in 994 ml water

Basic buffer: 13.6 g sodium acetate made up to 1000 ml with water

Mix 60 ml stock dye, 470 ml acetate buffer, and 30 ml basic buffer. Adjust to pH 3.5.

Permount

Microscope slides and coverslips

PROCEDURE

Place slides in the following solutions for the specified amount of time. The time required for staining and differentiation will depend upon the type of tissue and the strength of the dye.

Solution	Time of incubation
1. Cresyl violet (staining step)	30 min*
2. Double-distilled water	7 dips
3. 50% ethanol	6 dips
4. 70% ethanol	5 dips
5. 95% ethanol	5 dips
6. 95% ethanol, adjusted to pH 3.5 with acetic acid (differentiation step)	3 min*
7. 95% ethanol	3 min
8. 100% ethanol	3 min
9. 100% ethanol	3 min
10. 100% N-butanol	3 min
11. Xylene	5 min
12. Xylene	5 min
13. Xylene	5 min

Place coverslips over the slides with Permount and allow to dry for 24 hours. The slides are now ready to be examined with a light microscope.

REFERENCE

Rogers, A. W. 1973. *Techniques of Autoradiography*. Elsevier Scientific Publication Co., Amsterdam.

* The exact amount of time should be determined with test slides.

II

CELL SEPARATION

Progress in understanding cellular immunology has occurred in large part through the identification of subpopulations of cells and the analysis of their function. During the 1970s, research uncovered a great deal of heterogeneity among lymphocytes and accessory cells* and established criteria for distinguishing subpopulations. The existing categories of cells will most likely be subdivided further. Towards this end, the development of cell separation techniques will continue to be essential.

To analyze the functions of cellular subpopulations, a wide variety of cell separation procedures have been developed. Most procedures make it possible to remove one or more cell types from a heterogeneous population. Ideally, cell separation methods should result in high, representative yields of the desired cells with little or no contamination by other cell types. Moreover, the separation method should be reproducible, result in minimal effects on the subsequent behavior of the recovered cells, and permit recovery of sterile cells. In general, methods based on selection of cells by virtue of specific surface markers (Chapter 9) best meet these criteria. Heretofore, these methods had limited appli-

---

* The expression "accessory cells" refers to all cells, other than T and B lymphocytes, that have an immunoregulatory function. Macrophages are included in this category.

cation because antisera to only a few surface markers were available. Specific antibodies to many more surface markers should become available in the near future as a result of a widespread use of hybridoma technology to produce monoclonal antibodies (Chapter 17). These new reagents will greatly extend the range of cell types potentially separable by procedures employing antibodies to cell surface markers.

Several of the commonly used methods separate cells by their propensity to adhere to various surfaces (Chapter 7) or by their size and density (Chapter 8). Because functionally similar cells may be heterogeneous with respect to these properties, cell separation methods based on these characteristics are not likely to produce highly purified cell preparations. It has been particularly difficult to develop methods that adequately and reproducibly remove macrophages and other accessory cells from lymphocyte populations.

The methods described in Part II by no means include all useful cell separation procedures. They do, however, cover a number of the generally employed approaches and can be carried out in most conventionally equipped laboratories.

Adherence

7.1 INTRODUCTION

This chapter outlines three empirically developed cell separation methods that are based on the differential adherence properties of cells. The Sephadex G-10 and carbonyl iron procedures are commonly used to remove macrophages and other "adherent" accessory cells from lymphocyte populations. No direct comparisons of the relative effectiveness of the two procedures in removing macrophages have been reported. The nylon wool procedure is used primarily to obtain representative T cell populations largely free of B lymphocytes and macrophages. All three procedures are relatively simple to perform and are capable of processing large numbers of cells.

7.2 SEPHADEX G-10

Barbara B. Mishell, Robert I. Mishell, and June M. Shiigi

Sephadex preparations are a group of crosslinked dextran polymers that form gels when swelled in water. Although usually employed to separate

175

macromolecules, Sephadex G-10, which has the smallest pore size, can also be used to separate cells (Ly and Mishell 1974). When spleen cells are passed through a column of Sephadex G-10, the starting cell suspension is depleted of both adherent accessory cells and antibody-producing plaque-forming cells (PFC). The basis of the separation is not completely understood, but most likely involves cell adherence and size. We have found G-10 to be the most satisfactory Sephadex grade, probably because of the dimensions and elastic properties of the beads. The technique of passing cells through Sephadex G-10 is generally employed to remove macrophages and other large adherent accessory cells.

MATERIALS AND REAGENTS

Preparation of Sephadex G-10

Saline, 0.85% NaCl (w/v)
Sephadex G-10 (Pharmacia Fine Chemicals)
Flask, 6 liters
Centrifuge tubes, autoclavable, 50 ml (Falcon, #2074 or Corning Glass Works, #25330)

Preparation of Glass Beads

Sulfuric acid, concentrated
Nitric acid, concentrated
Sodium bicarbonate, 1% (w/v) in distilled water
Hydrochloric acid (1 : 100 dilution of concentrated HCl)
Class IV glass beads (Microbeads Subdivision of Cataphote Division, Ferro Corporation)
    Class IV-A #456 Unisphere beads, 250–350 μm
    Class IV-A #235.5 Unisphere beads, 500–710 μm
Drying oven
Glass test tubes, 12 × 75 mm, with stainless steel closures (Bellco Glass, #2005-00013)

Cell Separation

Spleen cell suspension in balanced salt solution (BSS; Appendix A.3), 4–6 × 10^8 cells/column (1.5 × 10^8 cells/ml)
Balanced salt solution containing 50 units/ml penicillin, 50 μg/ml streptomycin, and 5–10% heat-inactivated (56°C, 30 min) fetal calf serum (BSS-FCS)
Sephadex G-10, prepared for separation
Glass beads (approximately 5 g of each size)
Centrifuge tube, 50 ml (Falcon, #2074 or Corning Glass Works, #25330)

Syringe, disposable, 50 ml
Glass beaker, 150 ml
Ring stand and clamp
3-way stopcock (Pharmaseal Laboratories, #K-75)
Pasteur pipettes with rubber bulbs
Pipettes: 10 ml, 5 ml, 1 ml
Tissue culture dish, 60 mm; one per column
Centrifuge tubes, graduated; for collection of effluent

PROCEDURE

Preparation of Sephadex G-10

1. Place 1500–2000 ml of saline in a 6-liter flask and add approximately 250 g of Sephadex G-10. Stir gently to wet Sephadex completely. Cover the flask and allow the Sephadex to swell overnight at 4°C.

2. Remove the saline from the settled Sephadex by suction. Add a volume of saline that is approximately 3–4 times the estimated bed volume and resuspend the gel by gently swirling the flask. When most of the Sephadex has settled, remove the saline and unsettled fine Sephadex particles by suction. Repeat 3 times, each time removing the fine particles that do not settle. Finally, add a volume of saline equal to 30–50% of the estimated bed volume.

3. Adjust the ratio of packed Sephadex to saline such that 40–45 ml of slurry contain 30–35 ml of packed Sephadex. The ratio can be determined by centrifuging 40–45 ml of slurry at low speed (just enough to pack the gel); add or remove saline accordingly.

4. Aliquot the slurry in 40–45-ml volumes into 50-ml tubes and cap loosely. Place the rack of tubes in a container large enough to contain any spillage during sterilization. Autoclave for 40 minutes at 110°C (slow exhaust). Cap the tubes tightly and store at room temperature.

Preparation of Glass Beads

Prepare each bead size separately.

1. Soak beads in a 50:50 mixture of concentrated sulfuric and nitric acid for 24 hours (in a fume hood).

2. Place beads under gently running tap water for 8 hours to wash.

3. Soak the beads in a large volume of 1% sodium bicarbonate for 24 hours.

4. Rinse beads 10 times with double-distilled water.

5. Soak beads in diluted hydrochloric acid for 24 hours.

6. Rinse in double-distilled water until pH of rinse water is above 6. Dry beads in a drying oven.

7. Aliquot approximately 5 g of beads per tube and autoclave 20 minutes at 121°C (fast exhaust). Store at room temperature.

Cell Separation

The column separation is done at room temperature, or 37°C.

1. Attach the 50-ml plastic syringe to a ring stand. Remove and discard the plunger. Cover the top of the syringe with the lid of a 60-mm culture dish (sterile). Attach the stopcock to the syringe tip in closed position.

2. Pour the larger glass beads into the syringe, followed by the smaller beads. (If necessary, loosen the packed beads with a 1-ml plastic pipette.)

3. Add approximately 10 ml of BSS-FCS to the syringe, rinsing the beads from the sides of the syringe.

4. Gently pipet Sephadex on top of the glass beads, and let the gel settle in the column (40–45 ml of slurry/50-ml syringe).

5. Place a beaker under the column. Open the stopcock and allow the BSS-FCS to pass through the column.

6. Wash the Sephadex with 100–150 ml of BSS-FCS. During the last wash stir the top of the Sephadex bed with a 1-ml pipette to ensure an even, level top layer. Let all the fluid penetrate the column.

7. With a Pasteur pipette, quickly load the cells onto the Sephadex without disturbing the top of the column bed, and allow cells to penetrate the column. Continually add small amounts of BSS-FCS to the column until the cells are approximately halfway down the column and then add 15–20 ml of BSS-FCS. Begin collecting the effluent when the cells reach the glass bead layer. Collect 10–15 ml.

8. Allow any Sephadex contamination to settle for 2–3 minutes and then transfer the cells to another tube. Centrifuge at 200 × g for 10 minutes.

COMMENTS

1. Although Sephadex filtration is a convenient method for removing macrophages, it is important to interpret data obtained with this procedure cautiously because of the possibility that cells with functions similar to macrophages may be present in the filtered

population. The capacity of some preparations of depleted cells to generate responses in the presence of 2-mercaptoethanol may be due to the presence in the effluent cell fraction of a functionally significant number of small, nonadherent accessory cells. Precise characterization of such small, nonadherent accessory cells and the development of methods for removing them from lymphocyte populations is an objective of contemporary research.

2. Recently, C. Cowing (personal communication) reported that different samples of Sephadex G-10 differed in their capacity to remove accessory cells from spleen cells. Surprisingly, samples that gave higher yields of filtered cells appeared better able to remove accessory cells. Based on this report, we suggest that sample lots of Sephadex G-10 be screened prior to general use for cell separation.

REFERENCE

Ly, I. A., and R. I. Mishell. 1974. Separation of mouse spleen cells by passage through columns of Sephadex G-10. *J. Immunol. Meth.* **5:**239.

7.3 CARBONYL IRON POWDER

Kwok-Choy Lee

Macrophagelike, adherent, accessory cells are efficiently removed from cell suspensions by treatment with carbonyl iron powder (Sjöberg et al. 1972; Lee et al. 1976). Originally, it was believed that carbonyl iron particles were phagocytosed by the accessory cells, which were then removed together with the iron particles by means of a magnet. However, more recent evidence suggests that adherence is probably the basis of cell depletion especially when the iron particles are considerably larger than the cells (Sjöberg et al. 1972). For this reason, it is imperative to ascertain that moderately adherent lymphocytes (e.g., B cells) are not inadvertently removed. This can be readily checked in two ways:

1. By using fluorescent antibody directed at B cell surface immunoglobulin and Thy 1 alloantigen to enumerate the proportions of B and T cells. Using this method, we found that carbonyl iron treatment of mouse spleen cells produced a small (10%) depletion of B cells.

2. By making sure that the immune responses of lymphocytes depleted of A cells are fully restored by macrophages (irradiated and treated with anti–Thy 1).

MATERIALS AND REAGENTS

Mouse spleen cell suspension in medium at 10^7 cells/ml

Eagle's minimum essential medium or RPMI 1640 containing 10% fetal calf serum (FCS) and 3.5 g sodium bicarbonate/liter.

Saline, 0.85% NaCl (w/v)

Carbonyl iron powder (Atomergic Chemetals) or iron powder, 99+% pure, particle size <60 μm (Goodfellow Metals, #CB4 4DJ)

Screw-cap bottles, 100 ml

Pipettes: 5 ml, 10 ml

Glass centrifuge tubes, 50 ml

One powerful large magnet (horseshoe, approximately 4 in. across ends), one small bar magnet (approximately 1 in. long)

Gas mixture: 5% CO_2, 5% O_2, and 90% N_2

Water bath at 37°C

PROCEDURE

Pretreatment of Iron Powder

On the day of the experiment, the carbonyl iron powder should be washed, distributed into bottles, and sterilized.

1. Wash a weighed quantity of iron powder (usually 10 g) with 100 ml of saline 4 times to remove any soluble toxic material. Use the powerful magnet to retain the iron while pouring off the saline.

2. Finally, suspend the iron in 50 ml of saline (0.2 g iron powder/ml saline).

3. Pipet appropriate aliquots (usually 2–5 ml) into 100-ml screw-cap bottles. This should be done immediately after suspending the iron powder and before it settles.

4. Sterilize the bottles by autoclaving at 18 lb/sq. in. for 20 minutes. Disperse the iron immediately afterwards to discourage clumping.

5. Alternatively, sterilize the iron powder by extensive washing with sterile saline before dispensing it into bottles.

Cell Separation

1. Prepare a single-cell suspension of mouse spleen cells in medium at 10^7 cells/ml. Care should be taken to remove clumps by allowing the suspension to settle for 15 minutes. Make sure that the pH of the medium is between 7.1 and 7.3 (as indicated by the color of the phenol red in the medium).

2. Aspirate off the saline in which the iron powder is suspended.

3. To each bottle, add 8 ml of spleen cell suspension (8×10^7 cells/bottle).

4. Fill the bottles with the gas mixture of 5% CO_2, 5% O_2, and 90% N_2 so that the pH will be maintained.

5. Incubate the bottles in the 37°C water bath for 45 minutes.

6. Every 5 minutes, shake each bottle with just enough force to suspend the iron powder completely.

7. At the end of the incubation period, place the small magnet under each bottle to retain iron and adhering cells and pour off the cell suspension. Pool the suspensions from all the bottles in a single container.

8. Place a powerful magnet under this container, wait a few minutes, and then pour the contents into 50-ml centrifuge tubes. This should remove all residual iron powder.

9. Recover the cells by centrifugation.

COMMENTS

1. The yield of nonadherent cells varies with the amount of iron powder used, which in turn depends on the degree of accessory cell depletion desired. With 0.6 g or 1.0 g iron/bottle, the yields are about 50% and 33%, respectively. These yields are quite respectable when compared with those of other methods. We have found that for the effective reduction of the anti–sheep erythrocyte response, 0.6 g is sufficient, whereas 1.0 g is necessary for any significant reduction of the response to the T-independent antigen, bacterial flagellin (Lee et al. 1976).

2. Certain batches of carbonyl iron powder react with the culture medium, producing a brownish yellow color and a pungent odor. Such batches should not be used.

3. All steps must be performed under aseptic conditions if the cells are to be used for tissue culture.

4. The method described here applies only to coarse grades of iron whose particles are larger than cells.

REFERENCES

Lee, K. C., C. Shiozawa, A. Shaw, and E. Diener. 1976. Requirement for accessory cells in the antibody response to T cell-independent antigens *in vitro. Eur. J. Immunol.* **6**:63.

Lundgren, G., C. H. F. Zukoski, and G. Möller. 1968. Differential effects of human granulocytes and lymphocytes on human fibroblast. *Clin. Exp. Immunol.* **3**:817.

Sjöberg, O., J. Andersson, and G. Möller. 1972. Requirement for adherent cells in the primary and secondary immune responses *in vitro. Eur. J. Immunol.* **2**:123.

7.4 NYLON WOOL

Claudia Henry, with contributions from Yu-hua Una Chen,
Robert Stout, and Susan L. Swain

The passage of cells over a nylon wool column as described by Julius et al.
(1973) is an effective means of obtaining a population enriched with T
cells. B cells, plasma cells, and some accessory cells preferentially adhere
to the nylon wool, while many T cells (and some null cells) pass through
the column. Yields are often low, in the range of 15–25%. Most investigators have found that the T cells present in the effluent are representative of all T cell subpopulations. However, other studies suggest that T
cell subpopulations are selectively retained on nylon wool. Such selective
retention may, if confirmed, be due to variations in nylon wool lots, the
degree to which the column is packed, and/or the preparative washing
procedures used. With this in mind, we include an alternative washing
procedure for preparing nylon wool (see comment 6); however, we have
not performed comparative studies on the effluent cells.

MATERIALS AND REAGENTS

Washing and Drying of Nylon Wool

Nylon wool (Fenwall Laboratories, LP-1 Leuko-Pak Leukocyte Fil-
  ters)
Beaker, 4 liter
Aluminum foil
Disposable gloves
Stainless steel basket or large funnel
Large tray covered with absorbent paper

Packing of Nylon Wool Columns

Disposable syringes, 10–12 ml or 35 ml (save outer case and caps;
  plunger should also be saved if adherent cells are to be recovered)
Autoclaving bags

Cell Separation

Medium (Eagle's minimum essential medium or RPMI 1640) or bal-
  anced salt solution (BSS; Appendix A.3), supplemented with 5%
  heat-inactivated fetal calf serum (FCS; 56°C for 30 min). See
  Comment 1.
Nylon wool column
3-way stopcocks (Pharmaseal Laboratories, #K-75)
Cheese cloth
Needle, disposable, 22 gauge (1 per column)

Ring stand and clamps
Water bath and incubator at 37°C
Cap of syringe case to cover column
Centrifuge tubes, 50 ml, to collect effluent

PROCEDURE

Washing and Drying of Nylon Wool

1. Wear disposable gloves that have been rinsed free of powder. Remove nylon wool from one or two bulk packages (35 g each) and place in a beaker of deionized or distilled water. Cover the beaker with aluminum foil and boil the nylon wool for approximately 10 minutes.

2. Allow the water and nylon wool to cool to room temperature. Decant water and drain the nylon wool in a stainless steel basket or funnel.

3. Repeat the washing procedure a total of 6 times, with the last 2 washes in double-deionized or double-distilled water.

4. Wrap washed wool in cheese cloth, squeeze out excess water, and spread the wet nylon wool on a tray covered with absorbent paper or cheese cloth. Dry nylon wool in a 37°C incubator or in a laminar flow hood for 2–3 days. Store in a covered container.

Packing of Nylon Wool Columns

1. Determine the total number of cells to be passed through a column (yields are 15–25%). Use the information from Table 7.1 to determine the size of syringe and the weight of nylon wool required.

2. Weigh nylon wool. Tease apart, separating the strands until the piece is loosely connected yet free of tangles and knots. Loosely fold nylon wool so that it will fit the diameter of the syringe and pack the syringe to the volume indicated in Table 7.1.

3. For sterile work, replace syringes in the outer syringe cases, pack individual syringes into autoclaving bags, and autoclave at 110°C

TABLE 7.1
Size of syringe and weight of nylon wool required for nylon wool column

No. of cells	Capacity of syringe	Nylon wool/ syringe	Syringe packed to
1×10^8	10–12 ml	0.6 g	6 ml
3×10^8	35 ml	1.8 g	18 ml
4×10^8	35 ml	2.4 g	24 ml

for 15 minutes. Autoclave plungers separately if they are to be used also (see comment 2).

Cell Separation

1. Warm FCS-supplemented medium to 37°C in a water bath.
2. Mount syringe onto a ring stand and attach the 3-way stopcock and a capped 22-gauge needle to the syringe. Remove the needle cap, open the stopcock, and thoroughly rinse the nylon wool with 50–100 ml of prewarmed medium. Close the stopcock, add medium to cover the nylon wool, and free column of air bubbles by agitation with a pipette.
3. Replace needle cap and cover the column with the syringe case cap. Incubate the column at 37°C for 1 hour (an incubator room is most convenient since it permits a constant temperature of 37°C throughout the whole procedure).
4. While the column is incubating, prepare the cell suspension and adjust the concentration to approximately 5×10^7 cells/ml in medium or BSS supplemented with FCS and prewarmed to 37°C.
5. Just before adding the cell suspension, rinse the wool with 5–10 ml of prewarmed medium, let column run dry, and close stopcock. Add the appropriate number of cells (see Table 7.1), allow cells to penetrate the column, and close the stopcock. Add an additional 0.5 ml of medium-FCS (or BSS-FCS), cover the column with the syringe case cap, and replace needle cap. Maintain the column at 37°C for 45 minutes more.
6. Collect nonadherent cells into a graduated centrifuge tube by washing the 10–12-ml column with 20 ml of prewarmed medium and the 35-ml column with 60 ml of medium. Elute at about 1 drop per second. Centrifuge cells ($200 \times g$, 10 min) and resuspend in the appropriate medium.

COMMENTS

1. When using MEM or RPMI 1640 instead of BSS, it is necessary to add 25 mM HEPES to prevent the medium from becoming alkaline.
2. To recover adherent cells from the column, add cold saline (0.85% NaCl, w/v) to the column and forcibly push fluid out with the plunger.
3. It is possible to recycle nylon wool. After use, rinse the nylon in saline and then place in 0.1 M HCl at least overnight. Repeat the

washing procedure as before. Some lots may work at least as well, if not better, after recycling (R. Stout, personal communication).

4. The loss of Fc-receptor positive T cells on nylon wool is variable. The loss is increased by tightly packing the nylon but is rarely complete; it may vary with the batch (R. Stout, personal communication).

5. In general, T cells pass through nylon wool while B cells and macrophages are retained. However, some functional subpopulations of T cells may adhere to the columns. Functional subpopulations of T cells reported to pass through the columns include primed and unprimed antigen-specific helper cells, T cells that are the precursors of cytotoxic effectors, and T cells that proliferate in response to both alloantigens and soluble antigens. At least one subpopulation of T cells is reportedly retained by these columns (Tada 1977, 1978).

6. An alternative washing procedure follows: Wash nylon wool in 4 liters of freshly boiled distilled water containing 0.2% sodium bicarbonate (2 g/liter) and 0.2% EDTA (2 g/liter). Soak overnight at 37°C; wash with boiling distilled water as described above. Approximately 50% of total T cells are recovered when this procedure is used (S. Swain, personal communication).

REFERENCES

Julius, M. H., E. Simpson, and L. A. Herzenberg. 1973. A rapid method for the isolation of functional thymus-derived murine lymphocytes. *Eur. J. Immunol.* **3:**645.

Tada, T. 1977. Regulation of the antibody response by T cell products determined by different I subregions. In E. E. Sercarz, L. A. Herzenberg, and C. F. Fox (Eds.), *Immune System: Genetics and Regulation.* Academic Press, New York.

Tada, T., T. Takemori, K. Okumura, M. Nonaka, and T. Tokuhisa. 1978. Two distinct types of helper T cells involved in the secondary antibody response: Independent and synergistic effects of Ia$^-$ and Ia$^+$ helper T cells. *J. Exp. Med.* **147:**446.

Trizio, D., and G. Cudkowicz. 1974. Separation of T and B lymphocytes by nylon wool columns: Evaluation of efficacy by functional assays *in vivo*. *J. Immunol.* **113:**1093.

8

Size and Density

8.1 INTRODUCTION

John North

Subsets of cells with different biological characteristics can frequently be separated on the basis of their size and density, since the sedimentation rate of cells in suspension is proportional to both cell diameter and the difference between the density of the cell and that of the surrounding medium. Stokes Law gives the rate of sedimentation (v) of a sphere of diameter d in a gravitational field g:

$$v = \frac{d^2(\rho_P - \rho_L)}{18\eta} g$$

where ρ_P and ρ_L are the densities of the spherical particle and the liquid, respectively, and η is the viscosity of the liquid. Stokes Law is applicable in three different cell separation methods, each of which takes advantage of differences in size and density.

Isopyknic Centrifugation: Separation on the Basis of Density

In separation by isopyknic linear density gradients (Section 8.2), cells are sedimented at high g through increasingly dense medium. The cells eventually reach a point where the densities of the cell and the medium are equal. At this point $(\rho_P - \rho_L) = 0$, making $v = 0$, and the cells float in an equilibrium position. Since the buoyant densities of murine leukocytes range from 1.04 to 1.09 g/cm³, they can be separated on an appropriate gradient. Cells of densities greater than the most dense solution used in constructing the gradient sediment to the bottom of the tube and are subjected to large compression forces which frequently kill them. Dead cells, which are typically very dense, also sediment to the bottom of the tube. Discontinuous density gradients (Sections 8.3 and 8.4) separate cells on the same basis as linear gradients, but the cells collect at the appropriate interface between medium of $\rho_L < \rho_P$ and medium of $\rho_L > \rho_P$.

The high g forces usually employed in isopyknic separation serve simply to increase the rate at which equilibrium is achieved and to reduce the mixing effect of diffusion. Although cell size influences the rate of establishing equilibrium, it does not influence the point on the gradient at which a cell will remain at equilibrium. Because the rate of establishing equilibrium is inversely related to the viscosity of the medium, use of media with low viscosity, such as those made with silica gel (Section 8.4), allows equilibrium to be established in a short time at relatively low g.

Velocity Sedimentation: Separation Primarily on the Basis of Size

In velocity sedimentation, cells settle either through a low density medium (~1.01 g/cm³) at unit gravity (Section 8.5) or through a density gradient at low centrifugal force ($100 \times g$; Section 8.6). Since v is proportional to the square of the diameter of the cells and the diameter of mouse leukocytes varies from 5–15 μm, a maximum of a 9-fold range in sedimentation rates may be obtained on the basis of differences in cell size. In contrast, the densities of the majority of mouse leukocytes varies from 1.04 to 1.09 g/cm³, generating $(\rho_P - \rho_L)$ values of 0.03 to 0.08. Thus, slightly less than a 3-fold range of sedimentation rates is obtained on the basis of differences in cell densities. Size is, therefore, the chief determinant of differences in velocity: Larger cells settle through the medium at a higher rate than smaller cells.

Single-Step Gradient: Separation on the Basis of Size and Density

A suspension of cells is layered onto a high density medium (1.09 g/cm³ for mouse cells)* and centrifuged at low speed. Most mouse lymphocytes

---

* For human cells, the high density medium has a density of 1.075 g/cm³.

(with $\rho < 1.09$ g/cm^3) will not move into the denser medium. Red blood cells ($\rho = 1.095$–1.10 g/cm^3), dead cells, and cellular debris move through the denser material and form a pellet.

Single-step gradient methods employing Ficoll-Hypaque or silica gel are commonly used to separate lymphocytes on the basis of rosetting (Section 8.7). Rosette formation is induced by coupling (with suitable reagents) red blood cells to lymphocyte subpopulations carrying specific surface markers (see Sections 9.3, 9.4, and 9.5). The rosetted lymphocytes (which have the specific markers) are then separated from the free lymphocytes on a single-step gradient. Most rosettes have densities greater than 1.09 g/cm^3 and thus move rapidly through the dense medium, forming a pellet. The low density free lymphocytes stay at the interface; free lymphocytes with densities of 1.09 g/cm^3 or greater will move into the dense medium, but will not pellet during the centrifugation since their diameters are much smaller than those of the rosettes and the values for ($\rho_P - \rho_L$) are small. Thus, both the low and higher density unrosetted lymphocytes are recovered essentially free of those lymphocytes that form rosettes.

8.2 LINEAR ISOPYKNIC BSA GRADIENTS

John Marbrook

This method was developed by Shortman (1968) for generating a linear gradient of bovine serum albumin (BSA) at pH 5.1. The advantages of the system and the rationale for adopting some of the procedures are clearly described in the references and in other papers to which Shortman refers. In brief, cells are suspended in an isotonic linear gradient of BSA and centrifuged until they reach equilibrium in that region of the gradient which corresponds to their buoyant density.

MATERIALS AND REAGENTS

Preparation of Bovine Serum Albumin

Bovine serum albumin (BSA)
Chloroform
Dialysis tubing (Appendix D)
Freeze-drying apparatus
Desiccator with phosphorus pentoxide

Preparation of Dense BSA Stock Solution

Balanced salt solution, unbuffered (unbuffered BSS; Appendix A.7)
Magnetic stirrer, stirrer bar
Membrane filtration apparatus, 0.45 μm filter (sterile)

Determination of the Density of the BSA Solution

Refractometer
Accurate container, such as a 250-μl Carlsberg constriction pipette

Preparation of a Linear Gradient and Separation of Cells

Spleen cell suspension (Section 1.2) or other cell population
Chlorhexidine digluconate: 0.05% solution (w/v) (Accurate Chemical
  & Scientific Corp.)
Mixing chambers (see Figure 8.1)
Peristaltic pump (3 channels)
Refrigerated centrifuge (e.g., Sorvall with an HB-4 swinging bucket,
  distributed by Dupont)
Glass centrifuge tube
Stainless steel tubing attached to tygon tubing (for removal of cells
  from centrifuge tube after gradient separation)
Pasteur pipette

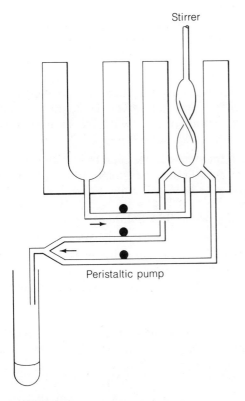

FIGURE 8.1
Schematic diagram of mixing chambers
and peristaltic pump.

PROCEDURE

Preparation of Bovine Serum Albumin

1. Dissolve two 75-g batches of BSA in separate 500-ml volumes of double-distilled water. Place each batch of the BSA solution in dialysis tubing and dialyze separately against 6 liters of glass-distilled water for 48 hours, changing the water at least four times. Dialyze at 4°C in a cold room and add a drop of chloroform to the water to prevent bacterial growth.

2. After the dialysis step, lyophilize the BSA solution. Store the dried BSA in beakers placed in a desiccator containing phosphorous pentoxide.

Preparation of Dense BSA Stock Solution

1. Weigh out 100 g of lyophilized BSA into a suitable flask (if conditions are humid, work swiftly to avoid introducing errors due to the absorption of water).

2. Add 132 ml unbuffered BSS followed by 4 ml of glass-distilled water (the water compensates for the contribution of the albumin to the final osmolarity). Add another 50 ml of BSS to assist in dissolving the protein.

3. Seal the flask tightly with Parafilm and place on magnetic stirrer in a cold room. The protein may take over 48 hours to dissolve completely. The stock solution of BSA will have an osmolarity of 308 mOsm (isotonic with mouse serum) and a pH of 5.1.

4. If the BSA will be used for sterile work, membrane filter the stock solution (Appendix C.2). Aliquot the stock solution and store frozen.

Determination of the Density of the BSA Solution

The simplest way to determine the density of the BSA stock solution and to check the linearity of the gradients is by measurement of the refractive index of the solution in a refractometer. Two methods may be used to correlate density with the refractive index of a solution:

Calibration Curve

1. Make up a series of dilutions of the BSA stock in unbuffered BSS. A suitable range of dilutions is obtained by mixing 6, 5, 4, 3, and 2 parts of the BSA stock to obtain 6 parts of final solution (e.g., 4 ml stock BSA plus 2 ml BSS).

2. Measure the refractive indices of the series of dilutions; they should be between 1.370 and 1.400.

3. Determine the density of the BSA dilutions by measuring the weight of a known volume of the solution. Use a micropipette (about 200 μl) as an accurate container and determine the weight of the solution by difference:

$$\text{Density} = \frac{\text{weight of solution in g}}{\text{volume of solution in ml}}.$$

The density of the stock BSA solution is about 1.100 g/ml.

4. Construct a calibration curve by plotting density versus refractive index.

Formula of Leif and Vinograd

An alternate method of determining the density of the BSA solution from refractive index measurements is by the formula of Leif and Vinograd (1964):

$$\text{Density} = (1.543 \times \text{refractive index}) - 1.0553.$$

Preparation of a Linear Gradient and Separation of Cells

The following procedures are devised for preparing a linear gradient of 12 ml from $\rho = 1.065$ to $\rho = 1.085$. Keep all solutions at 4°C and carry out all manipulations in a cold room.

1. Set up the mixing chambers, stirrer, and peristaltic pump according to the diagram in Figure 8.1.

2. If sterile work is being performed, fill the chambers (including the tygon tubing and the stirrer) with 0.05% chlorhexidine digluconate solution and leave for 24 hours. Soak the stainless steel-tygon tubing in the same solution. Before use, pump out the chlorhexidine solution and wash the chambers 2 times by filling them with sterile BSS and pumping the BSS out. Remove any BSS remaining in the chambers with a sterile Pasteur pipette. Rinse the stainless steel-tygon tubing out with sterile BSS.

3. Prepare a suspension of mouse spleen cells (Section 1.2). Up to 6×10^8 cells can be separated on one 12-ml gradient. The cells must be centrifuged down to a pellet in preparation for the run.

4. Calculate the amount of stock BSA needed to make 6-ml solutions at densities 1.085 and 1.065. The volume of BSA stock in milliliters is determined by the formula:

$$X = \frac{(A \times B) - B}{C - 1}$$

where:

$$X = \text{ml BSA stock}$$
$$A = \text{desired density}$$
$$B = \text{volume of final solution}$$
$$C = \text{density of stock solution}$$

5. Make up the $\rho = 1.065$ solution using the unbuffered BSS as the diluent.

6. To make the $\rho = 1.085$ solution, suspend the pelleted cells (up to 6×10^8 cells) in the amount of unbuffered BSS calculated to be needed to make the $\rho = 1.085$ BSA solution; then add the required amount of BSA stock. Care must be taken in dispersing the cells as any aggregates will cause a loss of resolution of the cells during the separation procedure.

7. Place the 6 ml of $\rho = 1.065$ BSA solution into the chamber without the stirrer (left side in Figure 8.1). Turn on the peristaltic pump until the tubing connecting the two chambers is filled with the BSA solution. Stop the pump.

8. Transfer the 6 ml of $\rho = 1.085$ BSA solution (which contains the cells) into the chamber with the stirrer. Turn the stirrer on.

9. Turn the peristaltic pump on and collect the gradient into a centrifuge tube. Let the BSA solution run down the side of the tube.

10. After the gradient is formed, place a cap on the centrifuge tube and accelerate the centrifuge slowly to $3000 \times g$ and centrifuge for 45 minutes at 4°C.

11. Collect the fractionated cells as follows: Attach the stainless steel-tygon tubing apparatus onto a peristaltic pump set to withdraw approximately 1–2 ml/minute. With the pump off, carefully place the steel tubing down to the bottom of the centrifuge tube without disturbing the cells. Turn the pump on and collect fractions of about 0.4 ml into each centrifuge tube. Remove 15- to 20-μl aliquots from each tube and measure the refractive index to determine the density of each fraction. (Plot the density of each fraction against the fraction number to check the linearity of the gradient.)

12. Add 5 ml of BSS to each fraction, mix, and centrifuge to sediment the cells ($200 \times g$, 10 min). Repeat this washing step.

13. Resuspend the cells in a suitable volume of buffered BSS (Appendix A.4) or medium. The density distribution of nucleated

cells can be determined by removing an aliquot from each fraction and determining the concentration of nucleated cells by procedures described in Section 1.10 or with an electronic cell counter.

14. The washed cells can be assayed for various activities.

REFERENCES

Leif, R. C., and J. Vinograd. 1964. The distribution of buoyant density of human erythrocytes in bovine albumin solutions. *Proc. Natl. Acad. Sci.* (USA) **51**:520.

Haskill, J. S., and J. Marbrook. 1972. The *in vitro* immune response to sheep erythrocytes by fractionated spleen cells: Biological and immunological differences. *J. Immunol. Meth.* **1**:43.

Shortman, K. 1968. The separation of different cell classes from lymphoid organs. II. The purification and analysis of lymphocyte populations by equilibrium density gradient centrifugation. *Aust. J. Exp. Biol. Med. Sci.* **46**:375.

Shortman, K. 1974. Separation methods for lymphocyte populations. *Cont. Top. Mol. Immunol.* **3**:161.

Shortman, K., N. Williams, and P. Adams. 1972. The separation of different cell classes from lymphoid organs. V. Simple procedures for the removal of cell debris, damaged cells, and erythroid cells from lymphoid cell suspensions. *J. Immunol. Meth.* **1**:273.

8.3 DISCONTINUOUS BSA GRADIENTS

Donald J. Raidt

The procedure described here can separate a population of cells into four subpopulations (or bands), which form at the interfaces between albumin layers of different densities during centrifugation. It is easy to modify the procedure to suit particular needs by changing the concentrations of the albumin solutions and/or the number of layers of albumin of differing densities.

Because batches of bovine serum albumin (BSA) vary considerably in their usefulness for this technique, they must be screened and evaluated prior to experimental use. The basis for the differences among lots is not precisely known, but it is thought to be related to the composition and concentrations of cations in the salts found in various albumin preparations and unrelated to the osmolarity (D. J. Raidt, unpublished observations). Screening is most easily accomplished by performing gradient separations on spleens from mice that have been primed with SRBC two to three days earlier (0.2 ml of a 1% SRBC suspension, v/v, intravenously).

Batches of BSA that yield at least a 20-fold enrichment of plaque-forming cells (PFC) per 10^6 recovered viable spleen cells in the A and B bands when compared to that of the cells recovered in the C and D bands (Figure 8.2) will yield reasonably consistent separations; some lots are capable of giving as much as 120-fold enrichments of antibody-forming cells.

MATERIALS AND REAGENTS

Sterilization of Centrifuge Tubes and Swinging Buckets

Cellulose nitrate centrifuge tubes, $\frac{1}{2} \times 1$ in., 5 ml or $1 \times 3\frac{1}{2}$ in., 35 ml (Beckman Instruments)
Ethanol, 70% and 95%
UV source in sterile hood
Swinging bucket rotor for cellulose nitrate tubes
Centrifuge tubes, 50 ml (Falcon, #2074 or similar)

Preparation of Stock BSA Solutions

35% bovine serum albumin (BSA), sterile (Path-O-Cyte-4 sterile buffered albumin, Miles Research Products or similar); see comment.
Balanced salt solution (BSS; Appendix A.3)
Graduated cylinders
Culture flasks, 250 ml (Falcon, #3024 or similar)

Preparation of Discontinuous Gradients and Separation of Cells

Spleen cell suspension (Section 1.2) or other cell population
Syringes, 3 ml for smaller gradients, 20 ml for larger gradients

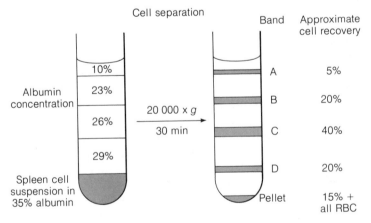

FIGURE 8.2
Diagram of cell separation with discontinuous BSA gradients, showing approximate cell recoveries per band. (After Raidt, Mishell, and Dutton 1968.)

Needles, 15 gauge and 26 gauge

Centrifuge tubes, conical graduated, 12 ml (Bellco Glass, #3041-00012) and stainless steel closures (Bellco Glass, #2005-00016)

Pasteur pipettes and bulbs

Cellulose nitrate centrifuge tubes

Ultracentrifuge

Swinging bucket rotor for cellulose nitrate tubes

PROCEDURE

Sterilization of Centrifuge Tubes and Swinging Buckets

1. Rinse the swinging buckets and their caps with 95% ethanol and allow them to dry under UV light in a sterile hood if sterile conditions are required.

2. Place cellulose nitrate centrifuge tubes in 70% ethanol for 30 minutes. Using sterile forceps, rinse cellulose nitrate tubes in 95% ethanol and place them on sterile gauze. Allow them to dry under UV light in a sterile hood. Store cellulose nitrate tubes in sterile containers until needed. (Three 5-ml tubes fit conveniently in a plastic 50-ml centrifuge tube.)

Preparation of BSA Dilutions

Prepare dilutions of 35% albumin stocks on a volumetric basis using sterile BSS as diluent. For example, to prepare 100 ml of 29% BSA from the 35% stock BSA,

$$\text{Volume of 35\% BSA} = 100 \text{ ml} \times \left(\frac{29}{35}\right) = 82.86 \text{ ml}$$
$$\text{Volume BSS} = 100 \text{ ml} - 82.86 \text{ ml} = 17.14 \text{ ml}$$

These dilutions can be stored indefinitely at 4°C. Solutions of 29% 26%, 23%, and 10% BSA are required for the separation described below.

Preparation of Discontinuous Gradients and Separation of Cells

1. Prepare a suspension of mouse spleen cells and wash the cells twice in BSS ($200 \times g$, 10 min). Use a conical graduated centrifuge tube.

2. To 1 part of packed cells, add 9 parts of 35% BSA. Resuspend the cells carefully with a syringe and 15-gauge needle to avoid the formation of bubbles. This is best done if all air is excluded from the syringe and needle. The final concentration will be approximately 2×10^8 cells/ml.

3. Using the syringe and 15-gauge needle, carefully load the cells suspended in albumin in the bottom of the cellulose nitrate tube. 5-ml tubes should receive 1 ml, and 35-ml tubes should receive 5 ml.

4. Overlay the cell suspension with equal volumes (1 ml or 5 ml, depending on the size of the tube) of 29%, 26%, 23%, and 10% BSA solutions (see Figure 8.2). Add the albumin dilutions, using a syringe and a 26-gauge needle, by slowly allowing the albumin to flow down the side of the centrifuge tube.

5. Load the tubes aseptically into the rotor buckets and secure the caps. Accelerate gently and centrifuge at 20 000 $\times$ g for 30 minutes at 4°C.

6. With a sterile Pasteur pipette, harvest the discrete bands of cells that form at the interfaces of different densities of BSA. Add excess BSS to dilute the BSA and pellet the cells (200 $\times$ g, 10 min). Wash the cells 3 times in excess BSS before culture or assay.

COMMENT

Miles Research Products currently produces two additional 35% albumin solutions that differ in osmolarity. The capacity of these solutions to separate cells can be tested as described above. Small amounts of various salts can be added to the albumin of lowest osmolarity to enhance the separation of particular cell types.

REFERENCES

Dutton, R. W., M. M. McCarthy, R. I. Mishell, and D. J. Raidt. 1970. Cell components in the immune response. IV. Relationships and possible interactions. *Cell. Immunol.* **1**:196.

Mishell, R. I., R. W. Dutton, and D. J. Raidt. 1969. Methods for the study of *in vitro* immunization of mouse spleen cells. *In Vitro* **4**:83.

Mishell, R. I., R. W. Dutton, and D. J. Raidt. 1970. Cell components in the immune response. I. Gradient separation of immune cells. *Cell. Immunol.* **1**:175.

Raidt, D. J., R. I. Mishell, and R. W. Dutton. 1968. Cellular events in the immune response. Analysis of *in vitro* response of mouse spleen cell populations separated by differential flotation in albumin gradients. *J. Exp. Med.* **128**:681.

8.4 COLLOIDAL SILICA GRADIENTS

Geraldine L. Dettman and Stanley M. Wilbur

Density gradients made from colloidal silica coated with polymers (to stabilize the particles in suspension and make the silica nontoxic to cells) and adjusted to physiologic pH and osmolarity can be used as an alternative to BSA gradients to separate subpopulations of leukocytes and other cell types. Initially, preparations of colloidal silica using Ludox-HS were employed (Mateyko and Kopac 1959, 1963; Pertoft 1966, 1969; Pertoft et al. 1968). However, Ludox-HS is inconvenient to use because it gels upon storage after the preparative procedures. More recently, colloidal silica prepared from Ludox-AM (aluminum modified surface) has been used. When prepared according to the procedures described below, Ludox-AM can be stored for long periods without gelling (Dettman and Wilbur 1978). This Ludox-AM preparation has been used to separate human peripheral blood subpopulations (Nathanson et al. 1977) and mouse spleen cell subpopulations (Dettman and Wilbur 1978); it can also be used to separate red blood cells and cell debris from a leukocyte cell suspension.

In addition to its long-term stability, many other properties of the Ludox-AM colloidal silica preparation make it ideal for density gradients. First, after its initial preparation, the colloidal silica has a very high density, which varies between 1.16 g/cm^3 and 1.20 g/cm^3. Thus, there is a wide range of densities possible upon dilution, easily including the densities of most mammalian cells. Second, the colloidal silica particles contribute only slight intrinsic osmolarity; therefore isotonicity is maintained over the whole range of densities. Third, the colloidal silica preparation also has a low viscosity, even at the highest densities. As a result, cells separated with this medium reach buoyant density equilibrium in a short time under relatively low centrifugal forces; yet the medium is viscous enough to permit the easy construction of discontinuous gradients. Finally, Ludox-AM preparations are nontoxic to cells and are easily removed from the cells by washing.

MATERIALS AND REAGENTS

Hanks' balanced salt solution (HBSS), 10×, Mg^{2+}- and Ca^{2+}-free (Grand Island Biological)

HBSS, 1× (Grand Island Biological)

HEPES (N-2-hydroxyethylpiperazine-N-2-ethanesulfonic acid; Calbiochem)

Ludox-AM, technical grade colloidal silica (E. I. Dupont de Nemours)

Polyvinylpyrrolidone (PVP) K-30, average $M_r = 40\ 000$ (MCB Man-
ufacturing Chemists, #PX1300): Prepare a 50% (w/v) solution in
double-distilled water, adding the powder *slowly* into the water.
1 M HCl
Dialysis tubing
Freezing point depression osmometer (e.g., Osmette from Precision
System)
Specific gravity balance

PROCEDURE

1. Dialyze the Ludox-AM extensively with at least three 5X volumes
   of distilled water. The dialysis bags should be tight to prevent
   osmotic swelling of the bags during dialysis.

2. Adjust the pH of the dialyzed Ludox-AM to 7.4 with 1 M HCl.

3. Centrifuge the Ludox-AM at $9000 \times g$ for at least 30 minutes;
   decant and save the supernatant.

4. To the supernatant, slowly add the 50% (w/v) PVP aqueous solution to give a final concentration of 3.4% (w/v). The volume of
   concentrated PVP solution added to the Ludox-AM is determined
   by the formula:

$$X = \frac{3.4Y}{Z - 3.4}$$

   where:

   X = volume of the concentrated PVP added to the Ludox-
   AM
   Y = volume of the Ludox-AM
   Z = the concentration of the PVP solution in units of percent weight/volume

   Upon the addition of the PVP, the colloidal silica will become
   slightly opaque and very viscous. However, with continued mixing this suspension will clear to become a translucent solution of
   low viscosity.
   If a pH adjustment is necessary, this can be accomplished by
   the slow addition of 1 M HCl. A white precipitate will form, but it
   will redissolve with continued mixing. The pH should be about 0.2
   pH unit higher than that desired for the final preparation. At this
   point, autoclave the colloidal silica if sterility is desired.

5. To the 10X HBSS, add HEPES to a concentration of 0.2 M and
   PVP to a concentration of 3.4% (w/v). The pH of this solution
   should also be adjusted to 0.2 pH unit higher than that desired for
   the final preparation. Autoclave this solution if sterility is desired.

6. Titrate a sample of the dialyzed colloidal silica with the supplemented 10× HBSS (from step 5) until the mixture is isoosmotic with the cells to be centrifuged (mouse cells, 308 mOsm; human cells, 290–300 mOsm) when measured by a freezing point depression osmometer or similar instrument. The ratio of colloidal silica to 10× HBSS (from step 5) will be slightly less than 10 : 1. Mix the rest of the colloidal silica batch with the same ratio of 10× BSS and check the osmolarity. After mixing the colloidal silica and the 10× HBSS, the solution should be at the final desired pH. At this point it is no longer possible to adjust the pH or autoclave the solution. The density of this preparation is usually around 1.2 g/cm³. (We use a specific gravity balance to determine the densities.)

7. A penicillin-streptomycin solution can be added to this preparation if desired.

8. Dilute the colloidal silica-HBSS solution to the desired density with 1× HBSS (sterile if required) at the proper osmolarity that contains 3.4% PVP and has been adjusted to the proper pH. The density of the colloidal silica is linearly related to its concentration.

9. This preparation of colloidal silica can now be used to make density gradients. Mouse spleen cells usually vary in density from 1.04 g/cm³ to 1.09 g/cm³. Therefore, a discontinuous gradient can be made up of density steps within this range. For example, we have used a 5–6 step gradient from 1.030 g/cm³ for the top layer to 1.090 g/cm³ for the bottom layer. Cells are suspended in the bottom layer. The gradient is then centrifuged at 2000 × g for 30 minutes at 20°C and the banded cells collected with a Pasteur pipette.

COMMENTS

1. Prepared as described, the colloidal silica is extremely stable as long as physiological pH and osmolarity are maintained. If stored at acidic or alkaline pH, or at high salt concentrations, the colloidal silica will eventually gel and become unusable. It can be stored at either room temperature or at 4°C but is destroyed by temperatures approaching 100°C and by freezing.

2. This method of preparing the colloidal silica can be modified to suit particular needs. For example, another buffer, such as Tris, can be substituted for the HEPES buffer. Also, other polymers may be used in place of the polyvinylpyrrolidone.

3. A few words of caution regarding the use of colloidal silica:

    a. This material should not be used at high g forces. The density gradients are usually centrifuged at only 1000–2000 × g.

    b. Although no noticeable detrimental effect has been noted on mouse cells, a slight depression in monocyte migration has been reported with human peripheral blood cells after separation on colloidal silica gradients. This problem could possibly be overcome with higher PVP concentrations.

    c. The PVP causes hemagglutination of red blood cells and thus colloidal silica coated with PVP cannot be used to separate erythrocyte subpopulations.

REFERENCES

Dettman, G. L., and S. M. Wilbur. 1979. The preparation of colloidal silica-AM-PVP for density gradient centrifugation: Centrifuge tube wall cell adherence, cell aggregation, cell separation properties and comparison to BSA and Ficoll. *J. Immunol. Meth.* **27**:205.

Mateyko, G. M., and M. J. Kopac. 1959. Isopyknotic cushioning for density gradient centrifugation. *Exptl. Cell Res.* **17**:524.

Mateyko, G. M., and M. J. Kopac. 1963. Cytophysical Studies. *Ann. N.Y. Acad. Sci.* **105**:183.

Nathanson, S. D., P. L. Zamfirescu, S. I. Drew, and S. M. Wilbur. 1977. Two-step separation of human peripheral blood monocytes on discontinuous density gradients of colloidal silica-polyvinylpyrrolidone. *J. Immunol. Meth.* **18**:225.

Pertoft, H. 1966. Gradient centrifugation in colloidal silica-polysaccharide media. *Biochim. Biophys. Acta* **126**:594.

Pertoft, H. 1969. The separation of rat liver cells in colloidal silica-polyethylene glycol gradients. *Exptl. Cell Res.* **57**:338.

Pertoft, H., O. Bäck, and K. Lindahl-Kiessling. 1968. Separation of various blood cells in colloidal silica-polyvinylpyrrolidone gradients. *Exptl. Cell Res.* **50**:355.

8.5 VELOCITY SEDIMENTATION AT UNIT GRAVITY

Cells are allowed to sediment at unit gravity for several hours in a medium that is slightly less dense than the cells (Miller and Phillips 1969). Large cells (e.g., lymphoblasts, plasma cells, granulocytes) sediment rapidly and thus can be separated from small lymphocytes, which sediment more slowly. The advantages of this method are: (1) reproducibility; (2) good cell recoveries; and, (3) the large number of cells that can be separated. A major disadvantage is the time required for the separation.

Detailed instructions for performing sedimentation velocity separation are found in the review by Miller (1973) and in the instruction manual of the Sta-Put Apparatus (Johns Scientific, Toronto, Canada). Consult these references for further information.

REFERENCES

Miller, R. G. 1973. Separation of cells by velocity sedimentation. In R. H. Pain and B. J. Smith (Eds.), *New Techniques in Biophysics and Cell Biology,* Vol. 1. Wiley, New York.

Miller, R. G., and R. A. Phillips. 1969. Separation of cells by velocity sedimentation. *J. Cell. Physiol.* **73**:191.

8.6 VELOCITY SEDIMENTATION AT LOW-SPEED CENTRIFUGATION

Harley Y. Tse

This separation method (Tse and Dutton 1976) is a modification of the $1 \times g$ velocity sedimentation method described by Miller and Phillips (1969). The changes eliminate the use of large separation chambers such that as few as 10^7 cells can be applied to the gradient with good recoveries. Moreover, the time required for completion of the separation procedure is greatly shortened. In this system, successful cell separation depends on the correct determination of the following variables: (1) the appropriate concentration range of the supporting medium; (2) the centrifugal force; and (3) the centrifugation time. Suggestions for a quick determination of these parameters will be discussed later.

Ficoll is commonly used as a supporting medium for gradient separation because of its many unusual physical properties: (1) it is a chemically well-defined synthetic product; (2) unlike sucrose, Ficoll has low osmotic activity; (3) it is nontoxic to mammalian cells (Yu et al. 1973); and (4) there is an exponential relationship between the concentration and viscosity of Ficoll (Pretlow and Boone 1969). For the separation of activated T cells, we routinely use a 5–20% Ficoll gradient and centrifuge at $100 \times g$ for 25 minutes such that the fastest sedimenting cells have traveled the length of the centrifuge tube. It should be pointed out that the procedures and specifications described below have been adapted for use with equipment in our laboratory.

MATERIALS AND REAGENTS

Cell suspension: If cultured cells are used for separation, dead cells should be removed; see comment 3.

Fetal calf serum (FCS)

Hanks' balanced salt solution (HBSS)

Ficoll 400 (Pharmacia Fine Chemicals): Prepare a 20% Ficoll solution by slowly dissolving 20 g of Ficoll 400 in 100 ml HBSS. Sterilize solution by passage through a 0.45-μm filter (Appendix C.2), aliquot (40 ml), and store frozen.

70% ethanol

International centrifuge Model PR-6 with #269 bucket head (Damon/ IEC)

Cellulose nitrate centrifuge tubes, 1 × 3½ in. (Beckman Instruments)

Tube stand for centrifuge tubes

Adapters for centrifuge tubes (see comment 5)

Gradient maker, two chambers (Sargent-Welch Scientific or Beckman Instruments)

Magnetic stirrer (or stirrer device supplied with the gradient maker)

Test tubes for fraction collection

Parafilm

Pasteur pipettes with 1-ml mark, sterile

Hemostat

Filter unit, 0.45 μm (Falcon, #7102)

PROCEDURE

Sterilization of Equipment

1. Wet tissue paper with 70% ethanol and wipe the inside of the cellulose nitrate tube thoroughly.

2. Wash the tubes with a large volume of sterile HBSS and shake dry.

3. Fill the tubes with FCS at room temperature. Cover with caps until ready to use. This procedure coats the tubes with FCS proteins and prevents nonspecific sticking of cells to the wall of the tubes during centrifugation.

4. Sterilize the gradient maker with 70% ethanol-wetted tissue paper. Be sure to run alcohol through the connection between the two chambers and through the tubing that leads out from the chamber. Wash away any trace of alcohol with a large volume of sterile HBSS. Cover with Parafilm.

Making the Gradient

A 30-ml 5–20% Ficoll gradient has the capacity to separate from 10^7 to 7×10^7 cells. If more cells are needed, more than one gradient has to be prepared. The following specifications are for one gradient.

1. Pipette 5 ml from the stock of 20% Ficoll solution. Add 15 ml of sterile HBSS with 5% FCS to give a 5% Ficoll solution.

2. Close the stopcock between the chambers of the gradient maker. Use a hemostat to clip the outlet tubing.

3. Place 15.5 ml of the 20% Ficoll solution in the chamber with the outlet tubing.

4. Open the stopcock between the chambers and allow approximately 0.5 ml of solution to flow into the other chamber. Close the stopcock and suck out the liquid that flowed into the chamber. This procedure ensures that no air is trapped between the chambers.

5. Into the empty chamber, add 15.0 ml of the 5% Ficoll solution.

6. Pour off the FCS from the cellulose nitrate tube. Shake dry. Seal tube with Parafilm wax paper and stand it upright in a tube holder. Position the tube so that its top is about 0.5 cm below the bottom of the gradient maker chambers. This distance has been arbitrarily set and can be increased if a faster flow rate is desired.

7. Pierce a hole into the Parafilm on the cellulose nitrate tube with a 1-ml pipette. Direct the outlet tubing from the 20% Ficoll chamber through the hole until it touches the inside wall of the tube.

8. Before removing the hemostat and opening the stopcock, make sure that the *20% solution chamber* receives constant mixing with magnetic stirrer or other device.

9. Remove the hemostat. Liquid should start flowing out. If it does not, tap outlet tubing a little.

10. Quickly open the stopcock and allow the 5% solution to flow into the 20% solution chamber under atmospheric pressure.

11. The speed of the mixing may have to be adjusted from time to time as the volume of liquid in the chamber decreases.

12. After the gradient is made, slowly and carefully layer another 3 ml of 5% Ficoll on top of the gradient. This additional layer is intended to minimize "streaming effects" during centrifugation.

13. Layer 1 ml of the cells to be separated on top of the 5% Ficoll zone.

14. Seal the tube with a fresh piece of Parafilm.

Centrifugation

1. Place the gradient in an adapter which in turn goes into a centrifuge bucket.

2. Set the time to 25 minutes with the speed dial at zero, then slowly increase the speed to an rpm equivalent of $100 \times g$ (700 rpm with #269 bucket head in an International PR-6 centrifuge).

3. Our experiments were routinely done at 4°C.

4. No brake should be used.

Fractionation

1. Make a 1-ml mark on a sterile Pasteur pipette (if this was not done prior to sterilization). Position the pipette so that it just touches the surface of the liquid. Carefully remove a 1-ml volume each time from the top. Collect 34 fractions. The top 7 or 8 fractions usually contain very few cells.

2. For the first trial run, monitor each fraction for cell number and relative cell size (small, medium, or large) on a hemacytometer and, if the cells are labeled, also monitor for radioactivity. Once this information is known, pool fractions with cells of similar size.

3. The Ficoll in each pool has to be diluted before cells can be spun down. Determine the approximate concentration of Ficoll in each pool and dilute with HBSS until the final Ficoll concentration is about 5%. A final centrifugation at $400 \times g$ for 15 minutes will bring the cells down.

4. Finally, resuspend each pool to the appropriate concentration with culture medium.

COMMENTS

1. In early experiments, the linearity of the gradient should be checked. This can be done by performing the separation without any cells and measuring the refractive index of each fraction.

2. It is important to select the appropriate combination of speed and time of centrifugation. A simple method to determine these conditions is to use cells labeled with ^{3}H-thymidine as markers. After fractionation, locate the peak of radioactivity, which should indicate where the majority of the blast cells are. If the peak is not far enough down the gradient, increase the speed or time of centrifugation, or both.

3. Dead cells should be removed before applying the cells on the gradients. Centrifugation through Ficoll-Hypaque (Section 1.19) is recommended.

4. With practice the separation procedure can be performed in less than 4 hours, with a cell yield of 70–90%.

5. Adapters for fitting the cellulose nitrate tubes to the centrifuge buckets can be made in the following manner:

   a. Hold a Beckman cellulose nitrate tube inside a 50-ml Falcon (or similar) centrifuge tube such that the edge of the Beckman tube is about 0.5 cm above the edge of the Falcon tube.

   b. Fill the empty space between the two tubes with molten wax.

   c. Allow the wax to solidify and remove the Beckman tube.

   d. Finally, line the inside of the wax-well in the Falcon tube with aluminum foil so that the Beckman tube fits tightly. It is desirable to have adapters of the same weight if more than one is used.

REFERENCES

Miller, R. G., and R. A. Phillips. 1969. Separation of cells by velocity sedimentation. *J. Cell. Physiol.* **73:**191.

Pretlow, T. G., and C. W. Boone. Resolution of viable cell mixtures using Ficoll gradient centrifugation. *Fed. Proc.* **27:**545.

Tse, H., and R. W. Dutton. 1976. Separation of helper and suppressor T lymphocytes on a Ficoll velocity sedimentation gradient. *J. Exp. Med.* **143:**1199.

Tse, H. Y., and R. W. Dutton. 1977. Separation of helper and suppressor T lymphocytes. II. Ly phenotypes and lack of DNA synthesis requirement for the generation of concanavalin A helper and suppressor cells. *J. Exp. Med.* **146:**747.

Tse, H. Y., and R. W. Dutton. 1978. Separation of helper and suppressor T lymphocytes. III. Positive and negative effects of mixed lymphocyte reaction-activated T cells. *J. Immunol.* **120:**1149.

Yu, D. T. Y., J. B. Peter, H. E. Paulus, and H. I. Machleder. 1973. Lymphocyte populations: Separation by discontinuous density gradient centrifugation. *J. Immunol.* **110:**1615.

8.7 ONE-STEP GRADIENT SEPARATION OF ROSETTED CELLS

John North and Claudia Henry

A single-density step gradient separation using Ficoll-Hypaque was developed for the separation of rosetted mouse lymphocytes by Parish et al. (1974). Similar separations can be achieved using colloidal silica density gradients (Section 8.4). Both procedures depend upon cell size and density to separate rosetted from nonrosetted lymphocytes (Section 8.1). The rosetted cells pass through the dense medium and form a pellet during centrifugation. The nonrosetted cells either never enter the dense medium or enter the dense medium but do not form a pellet. Thus, the nonrosetted cells are recovered by taking all the medium above the pellet, diluting the medium to decrease its density, and centrifuging the suspended cells.

The following procedure describes the use of Ficoll-Hypaque; procedures describing the use of colloidal silica are outlined in Section 8.4.

MATERIALS AND REAGENTS

Minimum essential medium (MEM) or balanced salt solution (BSS; Appendix A.3), containing 5% fetal calf serum (FCS)

Ficoll 400 (Pharmacia Fine Chemicals)

Hypaque, 50% w/v (Winthrop Laboratories), or Isopaque, 32.8% w/v (Nyegaard or Accurate Chemical & Scientific): Occasional lots give poor separations; thus batches should be tested prior to general use and stored in a cool dark place.

Volumetric flask, 100 ml

Polycarbonate tubes, 16 × 125 mm (Nalge, #3117)

Centrifuge, swinging bucket rotor, with rapid acceleration (2000 × g within 20 seconds)

PROCEDURE

Preparation of Ficoll-Hypaque Solution

1. Prepare a 14% Ficoll solution: Weigh 14 g of Ficoll 400 and slowly add to a bottle or beaker containing 50–80 ml double-distilled water. Stir overnight or until Ficoll dissolves completely. Quantitatively transfer all the dissolved Ficoll into a 100-ml volumetric flask and bring the volume up to 100 ml. Mix the solution thoroughly.

2. Mix 12 parts of 14% Ficoll with 5 parts of 32.8% (w/v) Hypaque or Isopaque (dilute the 50% (w/v) Hypaque to 32.8% with double-distilled water). Sterilize the Ficoll-Hypaque (Isopaque) mixture by membrane filtration (Appendix C.2) and store at 4°C protected from light. The mixture should have a density of 1.09 g/cm³ (see Section 8.2 for general procedure for determining density) and an osmolarity of 280–308 mOsm. Since Hypaque has a high density and osmolarity, small inaccuracies during preparation of the Ficoll-Hypaque produce large variations in the final density and osmolarity.

Separation of Rosetted from Nonrosetted Cells

1. Prewarm rosette suspension and Ficoll-Hypaque to 20°C in a waterbath. Prewarm the centrifuge to 20°C.

2. Add 4 ml of Ficoll-Hypaque to a 16 × 125-mm polycarbonate tube and gently layer 5 ml of rosette suspension onto the Ficoll-Hypaque. Add the suspension down the tube wall. (The use of polycarbonate tubes reduces cell losses due to adherence.)

3. Place tubes in a prewarmed centrifuge and centrifuge at 2000 × g for 20 minutes. Rapid acceleration of the samples to reach 2000 × g within 20 seconds is essential for clean separations.

COMMENTS

1. The pellet contains red blood cells, rosetted cells, dead cells, and cell debris. The interface and the Ficoll-Hypaque layer above the pellet contain viable nonrosetted lymphocytes and accessory cells.

2. To recover the nonrosetted cells, take all the medium above the pellet, add 10 ml of MEM or BSS (containing 5% FCS), and centrifuge at 300–350 × g for 10–15 minutes. Repeat the washing step twice before using the cells for functional studies.

3. To remove the red blood cells from the rosetted cells prior to functional studies, we have used either osmotic shock (Section 1.16) or treatment with hemolytic Gey's solution (Section 1.18). After the treatment, pass the cell suspension through a glass wool column (Section 1.21) to remove dead cells and cell debris. Centrifuge the cell suspension (200 × g, 10 min) and wash twice with MEM or BSS (plus 5% FCS).

4. Commercially available Ficoll-Hypaque mixtures (Pharmacia Fine Chemicals, "Ficoll-Paque R" and Sigma Chemical, "Ficoll F P") are similar to the Ficoll-Hypaque described here, but have a lower density, being designed for human lymphocyte separations. When the commercial mixtures are used with mouse lymphocytes, live nonrosetted cells tend to move faster into the separation medium and thereby contaminate the pellet and give lower yields of unrosetted cells. This effect is partially mitigated by centrifugation at 500–1000 × g for only 10–15 minutes, but the resulting separations are nevertheless less satisfactory than those obtained with the Ficoll-Hypaque described here.

5. A few rosettes formed by lymphocytes of low densities (about 1.05 g/cm³) containing few red blood cells (less than 4) will not sediment unless a lower density separating medium is employed. However, if a lower density medium is used, some high-density lymphocytes will accumulate in the pellet.

REFERENCES

Parish, C. R. 1975. Separation and functional analysis of subpopulations of lymphocytes bearing complement and Fc receptors. *Trans. Rev.* **25**:98.

Parish, C. R., S. M. Kirov, N. Bowern, and R. V. Blanden. 1974. A one-step procedure for separating mouse T and B lymphocytes. *Eur. J. Immunol.* **4**:808.

9

Cell Surface Markers

9.1 INTRODUCTION

Robert I. Mishell and Claudia Henry

Separation procedures based on differentially expressed cell surface markers constitute the most promising techniques for the reliable preparation of cell subpopulations with defined characteristics. Most of the current methods result in the recovery of a heterogeneous population of cells from which a subpopulation carrying a specific marker has been removed (*negative selection*). These methods have been very useful for obtaining information about the functions of the depleted cell subpopulations. Complementary *positive selection* procedures permitting the isolation and recovery of the cells that carry markers are not yet generally available. The continued development of generally applicable positive selection methods will greatly enhance the use of surface markers as tools for defining cellular functions.

The principal historic method of depleting cells bearing a particular marker has been to bring about their lysis by treatment with specific antisera and complement (Section 9.2). Although effective for many studies, this approach has two main disadvantages: (1) Finding a source of complement for use with certain types of antisera can be a problem; and

(2) in some situations, the relevant marker-bearing cells are not adequately eliminated.

Recently developed methods employ antisera specific for cell surface markers, that do not require the use of complement. Procedures of this type, based on a hapten-sandwich modification (Wofsy et al. 1978) of the rosetting technique of Parish et al. (1974), are described in Sections 9.3 and 9.4. We have found that these techniques deplete more than 95% of cells bearing Ig, Thy 1, or Ia markers. During the preparation of this manuscript, a new procedure using antibodies bound to the flat plastic surfaces of tissue culture Petri dishes and flasks was introduced for separating cells (Mage et al. 1977; Wysocki and Sato 1978). This method appears to have several advantages: Cell recovery rates are high; the method is less complex than others; and it has been used with some success for positive as well as negative selection. Its use as a negative selection procedure for the removal of Ig positive murine splenic B cells is described in Section 9.7.

Other differentially expressed surface constituents, such as those that function as receptors for macromolecules and those containing carbohydrate that bind to specific plant lectins, have been used to separate cells. Rosetting procedures for separating cells bearing receptors for complement (Bianco et al. 1970) and for Fc (Parish and Hayward 1974) are described in Section 9.5. Separations based on the agglutination of appropriate cells with peanut and soybean lectins are described in Section 9.6. The lectin agglutination methods are particularly interesting because they permit recovery of both the nonagglutinated and the agglutinated cell populations.

REFERENCES

Bianco, C., R. Patrick, and V. Nussenzweig. 1970. A population of lymphocytes bearing a membrane receptor for antigen-antibody-complement complexes. I. Separation and characterization. *J. Exp. Med.* **132:**702.

Mage, M. G., L. L. McHugh, and T. L. Rothstein. 1977. Mouse lymphocytes with and without surface immunoglobulin: Preparative scale separation on polystyrene tissue culture dishes coated with specifically purified anti-immunoglobulin. *J. Immunol. Meth.* **15:**47.

Parish, C. R., and J. A. Hayward. 1974. The lymphocyte surface. I. Relation between Fc receptors, C'3 receptors, and surface immunoglobulin. *Proc. R. Soc. Lond. B.* **187:**47.

Parish, C. R., S. M. Kirov, N. Brown, and R. V. Blanden. 1974. A one-step procedure for separating mouse T and B lymphocytes. *Eur. J. Immunol.* **4:**808.

Wofsy, L., C. Henry, and S. Cammisuli. 1978. Hapten-sandwich labeling of cell surface antigens. In R. A. Reisfield and F. P. Inman (Eds.), *Contem-*

porary Topics in Molecular Immunology, Vol. 7. Plenum Press, New York.

Wysocki, L. J., and V. L. Sato. 1978. "Panning" for lymphocytes: A method for cell selection. *Proc. Natl. Acad. Sci.* (USA) **75**:2844.

9.2 SPECIFIC ANTISERA AND COMPLEMENT

Claudia Henry

The most commonly employed method for depleting a heterogeneous cell suspension of a subpopulation bearing a specific marker is to treat the suspension with appropriate antisera and complement, thereby killing the relevant cells. Variations in technique are frequently required to obtain satisfactory cytolysis. Although empirical testing of conditions with particular reagents is often necessary, certain general guidelines apply.

1. If the antiserum is anticomplementary (usually obvious in a preliminary titration), it is unwise to use a single-step procedure in which cells, antiserum, and complement are incubated together. A two-step procedure should be adopted: Incubate antisera and cells first and remove excess antiserum; then add complement.

2. For heteroantisera, guinea pig serum absorbed with agarose (Appendix A.2) is usually a good source of complement. For alloantisera, rabbit complement is normally preferable; however each lot must be tested for toxicity. It is best to use rabbits 1 month old or younger because serum from older rabbits is usually toxic.

3. With potent antisera (e.g., rabbit anti–mouse brain), it is possible to treat cells at densities of 1.5×10^7 cells/ml. With weak antisera, the cell concentration should not exceed 5×10^6 cells/ml.

4. Some surface markers (e.g., B cell Ig) modulate on exposure to antiserum. In this case, sodium azide at a final concentration of 0.02% should be included in the incubation mixture.

5. Some investigators believe that exposing T cells to low temperature (e.g., 4°C) interferes with their subsequent lysis. These investigators recommend that cell suspensions be maintained at 20°C or more during the preparative phase preceding attempts to eliminate T cells with antiserum and complement.

6. Appropriate controls should always be included (i.e., assays with complement plus normal sera).

In the following outline, we describe one- and two-step procedures with the understanding that appropriate modifications must be made for each particular case.

MATERIALS AND REAGENTS

Cell suspension
Specific antiserum
Normal serum for control
Source of complement, nontoxic (for agarose absorption see Appendix A.2)
Balanced salt solution (BSS; Appendix A.3)
Water bath at 37°C

PROCEDURE

One-Step Procedure

1. Suspend cells to 5×10^6–1.5×10^7 cells/ml in BSS containing the appropriate dilution of antiserum and complement (determined by prior titration of both reagents).
2. Incubate for 45 minutes in a 37°C water bath, shaking the reaction mixture periodically.
3. Centrifuge cells at $200 \times g$ for 10 minutes and wash 2 times in BSS.

Two-Step Procedure

1. Suspend cells to 5×10^6–1.5×10^7 cells/ml in BSS containing antiserum at the appropriate dilution.
2. Incubate for 30 minutes (4°C, room temperature, or 37°C), shaking reaction mixture periodically.
3. Centrifuge cells at $200 \times g$ for 10 minutes and resuspend the pellet to the original volume in BSS containing the appropriate dilution of complement.
4. Incubate for 30–45 minutes in a 37°C water bath, shaking the reaction mixture periodically.
5. Pellet the cells and wash two times in BSS.

9.3 HAPTEN-SANDWICH ROSETTING

Material for this section was provided by Maxwell Slomich, Elaine Kwan, Leon Wofsy, and Claudia Henry

The hapten-sandwich method, described in Chapter 13, has proven particularly useful when applied to rosetting procedures for cell separation. Lymphocytes coated with hapten-conjugated anti–cell surface antibodies are rosetted with red blood cells coated with purified anti-hapten antibodies. The procedures are based on those originally developed by Parish and coworkers (1974), who formed rosettes by mixing red blood cells coated with antisera to rabbit IgG and lymphocytes that had reacted with rabbit antiserum to cell surface determinants. The hapten-sandwich modification employs purified anti-hapten antibodies rather than crude antibody preparations, thus providing better control of the amount of effective binding antibody that is coupled to the red blood cells. Moreover, hapten-modified antibodies against cell surface markers present more determinants capable of being bound by the antibodies on the red blood cells than do unmodified antibodies to the cell surface determinants. Consequently, the hapten-sandwich technique results in the rapid formation of stable rosettes. The hapten-sandwich technique is especially appropriate for separations based on the recognition of alloantigens because it avoids the complication of the mouse immunoglobulin present on B lymphocytes and macrophages.

MATERIALS AND REAGENTS

Preparation of Anti-Ars Sheep Red Blood Cells

Sheep red blood cells (SRBC)

Affinity purified rabbit anti-phenylarsonate antibody (anti-Ars), stored at 2 to 5 mg/ml (see Section 11.3 for the preparation of antiserum and Section 12.4 for its purification)

Saline: 0.85% NaCl (w/v)

$CrCl_3 \cdot 6\ H_2O$: 6.67 mg/ml in saline

Phosphate-buffered saline (PBS; Appendix A.8)

RPMI 1640, without bicarbonate, containing 10% heat-inactivated (56°C, 30 min) fetal calf serum (RPMI-FCS)

Pasteur pipettes and rubber bulb

Sero-Fuge II centrifuge (Clay Adams) for washing red blood cells (optional)

Polypropylene tube, 17 × 100 mm (Falcon, #2059) for use with Sero-Fuge II

Conical, graduated tube

Balance accurate to 0.1 mg

Rotator (Scientific Products, #R4193-1)

30°C incubator

Coating of Spleen Cells with Hapten-Modified
Anti–Cell Surface Antibody

Spleen cell suspension (Section 1.2)

RPMI 1640 without bicarbonate

RPMI-FCS

FCS, heat-inactivated

Hapten-modified anti–cell surface antibody (e.g., Ars-rabbit anti–mouse brain for T cell rosettes, Ars-anti–mouse Ig for B cell rosettes, Ars-anti-Ia for Ia positive cells) stored at approximately 1 mg/ml (see Chapter 11 for the preparation of antisera and Section 13.2 for hapten modification)

Glass and plastic graduated, conical tubes

Glass wool columns (Section 1.21)

Preparation of Rosettes

SRBC modified with rabbit anti-Ars antibody

Spleen cells modified with hapten-modified cell surface antibody

RPMI-FCS

Ficoll-Hypaque (Section 8.7)

Crystal violet, 1% (w/v) in double-distilled water

Conical, graduated centrifuge tubes

Vortex mixer

Hemacytometer

Hand counter

PROCEDURE

Preparation of Anti-Ars Sheep Red Blood Cells

1. Wash SRBC four times with saline in a Sero-Fuge II using 17 × 100-mm polypropylene tubes. (A Sero-Fuge, while not necessary, is convenient since RBC will pellet after $1\frac{1}{2}$ to 2 minutes of centrifugation. It is not satisfactory for spleen cells.) Transfer SRBC into a conical, graduated tube for the fifth wash to determine the packed volume. Pellet the cells at $400 \times g$ for 10 minutes.

2. Immediately before use, weigh 3–6 mg $CrCl_3 \cdot 6H_2O$ and adjust to 6.67 mg/ml in saline. Dilute 1 : 100 in saline (2.5×10^{-4} M).

3. To each 0.1 ml packed SRBC, add 50–100 μl rabbit anti-Ars (2–5 mg/ml) in saline and 1 ml of diluted chromic chloride.

4. Rotate mixture at 30°C for 1 hour.

5. Add twice the volume of PBS to the mixture to quench coupling. Pellet the cells at $250 \times g$ for 10 minutes (or 2 minutes in a Sero-Fuge II).

6. Wash twice with the same volume of PBS and then once in RPMI-FCS. Resuspend red blood cells to $1-2 \times 10^9$ cells/ml in RPMI-FCS (0.1 ml packed SRBC contains approximately 2×10^9 cells). Check a diluted aliquot microscopically to verify that red blood cells have not agglutinated.

Coating of Spleen Cells with Hapten-Modified Anti–Cell Surface Antibody

1. Pass a spleen cell suspension through a short glass wool column (Section 1.21) and centrifuge cells at 200 × *g* for 10 minutes.

2. To remove dead cells resuspend cells in 3 ml of RPMI 1640 and remove any debris and agglutinated dead cells by centrifuging at 45–50 × *g* for about 30 seconds (turn centrifuge off when speed is reached). Transfer supernatant to another tube and repeat the process 3 times.

3. Pellet spleen cells at 200 × *g* for 10 minutes.

4. To 0.1 ml packed spleen cells, add 0.1 ml of Ars-modified anti–cell surface antibody at a concentration previously determined to be optimal (see Comment 3). Antibody should be diluted in RPMI-FCS. Resuspend cells and place at 4°C for 20 minutes.

5. Add approximately 1 ml of RPMI (without FCS) to the mixture and layer the cell suspension onto 2 ml of heat-inactivated FCS. Centrifuge at 300 × *g* for 10 minutes and wash pelleted cells twice in RPMI-FCS.

Preparation of Rosettes

Satisfactory rosettes are produced with 20 : 1 to 50 : 1 ratios of SRBC to spleen cells.

1. Resuspend modified spleen cells to $2–10 \times 10^7$ cells/ml in RPMI-FCS.

2. Add the spleen suspension dropwise to the red cell suspension, mixing *gently* with a vortex mixer. (Add the appropriate volume of spleen cells to attain a red cell : spleen cell ratio of 20 : 1 to 50 : 1, depending on preference.)

3. Place the mixture on ice for approximately 20 minutes, gently shaking periodically to keep cells in suspension.

4. Check microscopically for rosettes with a sample adjusted to 2×10^6 lymphocytes/ml. Discrimination between rosettes and red cell clumps is facilitated by adding 1 drop of 1% crystal violet to 1.0 ml of the suspension; allow 5 minutes for the lymphocytes to become stained (violet lymphocytes are evident in the rosettes). Any lymphocyte with more than 5 bound red blood cells is classified as a rosette.

5. To separate rosettes from single lymphocytes, dilute to 10^7 lymphocytes/ml in RPMI-FCS and centrifuge through Ficoll-Hypaque (Section 8.7).

COMMENTS

1. Phosphate-containing buffer must be avoided in the chromic chloride coupling of the red blood cells; in fact, it is used to quench the coupling.

2. The above method uses freshly prepared chromic chloride. Many prefer to use aged chromic chloride. The aging protocol is as follows: a 1% (w/v) $CrCl_3 \cdot 6H_2O$ solution in saline is immediately adjusted to pH 5 with 1 M NaOH. The solution is stored at room temperature for 3 weeks, its pH being readjusted to 5.0 with 1 M NaOH thrice weekly. It is then ready for use as a coupling reagent. At this time it must be titrated with washed red blood cells in saline; it is used at the concentration just below that giving aggregates of the red blood cells in the absence of antibody. The solution is stable for at least 6 months without further pH readjustment. Eventually it aggregates red blood cells rather than conjugating them with protein. The chemical basis of the aging is poorly understood as is the mechanism of chromic chloride coupling of proteins.

3. For coating spleen cells with Ars-modified anti–cell surface antibody, it is very important that each pool of antiserum be titrated to determine the concentration that gives a maximal number of rosettes without causing clumping.

4. Controls consisting of coated red blood cells and uncoated lymphocytes or lymphocytes coated with unmodified antibody should be devoid of rosettes.

5. If the spleen cell suspension is to be depleted of two cell types (e.g., B and T cells), react the spleen cells in sequence with each Ars-modified antibody (washing once in between), then add anti-Ars-modified red blood cells, and proceed as above.

REFERENCES

Parish, C. R., and J. A. Hayward. 1974. The lymphocyte surface. I. Relation between Fc receptors, C'3 receptors, and surface immunoglobulin. *Proc. R. Soc. Lond. B.* **187**:47.

Parish, C. R., S. M. Kirov, N. Brown, and R. V. Blanden. 1974. A one-step procedure for separating mouse T and B lymphocytes. *Eur. J. Immunol.* **4**:808.

Wofsy, L., C. Henry, and S. Cammisuli. 1978. Hapten-sandwich labeling of cell surface antigens. In R. A. Reisfeld and F. P. Inman (Eds.), *Contemporary Topics in Molecular Immunology*, Vol. 7. Plenum Press, New York.

9.4 ROSETTE REMOVAL BY AGGLUTINATION

Elaine Kwan, Robert I. Mishell, and Barbara B. Mishell

The agglutination of rosettes with antisera provides an alternative to the use of density gradients for separating rosettes from nonrosetted lymphoid cells. The technique employs human A_1 red blood cells for rosette formation and commercial anti–A typing sera, a combination of reagents that fosters particularly strong agglutination reactions. This modification (Mishell and co-workers, manuscript in preparation) of the hapten-sandwich technique (Wofsy et al. 1978) has been used for preparing large quantities of cells because it avoids the labor involved in the preparation and use of sterile density gradients.

MATERIALS AND REAGENTS

Human red blood cells (HuRBC), type A_1, no older than one week
Anti–A blood typing serum
Fetal calf serum (FCS), heat inactivated (56°C, 30 min)
Balanced salt solution (BSS; Appendix A.3)
BSS containing 5% heat-inactivated FCS (BSS-5%FCS)
BSS containing 25% heat inactivated FCS (BSS-25%FCS)
$CrCl_3 \cdot 6H_2O$: 6.67 mg/ml in saline (0.85% NaCl, w/v); see Section 9.3
Plastic conical centrifuge tubes, 15 ml, disposable (Corning Glass Works, #25310 or similar)

PROCEDURE

1. Prepare hapten-sandwich rosettes as described in Section 9.3 using HuRBC instead of SRBC and making these other changes: Dilute the 6.67 mg/ml solution of $CrCl_3 \cdot 6H_2O$ in saline 1 : 75 rather than 1 : 100. Hold the HuRBC in saline until just prior to the formation of rosettes (see comment 5).

2. Centrifuge the cell mixture at $200 \times g$ for 10 minutes in a plastic conical tube (using plastic conical tubes from this point on allows the recovery of a larger percentage of cells).

3. Remove and discard the supernatant. Add undiluted anti–A serum to the pellet (0.5 ml antiserum for a rosette mixture containing 2×10^9 HuRBC). Pipet the mixture up and down 4 or 5 times.

4. Agglutinated cells will immediately begin to settle to the bottom of the tube. After 5 minutes, most (if not all) clumps will have settled. Add approximately 4 ml of BSS-5%FCS to dilute the antiserum and gently resuspend so as to free the white blood cells without breaking up the clumps. Allow clumps to settle again for approxi-

mately 5 minutes. Transfer the supernatant (free of agglutinated clumps) to another plastic conical tube, and pellet the cells (200 × g, 10 min).

5. Resuspend the cells in 2 ml BSS-5%FCS. If small clumps are visible, gently layer the cells on top of 8 ml of BSS-25%FCS in a 15-ml plastic conical tube. Incubate at room temperature for 15 minutes to allow clumps to settle to the bottom of the tube. Harvest the nonagglutinated cells on top of the gradient. Pellet cells again (200 × g, 10 min).

COMMENTS

1. Approximately 10–25% of the cells are lost nonspecifically through centrifugation, trapping, and proximity to the agglutinated cells at the bottom of the tube.

2. A_1 type cells provide the "tightest" agglutination and the least possibility of recovering any rosetted lymphocytes from the pellet. Type B human red cells also agglutinate rapidly but the agglutination is more easily disrupted into smaller aggregates. Other type A (or type B) subgroups seem to offer the best possibility for recovery, although we have not yet attempted to verify that assumption.

3. The commercial antisera contain a dye; however, functional studies of the depleted populations indicate that it is not toxic.

4. The small percentage of human red blood cells that remain in the supernatant can be removed by one of the methods described in Sections 1.16 to 1.19.

5. The HuRBC should be kept in saline until just prior to rosette formation; they will undergo crenation if suspended in BSS for longer than 20 minutes. However, by this time, the rosettes will have formed. Forming rosettes in saline is not as suitable since the modified mouse spleen cells exhibit a tendency to aggregate in saline.

REFERENCE

Wofsy, L., C. Henry, and S. Cammisuli. 1978. Hapten-sandwich labeling of cell surface antigens. In R. A. Reisfeld and F. P. Inman (Eds.), *Contemporary Topics in Molecular Immunology,* Vol 7. Plenum Press, New York.

9.5   Fc AND COMPLEMENT RECEPTORS

Elaine Kwan and Robert I. Mishell

A large proportion of B lymphocytes and accessory cells possess receptors for the Fc region of IgG and for the activated form of the third component of complement. Cells bearing these two kinds of receptors (FcR^+ and CR^+, respectively) can be separated from cells that do not possess them by rosette formation and subsequent separation on density gradients. Fc rosettes are formed with sheep red blood cells (erythrocytes, E) coated with IgG antibodies (EA). Complement receptor (CR) rosettes are formed with sheep red blood cells coated with nonhemolytic amounts of IgM antibodies and reacted with mouse complement (EAC). The procedures described below are based on those of Bianco et al. (1970) and Parish and Hayward (1974). When combined with other cell separation methods, separation of cells by virtue of receptors for either Fc or complement can be used to obtain restricted subpopulations of cells.

The reagents and procedures for forming Fc rosettes and CR rosettes are similar. The principle difference is that the Fc rosette procedure employs antiserum that contains mainly IgG at sufficiently high concentrations to form rosettes in the absence of complement; whereas the CR rosette procedure employs antiserum containing mainly IgM at concentrations that form no rosettes in the absence of complement and a maximum number when complement is also adsorbed onto the EA cells. Although commercially prepared antisera can be used, we recommend making different antisera specially for the two procedures, using the immunization protocols suggested by Parish and Hayward (1974).

A.   Fc Rosetting

MATERIALS AND REAGENTS

Preparation of 10% E (Sheep Red Blood Cells)

Sheep red blood cells (SRBC)
Balanced salt solution (BSS; Appendix A.3)
Graduated, conical tubes, 15 ml (Corning Glass Works, #25310 or
  similar)

Preparation of 5% EA$_{Fc}$ (Erythrocyte-Antibody)

Antiserum to SRBC, 2× concentration (the appropriate dilution of
  antiserum for Fc rosetting must be predetermined experimentally
  as described below in procedure for titration of anti-SRBC serum)

BSS
Clear tubes, 17 × 100 mm

Preparation of Fc Rosettes

5% EA$_{Fc}$ (v/v)
Spleen cell suspension (Section 1.2)
BSS
Clear tubes, 17 × 100 mm, with caps
Rotator (Scientific Products, #R4193-1)

Counting Rosettes

BSS
5% acetic acid
Crystal violet, 0.5% (w/v) in double-distilled water
Glass tubes, 12 × 75 mm
Parafilm
Hemacytometer and hand counter

Separation of Rosetted from Nonrosetted Cells

As described in Section 8.7.

Titration of Anti-SRBC Serum for Preparation of EA$_{Fc}$

Antiserum to SRBC (specially prepared for Fc rosetting; see proce-
dure below)
SRBC
Spleen cell suspension
BSS
Glass tubes, 12 × 75 mm
Hemacytometer and hand counter

PROCEDURE

Preparation of 10% E (Sheep Red Blood Cells)

1. Wash SRBC three times with BSS (400 × g, 10 min) in a graduated
   centrifuge tube.

2. Resuspend SRBC to 10% (v/v) in BSS (10% E).

Preparation of 5% EA$_{Fc}$ (Erythrocyte-Antibody)

1. Mix equal volumes of 10% E and 2× antiserum.

2. Incubate the mixture at 37°C for 30 minutes (the temperature and
   length of incubation are not critical).

3. Centrifuge the mixture (400 × g, 10 min) and wash once with BSS.
   Resuspend to 5% (v/v) with BSS (5% EA$_{Fc}$).

Preparation of Fc Rosettes

1. Adjust the spleen cell concentration to 2×10^7 cells/ml in BSS. Mix 2.5 ml of spleen cells with 2.5 ml of 5% EA_{Fc} in a 17×100-mm clear tube. For complete Fc rosette formation, the concentration of EA_{FC} must be kept at 2.5% during the rosetting procedure.

2. Cap the tube tightly and place on a vertical rotator. Rotate the tube at 30 rpm at 37°C for 15 minutes. The temperature of this step is critical. Place the tube on ice before counting the rosettes.

Counting Rosettes

1. Remove 0.1 ml of sample from the rosetted suspension and dilute with 0.4 ml of BSS. Add 1 drop of 0.5% crystal violet and wait 5 minutes to allow the white blood cells to stain. Count the total number of rosettes and the total number of white blood cells (count about 200 white blood cells from the rosetted suspensions). Express the results as the percentage of rosettes to the total number of white blood cells.

2. Alternatively, the total number of white blood cells and rosettes may be counted separately. Remove two 0.1 ml-aliquots from the rosetted suspension. To one aliquot, add 0.1 ml of 5% acetic acid in distilled water to lyse the red blood cells. Add 0.3 ml BSS and count the total number of white blood cells. Dilute the other aliquot with 0.4 ml BSS and count the number of rosettes.

Separation of Rosetted from Nonrosetted Cells

As described in Section 8.7.

Titration of Anti-SRBC Serum for Preparation of EA_{Fc}

Serum rich in IgG anti-SRBC antibodies should be used to prepare EA_{Fc}. Serum with high titer ($1:64$ to $1:512$) is obtained by immunizing rats subcutaneously with 10^8 SRBC in complete Freund's adjuvant and bleeding the rats 14 days later. Heat the antiserum (56° C, 30 min) to inactivate complement prior to use. To determine the dilution at which the antiserum is to be used, first prepare a series of EA_{Fc} using antiserum at various dilutions (in BSS). Then test each EA_{Fc} preparation for the ability to form rosettes with lymphocytes from a test pool of spleen cells. Finally, plot the percentage of rosettes against the antiserum dilution. The antiserum is used at the highest dilution (lowest concentration) that gives a maximum of rosettes. For convenience, dilute the antiserum to twice the concentration at which it will be used and store at -20°C.

B. Complement Receptor Rosetting

MATERIALS AND REAGENTS

Preparation of 10% E (Sheep Red Blood Cells)

Sheep red blood cells (SRBC)
Balanced salt solution (BSS; Appendix A.3)
Graduated, conical tubes, 15 ml (Corning Glass Works, #25310 or
  similar)

Preparation of 10% EA_{CR} (Erythrocyte-Antibody)

Antiserum to SRBC, 2× concentration (the appropriate dilution of
  antiserum for the preparation of CR rosettes must be predetermined experimentally as described below in procedure for titration
  of anti-SRBC serum)
BSS
Clear tubes, 17 × 100 mm

Preparation of 5% EAC (Erythrocyte-Antibody-Complement)

10% EA_{CR}
Mouse complement (mouse serum diluted 1 : 3 and stored at −70°C)
BSS

Preparation of Complement Receptor Rosettes

5% EAC
Spleen cell suspension (Section 1.2)
BSS
Clear tubes, 17 × 100 mm, with caps
Rotator (Scientific Products, #R4193-1)

Counting Rosettes

BSS
5% acetic acid
Crystal violet, 0.5% (w/v) in double-distilled water.
Glass tubes, 12 × 75 mm
Parafilm
Hemacytometer (Section 1.10) and hand counter

Separation of Rosetted from NonRosetted Cells

As described in Section 8.7.

Titration of Anti-SRBC Serum for Preparation of SRBC Appropriately Sensitized for Complement Receptor Rosetting

Antiserum to SRBC (specially prepared for CR rosetting; see procedure below); alternatively, commercial hemolysin (prepared in rabbits; Colorado Serum Co.)

SRBC

BSS

Saline: 0.85% NaCl (w/v)

Glass tubes, 12 × 75 mm

Hemacytometer and hand counter

PROCEDURE

Preparation of 10% E (Sheep Red Blood Cells)

1. Wash SRBC three times in BSS (400 × g, 10 min) in a graduated centrifuge tube.

2. Resuspend the SRBC to 10% (v/v) in BSS (10% E).

Preparation of 10% EA_{CR} (Erythrocyte-Antibody)

1. Mix equal volumes of 10% E and 2× antiserum.

2. Incubate the mixture at 37°C for 30 minutes (the temperature and length of incubation are not critical).

3. Centrifuge mixture (400 × g, 10 min) and wash once with BSS. Resuspend to 10% (v/v) with BSS (10% EA_{CR}).

Preparation of 5% EAC (Erythrocyte-Antibody-Complement)

1. Thaw mouse complement and mix with an equal volume of 10% EA_{CR}. Incubate the mixture at 37°C for one hour.

2. Centrifuge and wash once with BSS. Resuspend to 5% (v/v) in BSS (5% EAC).

Preparation of Complement Receptor Rosettes

1. Adjust spleen cell concentration to 5 × 10^7 cells/ml in BSS. Mix 1 ml of spleen cells and 1 ml of 5% EAC in a 17 × 100-mm clear tube. Add 3 ml of BSS to a total volume of 5 ml.

2. Cap the tube tightly and place on a vertical rotator. Rotate the tube at 30 rpm at 37°C for 15 minutes. The temperature for this step is critical. Place the tube on ice before counting the rosettes.

Counting Rosettes

The procedure for determining the percentage of rosettes in the cell suspension is the same as that described above in subsection A.

Separation of Rosetted from Nonrosetted Cells

As described in Section 8.7.

Titration of Anti-SRBC Serum for Preparation of SRBC Appropriately Sensitized for Complement Receptor Rosetting

1. To prepare EA for CR rosetting, it is important to use a concentration of antiserum too low to give Fc rosettes, yet high enough to give a maximum of CR rosettes. Moreover, the antiserum should not cause lysis of the SRBC when mouse complement is added. The most satisfactory antiserum for CR rosetting is rich in IgM. Such an antiserum is obtained by immunizing rats intraveneously with 10^8 SRBC in saline and bleeding the rats 7 days later. Heat the antiserum (56°C, 30 min) to inactivate the complement prior to use.

2. Titrate the antiserum in a manner similar to that described for Fc rosetting (subsection A). Use various dilutions of the antiserum to prepare EA. Then test each of the EA preparations for both Fc and CR rosetting by the procedures described above. After determining the percentages of Fc and CR rosettes for each preparation, plot the results against the dilutions of antiserum. The dilution of antiserum for use in CR rosetting is the highest dilution (lowest concentration) that gives a maximum of CR rosettes and no Fc rosettes. Dilute the antiserum to twice the concentration at which it will be used and store at $-20°C$.

REFERENCES

Bianco, C., R. Patrick, and V. Nussenzweig. 1970. A population of lymphocytes bearing a membrane receptor for antigen-antibody-complement complexes. I. Separation and characterization. *J. Exp. Med.* **132**:702.

Parish, C. R., and J. A. Hayward. 1974. The lymphocyte surface. I. Relation between Fc receptors, C'3 receptors, and surface immunoglobulin. *Proc. R. Soc. Lond. B.* **187**:47.

9.6 PEANUT AND SOYBEAN AGGLUTININS

Linda M. Bradley, with contributions from Yu-hua Una Chen

Two lectins, peanut agglutinin (PNA) and soybean agglutinin (SBA), can be used to separate lymphocyte subpopulations by differential agglutination. The method of separation is rapid, reproducible, and efficient for large numbers of cells.

PNA separates the immunologically immature cortical thymocytes from the functionally mature medullary thymocytes. PNA is specific for D-galactose residues, which are exposed on the cortical thymocytes but masked by sialic acid on the medullary thymocytes. Five to eight percent of thymocytes do not react with PNA; the rest agglutinate.

SBA separates splenic T and B cells, with 5–10% cross-contamination. SBA is specific for N-acetyl-D-galactosamine and D-galactose. The former (and possibly also the latter) is accessible on B cells but masked by sialic acid on T cells. Thus, SBA agglutinates B cells but not T cells.

In procedures with either lectin, agglutinated cells are efficiently separated from nonagglutinated cells by $1 \times g$ sedimentation. The agglutinated cells can then be dissociated by treatment with D-galactose. Both recovered subpopulations are viable and functional in a variety of tests. Thus, PNA and SBA can be used for depletion as well as enrichment. With either lectin, macrophages and other accessory cells are present in both the agglutinated and the nonagglutinated populations.

A. Peanut Agglutinin (PNA)

MATERIALS AND REAGENTS

Suspension of thymus cells (Section 1.5) from 6-week-old mice

PNA* (Vector Laboratories), lyophilized, salt free, 1 mg/ml in BSS (or PBS); sterilize by membrane filtration (Appendix C.2).

Balanced salt solution (BSS; Appendix A.3) or phosphate-buffered saline (PBS; Appendix A.8)

BSS (or PBS) containing either 20% heat-inactivated fetal calf serum (FCS) or 2% bovine serum albumin (BSA)

0.2 M D-galactose, crystalline (Sigma Chemical) in sterile BSS or PBS, $M_r = 180.2$

Graduated centrifuge tubes, conical, 12–15 ml

Conical centrifuge tubes, 50 ml (Falcon, #2074 or similar)

Fine-mesh, stainless steel screen

Syringe, 5 ml, with 18-gauge needle

PROCEDURE

1. Aseptically excise thymuses from 6-week-old mice. Carefully remove any connective tissue that adheres to the thymic capsule, to ensure removal of parathymic lymph nodes (see Section 1.5).

2. Dissociate thymocytes by teasing. To further dissociate large clumps, gently force the suspension through an 18-gauge needle

---

* It is advisable to prepare a fresh batch of PNA for each experiment to prevent loss in activity. However, we have successfully stored small aliquots at 1 mg/ml, $-20°C$ for periods of 2–3 weeks.

with the 5-ml syringe 3–5 times. Pass the cells through a fine-mesh stainless steel screen to obtain a single-cell suspension free of debris.

3. Wash the cells twice in BSS (or PBS) and resuspend in the same buffer to 8×10^8 cells/ml.

4. Mix 0.25–0.5 ml of the thymocyte suspension with an equal volume of PNA (1 mg/ml in the same buffer), and incubate for 5–10 minutes at room temperature.

5. Gently layer the cells on top of 10 ml of BSS (or PBS) containing 20% heat-inactivated FCS or 2% BSA, in a 12–15-ml centrifuge tube. Incubate at room temperature 15–30 minutes. Agglutinated cells begin to fall immediately and by 15–30 minutes have completely settled to the bottom. Nonagglutinated single cells remain on the top of the gradient.

6. To treat larger quantities of cells, following the procedure outlined above, mix 0.75–1.0 ml of thymocytes (8×10^8 cells/ml) with an equal volume of PNA (1 mg/ml). After agglutination, layer cells on 25–30-ml gradients.

7. If agglutinated cells are to be recovered, transfer the bottom layer of cells to a 50-ml centrifuge tube with a Pasteur pipette. Mix the cells with 10–15 ml of 0.2 M D-galactose (room temperature). After 5–10 minutes, pellet the cells ($200 \times g$, 10 min). Wash once with galactose as above, and once with BSS (or PBS) before use.

8. To recover the nonagglutinated cells, remove the top layer of the gradient. The cells may be treated with galactose, as described above, or simply washed twice with buffer before use. We have found that omission of the galactose treatment of this population has no effect on the subsequent functional capacity of the cells.

B. Soybean Agglutinin (SBA)

MATERIALS AND REAGENTS

Spleen cell suspension (Section 1.2)

SBA (Vector Laboratories), lyophilized, salt free, 2–4 mg/ml in BSS or PBS; sterilize by membrane filtration (Appendix C.2)

BSS or PBS containing either 50% heat-inactivated FCS or 2% BSA

0.2 M D-galactose, crystalline (Sigma Chemical) in sterile BSS or PBS, $M_r = 180.2$

Conical centrifuge tubes, 50 ml

PROCEDURE

The method is essentially identical to that described for PNA, except that a larger volume of the FCS (or BSA) solution is used for cell separation. Preparations of SBA are more variable in activity than those of PNA, because this lectin tends to aggregate or polymerize upon storage. It is advisable to titrate each lot of SBA for optimal agglutination. SBA is also more sensitive to freezing than PNA and must be freshly prepared for each experiment.

1. Prepare single-cell suspensions of spleen by teasing, and adjust concentration to 4×10^8 cells/ml in BSS (or PBS).

2. Mix 0.5 ml of cells with an equal volume of SBA (2–4 mg/ml in the same buffer). Incubate for 5–10 minutes at room temperature.

3. Gently layer the cells on top of 40 ml of BSS (or PBS) containing 20% heat-inactivated FCS or 2% BSA. Incubate at room temperature for 15–30 minutes to allow separation of agglutinated and nonagglutinated cells.

4. Remove the top and bottom layers of cells separately, and transfer into 50-ml centrifuge tubes with Pasteur pipettes. Suspend the cells in 10–15 ml of 0.2 M galactose and incubate 5–10 minutes at room temperature. Pellet the cells and wash twice with the galactose solution and once with buffer before use.

REFERENCES

Despont, J. P., C. A. Abel, and H. M. Grey. 1975. Sialic acid and sialyl-transferases in murine lymphoid cells: Indicators of T cell maturation. *Cell. Immunol.* **17**:487.

Reisner, Y., M. Linker-Israeli, and N. Sharon. 1976. Separation of mouse thymocytes into two subpopulations by the use of peanut agglutinin. *Cell. Immunol.* **25**:129.

Reisner, Y., A. Ravid, and N. Sharon. 1976. Use of soybean agglutinin for the separation of mouse B and T lymphocytes. *Biochim. Biophys. Res. Comm.* **72**:1585.

9.7 SEPARATION OF T AND B CELLS USING PLASTIC SURFACES COATED WITH ANTI-IMMUNOGLOBULIN ANTIBODIES ("PANNING")

George K. Lewis and Roberta Kamin

Polystyrene surfaces may be employed as insoluble matrices for the affinity reagents used to separate lymphocyte subpopulations (Mage et al.

1977; Wysocki and Sato 1978). In the procedure described below, antibodies to mouse Ig are used to separate B cells from T cells. Polystyrene culture flasks are first coated with affinity-purified rabbit anti–mouse immuno-globulin antibodies; mouse spleen cells are then added to the flasks. B cells bind to the antibody-coated plastic surfaces whereas T cells do not. The T cells are recovered by gently removing the nonadherent cell population. Although described for the selective binding of mouse B cells, this technique can be used for the purification of other murine cell types and of cells from other species. It is possible to use hapten-sandwich procedures (see Section 9.3) as well as other ligand-receptor systems. For example, Taniguchi and Miller (1977) and Lewis and Goodman (1978) have used plastic plates coated with antigen for the selective enrichment of antigen-specific suppressor T cells.

Although the technique is new and experience with it is therefore limited, the panning procedure appears to be especially promising because of its relative simplicity and high rate of cell recovery.

MATERIALS AND REAGENTS

Preparation of Rabbit Anti–Mouse Ig Antibodies

NZW rabbits
Normal mouse serum
Ammonium sulfate (Section 12.2) or sodium sulfate
Phosphate-buffered saline (PBS; Appendix A.8)
Complete Freund's adjuvant (CFA). Note: Freund's adjuvant is a potentially hazardous agent (see Appendix F).
Dialysis tubing (Appendix D)
Syringe, 3 ml, with Luer-lock. Note: If Luer-lock syringes are not available, protective glasses should be worn (see Appendix F).
Needle, 22 gauge

Conjugation of Mouse Ig to Sepharose

Sepharose 4B (Pharmacia Fine Chemicals)
Mouse Ig, ammonium sulfate precipitated: 2.5–7.5 mg/ml in 0.2 M NaHCO$_3$
2 M NaOH, M_r = 40.0: 80 g/liter
1 M acetic acid (glacial acetic acid is 17.4 M; therefore, make a 1 : 17.4 dilution of glacial acetic acid)
Cyanogen bromide (CNBr). Note: CNBr is extremely toxic and a potent lachrymator (tear gas); store CNBr in a desiccator at −20°C and handle only in a well-ventilated chemical hood.
0.2 M NaHCO$_3$, M_r = 84.0: 16.8 g/liter, ice cold
Balanced salt solution (BSS; Appendix A.3)

Borate-buffered saline, pH 8.0 (BBS; Appendix A.9)
Dimethylformamide
Beaker, 100 ml
Buchner funnel, filter paper, and aspirator flask
Magnetic stirrer and bar
pH meter
Ice cold, double-distilled water
Crushed ice, approximately 50 ml

Purification of Rabbit Anti–Mouse Ig by Affinity Chromatography

Mouse Ig conjugated to Sepharose 4B
0.1 M EDTA, M_r = 372 (for disodium EDTA·2H$_2$O: 37.2 g/liter)
Phosphate-buffered saline (PBS; Appendix A.8), tissue culture grade, prepared with double-distilled water
3.5 M sodium thiocyanate, M_r = 81, or 3.5 M ammonium thiocyanate, M_r = 76, pH 8.0. Sodium thiocyanate: 283.5 g/liter; ammonium thiocyanate: 266 g/liter. Adjust to pH 8.0 with 1 M NaOH or 1 M HCl as required.
Gentamycin (Microbiological Associates)
Small chromatographic column
UV spectrophotometer
Dialysis tubing (Appendix D)
Membrane filtration equipment (Appendix C.2)
Ultrafiltration equipment (Amicon or similar)

Coating of Plastic Flasks with Anti-Ig

Affinity-purified rabbit anti–mouse Ig antibodies, 1 mg/ml in PBS
PBS, tissue culture grade, prepared with double-distilled water
Culture flasks (Corning Glass Works, #25100 or similar)

T Cell Enrichment

Mouse spleen cell suspension (Section 1.2)
Fetal calf serum (FCS)
Bicarbonate-free medium or BSS
BSS containing 5% FCS (BSS-5%FCS)
Antibody-coated flasks

B Cell Enrichment (Adherent Cell Removal)

PBS, tissue culture grade, prepared with double-distilled water so that it is free of Ca^{2+} and Mg^{2+}
BSS-5%FCS
Lidocaine HCl (xylocaine HCl; Astra Pharmaceutical Products): 20 mg/ml in PBS

PROCEDURE

Preparation of Rabbit Anti-Mouse Ig Antibodies

1. Precipitate the immunoglobulin fraction of normal mouse serum using either ammonium sulfate (40% final saturation, Section 12.2) or sodium sulfate (18% final saturation).

2. Dialyze precipitated Ig against PBS. Dilute dialyzed Ig to 2 mg/ml in PBS and emulsify with an equal volume of CFA (Appendix F).

3. Immunize 3 NZW rabbits with 1.0 ml of the emulsified antigen distributed among several subcutaneous sites on days 0, 12, and 21. Test bleed the rabbits on day 28. If the antibody titer is above 1.5 mg/ml as determined by a precipitin test, bleed the animals out. If the titer is below 1.5 mg/ml, boost the rabbits again, and test bleed 7–10 days later. If the titer does not increase after the additional boost, discard the animal.

Conjugation of Mouse Ig to Sepharose 4B

Note: This part of the procedure *must* be performed in a functioning fume hood.

1. Wash 14 ml of packed Sepharose 4B with 20 volumes of distilled water in a Buchner funnel. Dry the Sepharose by suction and transfer it to a 100-ml beaker. Place the beaker in an ice bath on a magnetic stirrer.

2. Add a volume of water to the beaker equal to the packed volume of the Sepharose (14 ml). Also, place a magnetic stirring bar into the beaker.

3. Adjust the pH to 11.0 with 2M NaOH and stir Sepharose gently.

4. Dissolve 1.0 g of cyanogen bromide in about 1.0 ml of dimethyl-formamide and add the solution dropwise to the Sepharose while stirring.

5. Readjust the pH to 11.0 and maintain at pH 11.0 by the addition of 2 M NaOH. Allow the reaction to proceed until further addition of 2 M NaOH is no longer required to maintain pH (10–15 minutes). Add approximately 50 ml of crushed ice to the reaction mixture and transfer the slurry to a Buchner funnel. Wash the Sepharose with 250 ml of cold water and then with 250 ml of cold 0.2 M NaHCO$_3$.

6. After washing, dry the Sepharose by suction and transfer it to 20 ml of mouse Ig (2.5–7.5 mg Ig/ml) in cold 0.2 M NaHCO$_3$.

7. Allow the reaction to proceed overnight at 4°C with *gentle* stirring.

8. Sequentially wash the immunoadsorbent on a Buchner funnel with 500 ml water, 500 ml 1 M acetic acid, 500 ml water, and 500 ml BBS. The degree of conjugation may be estimated by determining the OD_{280} of the first wash that passes through the filter.

Purification of Rabbit Anti–Mouse Ig by Affinity Chromatography

1. Pack the immunoadsorbent into a small chromatographic column and wash with BBS until no UV-absorbing material is eluted (measured at 280 nm). Make the antiserum 0.01 M with EDTA.

2. Allow the BBS to run down to the top of the column bed; then gently apply 15 ml of antiserum and allow it to run into the column.

3. Clamp the column off and incubate it for 1 hour at room temperature.

4. Wash away nonbinding serum protein with BBS until the OD_{280} of the effluent is less than 0.03.

5. Allow the BBS to run down to the top of the column bed and clamp the column off.

6. Fill the column with 3.5 M sodium or ammonium thiocyanate solution, pH 8.0. Open the column and monitor the effluent for absorption at 280 nm.

7. Pool all fractions containing protein and immediately dialyze against 2 changes of tissue-culture-grade PBS.

8. Concentrate the anti-Ig to 1 mg protein/ml by ultrafiltration and sterilize by filtration through a 0.22-μm membrane filter (Appendix C.2). Also, add gentamycin (50 μg/ml, final concentration) to the protein solution at this point. The activity of the preparation may be determined by standard precipitin methods or, more simply, by Ouchterlony analysis (Ouchterlony and Nilsson 1978).

9. The anti-Ig may be stored for many months at 4°C without loss of activity.

Coating of Plastic Flasks with Anti-Ig

Note: Perform procedure under sterile conditions.

1. Pipet 2 ml of anti-Ig (at 1 mg/ml in PBS) into a culture flask.

2. Incubate the flask, broad side down, on a level table for 18 hours at 4°C. These flasks may be kept this way indefinitely to provide a ready source of anti–Ig-coated flasks (see comment 1).

3. Immediately before use, carefully draw off the anti-Ig and transfer the solution to another sterile flask for storage as described above.

Mark the number of times the anti-Ig has been transferred on the new flask. (We have reused some preparations of anti-Ig as many as 12 times with no difference in the depletion of B cells.)

4. Wash the flask 3 times with approximately 5 ml of PBS. These flasks are now ready for use and should not be stored for longer than 2–3 hours.

T Cell Enrichment

1. Prepare a single-cell suspension of spleen cells (Section 1.2) and resuspend cells to 1.5×10^7 cells/ml in either bicarbonate-free culture medium containing 5% FCS or BSS-5%FCS.

2. Add 3 ml (or less) of spleen cells per flask.

3. Place the flask on a level table at room temperature and incubate for 30 minutes. Gently swirl the flasks and incubate an additional 30 minutes.

4. After one hour, carefully resuspend the nonadherent T cells by rocking the flask, and remove the cells with a pipette. Take care not to dislodge the adherent cells from the bottom surface of the flask (i.e., avoid pipetting directly off the bottom surface of the flask).

5. The plates may be washed by carefully adding 3 ml of BSS-5% FCS and repeating step 4. However, the highest degree of purity of the nonadherent population is obtained by omitting the washing step and using the cells directly after step 4.

B Cell Enrichment (Adherent Cell Removal)

1. Prepare a 1 : 5 dilution of lidocaine HCl in Ca^{2+}/Mg^{2+}-free PBS (the final concentration is 4 mg/ml).

2. After pipetting off the nonadherent cells from the flask, wash the adherent cell layer 5 times with 4–5 ml of Ca^{2+}/Mg^{2+}-free PBS, taking care not to dislodge the adherent cells by touching the cell layer with the pipette.

3. Add 2–3 ml of the lidocaine solution to the washed cell layer and allow to stand undisturbed for 10–15 minutes at room temperature. Using a Pasteur pipette, remove the adherent cells by vigorously pipetting the overlaying solution onto the cells. This step can be repeated if necessary until all the attached cells have been dislodged. Rinse the flask with BSS-5%FCS. Centrifuge the cells ($200 \times g$, 10 min) and wash twice with BSS-5%FCS (see comment 6).

COMMENTS

1. This technique is limited to those situations in which the non-targeted cells do not stick spontaneously to plastic and in which enough ligand adsorbs to the plastic surface.

2. The procedure described above gives volumes required for 25-cm² flasks. For 60-mm culture dishes (28 cm²), use the same volumes. For dishes of other sizes (e.g., 100-mm dishes), adjust the volumes appropriately based on the surface area of the bottom of the dish. We prefer flasks to dishes because the protein-coated flasks are much easier to store than the dishes.

3. The procedure described above should give a 15–30% yield of T cells containing 5% or less Ig-positive cells. We should point out that some T cells may stick to the surface by virtue of their Fc receptors; this should be borne in mind when ascribing function to recovered T cells. To circumvent the binding of T cells by their Fc receptors, $F(ab')_2$ anti-Ig can be employed. This reagent has the additional advantage of eliminating the binding of macrophages by their membrane Fc receptors.

4. To minimize nonselective binding on the basis of adherence to solid substrates, incubation can be carried out at 4°C in Ca^{2+}/Mg^{2+}-free and serum-free medium. However, B cell binding is not as efficient under these conditions.

5. The requirement of affinity-purified or high-titer antibody for coating the flasks (or dishes) is a disadvantage when separating subpopulations other than B cells. This problem can be overcome by using indirect methods. For example, T cells coated with crude rabbit anti–mouse brain antibody will bind to plastic surfaces coated with affinity-purified goat anti–rabbit Ig antibodies. Preliminary experiments indicate that indirect hapten-sandwich "panning" works well with alloantisera. In this modification, plates are coated with purified anti-hapten antibodies and cells are coated with a preparation of hapten-modified crude antibody to cell surface antigens (see Section 13.2).

6. Lidocaine-recovered adherent cells have been found to be >80% viable by trypan blue exclusion. Additionally, such cell suspensions give an enhanced proliferative response to lipopolysaccharide stimulation compared to the response of unfractionated spleen cell suspensions, thereby suggesting the presence of an increased proportion of B cells (Kamin, unpublished observations). We anticipate that further enrichment for B cells in the

lidocaine-treated population can be achieved by additional selection procedures (e.g., using anti-Thy 1 and complement).

Editors' note

We have obtained comparable results using large (150 × 16 mm) bacteriological grade Petri dishes (Scientific Products, #D1937) and incubation at 4°C rather than room temperature. These conditions, based on those described by Wysocki and Sato (1978), may reduce nonspecific adherence. We have found the 150 × 16 mm dishes preferable because they allow a more uniform distribution of cells following settling than do the smaller dishes.

REFERENCES

Lewis, G. K., and J. W. Goodman. 1978. Purification of functional, determinant specific idiotype-bearing murine T cells. *J. Exp. Med.* **148:**915.

Mage, M. G., L. L. McHugh, and T. L. Rothstein. 1977. Mouse lymphocytes with and without surface immunoglobulin: Preparative scale separation on polystyrene tissue culture dishes coated with specifically purified anti-immunoglobulin. *J. Immunol. Meth.* **15:**47.

Ouchterlony, Ö., and L.-Å. Nilsson. 1978. Immunodiffusion and immunoelectrophoresis. In D. M. Weir (Ed.), *Handbook of Experimental Immunology,* 3rd edition. Blackwell Scientific Publications, Oxford.

Taniguchi, M., and J. F. A. P. Miller. 1977. Enrichment of specific suppressor T cells and characterization of their surface markers. *J. Exp. Med.* **146:**1450.

Wysocki, L. J., and V. L. Sato. 1978. "Panning" for lymphocytes: A method for cell selection. *Proc. Natl. Acad. Sci.* (USA) **75:**2844.

10

Functional Separation by Inactivation of Proliferating Cells

10.1 HOT THYMIDINE PULSE

Linda M. Bradley

Exposure of lymphocytes to antigens or mitogens *in vitro* induces DNA synthesis and cellular proliferation. When exogenous ^{3}H-labeled thymidine is supplied, it is incorporated into newly synthesized DNA. If the ^{3}H-thymidine is of sufficiently high specific activity, intranuclear irradiation due to radioactive disintegration and β particle emission results in cell death. The incorporation of additional ^{3}H-thymidine can be blocked by adding excess cold thymidine. As a consequence, only those cells that have proliferated during the pulse period are killed and any cells that had not been stimulated to divide remain intact.

This "hot pulse" technique has been used for the selective elimination of clones in studies of humoral immune responses *in vitro* (Dutton and Mishell 1967), of mixed lymphocyte reactions (Hirano and Nordin 1976), and of cell-mediated cytolytic responses to alloantigens (Peavy and Pierce 1975). It is an alternative procedure to treatment with 5-bromo-2-deoxyuridine and light (Section 10.2) for the selective elimination of proliferating cells.

A number of considerations must be kept in mind when utilizing the hot thymidine pulse technique (Cleaver 1967; Hendke 1973; Evans 1974):

(1) The radiation effects depend quantitatively on the number of ^{3}H-thymidine molecules incorporated into DNA. Incorporation of the radio-active label is determined by the total concentration of thymidine available, the specific activity of the reagent, and the duration of exposure. For a given irradiation dose (i.e., μCi), the specific activity and concentration of thymidine are inversely proportional. Therefore, in principle, for a given dose of ^{3}H-thymidine, increasing the specific activity would result in greater radiation damage. However, in practice, ^{3}H-thymidine having a very high specific activity may not provide sufficient exogenous thymidine to saturate the incorporation pathways for the specified pulse period. Thus, if proliferation is asynchronous and thereby necessitates long pulse periods to eliminate a particular cell population, late-dividing cells may receive inadequate thymidine. Consequently, it is preferable to hold the specific activity to the minimum that can successfully be employed. The specific activity, time of initiation, and duration of the pulse required for particular experimental purposes must be empirically derived.

(2) The specific activities of ^{3}H-thymidine used in experiments of this type are 10–20 Ci/mmol, at doses of 5–10 μCi/ml culture. At these specific activities, ^{3}H-thymidine is unstable when stored in aqueous solution because of self-radiolysis and self-decomposition. Many lots of high-specific-activity ^{3}H-thymidine in aqueous solution are toxic *in vitro*. However, ethanol (in concentrations of 50–70%) protects against self-decomposition (Evans 1974). Thus ^{3}H-thymidine with a specific activity of 20 Ci/mmol, stored in 70% ethanol at 4°C, is indefinitely stable and non-toxic at 10 μCi/ml.

(3) There is no evidence of ^{3}H-loss or -exchange from thymidine under physiological conditions or after incorporation into DNA. However, in experiments requiring long pulse periods because of asynchronous division, cell death and subsequent DNA breakdown can lead to reutilization of the label. Furthermore, subpopulations of proliferating lymphocytes can recruit other cells into division. Thus, a long pulse period and/or label reutilization can introduce "nonspecific" cell death.

(4) At the end of the pulse, removal of unincorporated ^{3}H-thymidine by washing is preferable to simply blocking with excess cold thymidine. High concentrations of thymidine reversibly inhibit proliferation and are widely used to synchronize cultured cells (thymidine block). Since the sensitivity of different cell types to this effect differs, the possibility of blocking the incorporation of ^{3}H-thymidine with unlabeled thymidine must be evaluated for each system. For example, the precursors of IgG plaque-forming cells (PFC) are considerably more sensitive to thymidine inhibition than the precursors of IgM PFC (Kemshead et al. 1977). If a washing procedure is selected to terminate the ^{3}H-thymidine pulse, it is necessary subsequently to include low concentrations (10 μg/ml) of thymidine in the

medium to prevent the reutilization of label. However, it is important to control for the possibility that this precaution may also affect culture performance, in view of the evidence that the P815 Y mastocytoma cell line shows a delayed inhibition of division in the presence of 10 μg/ml thymidine (Thomas and Lingwood 1975). Control cultures treated with thymidine only and with ^{3}H-thymidine and thymidine simultaneously should be included in each experiment.

MATERIALS AND REAGENTS

Materials and reagents as described in Section 2.2 with the following additions:

^{3}H-methyl-thymidine, specific activity 20 Ci/mmol, 1 Ci/ml (New England Nuclear, #NET 027E): Dilute to 100 μCi/ml with sterile BSS.
Thymidine, unlabeled (cold): 2000 μg/ml in BSS, sterilized by membrane filtration (Appendix C.2)

PROCEDURE

Note: Use established safety procedures when handling radioactive materials.

1. Establish cultures as described in Section 2.2.

2. To initiate the pulse, add 5–10 μCi of ^{3}H-thymidine (0.05–0.1 ml ^{3}H-thymidine).

3. To terminate the pulse, aseptically harvest the cultures with a sterile Teflon policeman. Pellet the cells (200 $\times$ g, 10 min), and wash 3 times with sterile BSS. Culture the cells in fresh medium containing 10 μg of cold thymidine (see introduction to this section).

4. Alternatively, the pulse may be terminated by the addition of 100 μg of cold thymidine without washing or medium change (see introduction).

REFERENCES

Cleaver, J. E. 1967. Thymidine metabolism and cell kinetics. *North Holland Research Monographs, Frontiers of Biology,* Vol. 6.
Dutton, R. W., and R. I. Mishell. 1967. Cell populations and cell proliferation in the *in vitro* response of normal mouse spleen to heterologous erythrocytes. Analysis by the hot pulse technique. *J. Exp. Med.* **126**:443.
Evans, E. A. 1974. *Tritium and Its Compounds.* Wiley, New York.

Hendke, W. R. 1973. *Radioactive Tracings in Biological Research.* Wiley, New York.

Hirano, T., and A. A. Nordin. 1976. Cell-mediated immune responses *in vitro.* I. The development of suppressor cells and cytotoxic lymphocytes in mixed lymphocyte cultures. *J. Immunol.* **116:**1115.

Kemshead, J. T., J. R. North, and B. A. Askonas. 1977. IgG anti-hapten antibody secretion *in vitro* commences after extensive precursor proliferation. *Immunology* **33:**485.

Peavy, D. L., and C. W. Pierce. 1975. Cell-mediated immune responses *in vitro.* III. Elimination of specific cytotoxic lymphocyte responses by ³H-thymidine suicide. *J. Immunol.* **115:**1521.

Thomas, D. B., and C. A. Lingwood. 1975. A model of cell cycle control: effects of thymidine on synchronous cell cultures. *Cell* **5:**37.

10.2 5-BROMO-2-DEOXYURIDINE (BUdR) PULSE

John North

5-bromo-2-deoxyuridine (BUdR) is incorporated into the DNA of dividing cells as an analog of thymidine and, when activated by ultraviolet (UV) light, breaks down causing DNA damage and subsequent cell death (Djordjevic and Szybalski 1960; Zoschke and Bach 1970). This reaction provides an alternative to the ³H-thymidine "hot pulse" method for the selective killing of dividing cells.

It is essential to recognize that treatment with BUdR without exposure to UV light can have many effects on cultured cells. Studies of cell differentiation have shown that BUdR interferes with a variety of cellular processes (Holtzer et al. 1972; Levitt and Dorfman 1974; Moroni et al. 1975). In summary:

1. The growth and viability of some undifferentiated cell lines may be reduced, although differentiated cells escape this effect.

2. The formation of macromolecules associated with the phenotype of a differentiated state can be reversibly suppressed, while the general synthesis of DNA, RNA, and protein remains unaffected. In principle, therefore, effects on the synthesis of immunoglobulin or the function of cytotoxic effectors might be found in the absence of the overt killing of cells.

3. When incorporated during critical periods of cell differentiation, BUdR interferes with specific developmental programs and may therefore prevent the subsequent appearance of functional effector cells.

4. The malignancy of cultured cells has been reported to be reduced.

5. Endogenous virus expression may be stimulated.

Despite the potential for alternative effects, it is frequently possible to select an appropriate concentration of BUdR to achieve the selective killing of dividing cells. Since different sensitivities to the drug are exhibited by different cell types, it is necessary to choose the appropriate concentration of BUdR for each experimental system.

The drug concentration of choice is that which gives maximal effect after UV irradiation but minimal effect when irradiation is avoided. This concentration should be determined by preliminary experiments. For suspension cultures (Section 2.5) assayed at day 5 for secondary IgG anti-TNP responses, 3 μg per ml (10 μM) in a 24-hour pulse is appropriate (Kemshead et al. 1977). To further ensure that the measured effects can be ascribed to the selective killing of dividing cells, controls of cultures treated with BUdR alone or with UV light alone and washed in parallel with experimental groups should be included in each experiment. Since bright laboratory fluorescent lighting may constitute sufficient irradiation for some BUdR activation, cultures should be maintained in the dark.

MATERIALS AND REAGENTS

Materials and reagents as described in Section 2.5 with the following additions:

5-bromo-2-deoxyuridine, M_r = 307.1 (Aldrich Chemical, #85,881-1): Prepare a 100 μg/ml solution in balanced salt solution (BSS; Appendix A.3) and sterilize by membrane filtration (Appendix C.2). Note: This reagent is a carcinogen; do not pipet by mouth or allow skin contact.

Tissue culture chamber (Bellco Glass, #7741-10005), darkened (either paint outside of chamber or cover with opaque material)

Source of UV light (BUdR is activated by 313 nm): A bright fluorescent tube may be sufficient, but a pair of Phillips 20W/08, 300–400 nm tubes (or equivalent) is best. Note: UV light can severely damage eyesight but is blocked by glass spectacles.

PROCEDURE

1. Initiate cultures as described in Section 2.5.

2. *Start of Pulse:* Add appropriate volume of sterile BUdR in BSS. From this time onward, these cultures must be kept in a dark chamber and exposed to fluorescent light or direct sunlight as little as possible.

3. *End of Pulse:* Expose cultures to intense UV light for 20–30 minutes, using tubes located 4–6 inches above the culture dishes. Wash cells free of excess BUdR by one centrifugation in 10–15 ml BSS/ml of culture. Resuspend in fresh, complete tissue culture medium and return to original dishes in darkened chamber.

REFERENCES

Djordjevic, B., and W. Szybalski. 1960. Genetics of human cell lines. III. Incorporation of 5-bromo- and 5-iododeoxyuridine into the deoxyribonucleic acid of human cells and its effect on radiation sensitivity. *J. Exp. Med.* **112**:509.

Holtzer, H., H. Weintraub, R. Mayne, and B. Mochan. 1972. The cell cycle, cell lineages, and cell differentiation. *Curr. Top. Dev. Biol.* **7**:229.

Kemshead, J. T., J. R. North, and B. A. Askonas. 1977. IgG anti-hapten antibody secretion *in vitro* commences after extensive precursor proliferation. *Immunology* **33**:485.

Levitt, D., and A. Dorfman. 1974. Concepts and mechanisms of cartilage differentiation. *Curr. Top. Dev. Biol.* **8**:103.

Moroni, C., G. Schumann, M. Robert-Guroff, E. R. Sauter, and D. Martin. 1975. Induction of endogenous murine C-type virus in spleen cell cultures treated with mitogens and 5-bromo-2'-deoxyuridine. *Proc. Natl. Acad. Sci.* (USA) **72**:535.

Zoschke, D. C., and F. H. Bach. 1970. Specificity of antigen recognition by human lymphocytes *in vitro*. *Science* **170**:1404.

10.3 MITOMYCIN C

Susan L. Swain

Functions that require cellular division are abolished by treatment with mitomycin C, which causes DNA cross-linking. Treated populations generate neither antibody-forming cells nor cytotoxic effectors from their respective precursors. Suppressor T cell functions are also eliminated by this procedure. Cells treated with mitomycin C can be used as a source of T help provided they are obtained from antigen-primed donors. Moreover, we have found that mitomycin treatment results in a higher retention of primed T help than occurs following x-irradiation (Swain et al. 1977).

MATERIALS AND REAGENTS

Materials and reagents as described in Section 2.2 with the following additions:

Mitomycin C, lyophilized (Sigma Chemical, #M-0503)
Balanced salt solution (BSS; Appendix A.3)
BSS containing 5% heat-inactivated (56°C, 30 min) fetal calf serum (BSS-5% FCS)

PROCEDURE

1. Dissolve mitomycin C in BSS at a concentration of 0.5 mg/ml and sterilize by membrane filtration (Appendix C.2). Store protected from light. (If a precipitate forms on storage, discard and prepare fresh reagent.)

2. Prepare cell suspension in BSS at a concentration of 1–6 × 10⁷ cells/ml.

3. Add 25 μg of mitomycin C (50 μl of 0.5 mg/ml stock) per ml of cell suspension.

4. Incubate for 20 minutes at 37°C, protected from light.

5. Wash 3 times in excess BSS-5% FCS.

COMMENTS

1. Some cell clumping usually occurs; expect 30–40% recovery.

2. The quality of the reagent can be checked in two ways: (a) Antibody-forming cells treated with mitomycin C should still produce plaques in the hemolytic plaque assay since protein synthesis is not inhibited; (b) treated spleen cells should not divide in response to mitogens.

3. While the predominant action of mitomycin is to inhibit cellular division, controls should be included where necessary to confirm that other effects are not influencing any experimental results.

REFERENCES

Bach, F. H., and N. K. Voynow. 1966. One-way stimulation in mixed lymphocyte cultures. *Science* **153**:545.

Swain, S. L., P. E. Trefts, H. Y. Tse, and R. W. Dutton. 1977. The significance of T-B collaboration across haplotype barriers. *Cold Spr. Harb. Symp. Quant. Biol.* **41**:597.

10.4 IRRADIATION

Eva Lee Chan

Ionizing radiation is used both in studies utilizing adoptive transfer and as a means to abolish selectively the functions of radiosensitive subpopulations of immunocompetent cells. The commonly used means of radiation are the x-ray machine and cobalt (^{60}Co) and cesium (^{137}Cs) gamma irradiators. These machines generate high-energy photons that ionize atoms in matter receiving radiation. When the recipient of radiation is a living organism, the radiation alters the biochemical and therefore the functional properties of the cells.

The effects of radiation on biological materials depend on the quality and quantity of the ionizing radiation. In describing irradiation conditions, one should specify the operating potential across the x-ray tube (which determines the ability of the photons to penetrate and transfer energy), the current (which determines dose rate), any filters used, the distance from the x-ray source to the object being irradiated, and the total amount of exposure. With an x-ray machine, a potential of 250 kV and 15 mA current are commonly used to alter the biological properties of cells. The biological effects of gamma irradiation are essentially the same as those of x-irradiation. Operating conditions for the gamma irradiators depend on the particular machine being used.

Ionizing radiation is quantitated in roentgen units (R) and measured by ionization instruments called dosimeters. A roentgen is the amount of ionizing radiation required to ionize 0.001293 g of dry air to produce one electrostatic unit of electricity. The amount of energy absorbed by an irradiated object is measured in rads, one rad being an absorption of 100 ergs per gram of material. For the common sources of radiation and the biological material commonly irradiated, 1 R translates to approximately 0.95 rad.

The results of irradiation also depend on the target organism. Species vary greatly in their radiosensitivity. Among laboratory animals, for example, the rabbit, hamster, rat, and mouse are relatively resistant while the guinea pig, dog, sheep, goat, and pig are much more sensitive. Variation from strain to strain also exists; BALB/cJ is the most sensitive of the common laboratory mouse strains. An animal's sex, size, and age also affect its sensitivity.

Extensive radiation of an animal (e.g., the laboratory mouse) causes various modes of death. A dose of 700 to 1000 rads of total body irradiation may cause the animal to die in 2 weeks because of hemopoietic failure. With higher doses of radiation, death may occur in 5 to 6 days due to intestinal damage. With doses of radiation above 10 000 rads, death may be instantaneous, resulting from brain injury. Since lymphocytes are extremely susceptible to radiation damage, the longevity of irradiated mice depends in part on the general health of the mouse colony and the environment. Mice maintained in germ-free conditions survive irradiation for longer periods.

LD_{50} is the dose of total body irradiation necessary to kill 50% of experimental animals within 30 days. The LD_{50} of a typical mouse strain is 940 R. Animals receiving a dose of radiation equivalent to the LD_{50} are said to be lethally irradiated. Such animals are often used in adoptive transfer experiments as inert *in vivo* culture vessels for maintaining desired cell populations for study.

The radiosensitivity of various subpopulations of lymphocytes differs. It has been reported that B cell and suppressor T cell functions are relatively radiosensitive, their function being abolished by exposure to 500 R (Kettman and Dutton 1971; Chan and Henry 1976). The primed T helper function, by contrast, is quite radioresistant.

PROCEDURE

Whole Animals

1. Animals should be individually confined in containers when receiving x-ray. This is to ensure that they are exposed to a constant dose rate.

2. Following irradiation, animals should be kept under clean conditions and supplied with acidic drinking water (Appendix A.17) to minimize death due to infection by environmental pathogens.

Single-Cell Suspensions

1. Wash and resuspend cell populations at 5×10^6 cells/ml in balanced salt solution (BSS; Appendix A.3).

2. Place the cells in the irradiation chamber and deliver the desired dosage of x-ray.

3. Wash cells at least once in BSS before use, to remove any toxic free radicals and their products resulting from irradiation.

COMMENTS

1. If the container of the material being irradiated lies in the path of the x-ray, it may reduce the effective dosage of x-ray by acting as a filter. The degree of interference depends on the material of the container. To assess accurately the irradiation dose received, the dosimeter should be placed inside the container when measuring the dose rate.

2. If a cell suspension must remain inside the irradiation chamber longer than several minutes, it is advisable to supply an ice bath to avoid undesirable changes in temperature.

REFERENCES

Chan, E. L., and C. Henry. 1976. Coexistence of helper and suppressor activities in carrier-primed spleen cells. *J. Immunol.* **117:**1132.

Kettman, J., and R. W. Dutton. 1971. Radioresistance of the enhancing effect of cells from carrier-immunized mice in an *in vitro* primary immune response. *Proc. Nat. Acad. Sci.* (USA) **68:**699.

Storer, J. B. 1966. Acute responses to ionizing radiation. In E. L. Green (Ed.), *Biology of the Laboratory Mouse.* McGraw-Hill, New York.

Taliaferro, H., and G. Taliaferro. 1976. Methods and applications of radiation in immunological research. In C. A. Williams and M. W. Chase (Eds.), *Methods in Immunology and Immunochemistry,* Vol. 5. Academic Press, New York.

PREPARATION OF IMMUNOGLOBULINS FOR CELLULAR STUDIES

Part III describes methods for preparing the immunoglobulin reagents required in many of the cellular procedures presented in this book. The production, testing, and storage of several kinds of antisera are described in Chapter 11. Included are antisera to T cell surface antigens and to immunoglobulins, both of which are used in the microscopic identification of cells and in various cell separation procedures; antisera to immunoglobulins are also used as reagents in indirect hemolytic plaque assays. Chapter 11 also outlines methods for producing antisera against azophenyl haptens conjugated to KLH. Antibodies from these sera are purified by affinity chromatography (Chapter 12) and used in the hapten-sandwich technique for cell identification (hapten-sandwich rosetting). Procedures for hapten-sandwich labeling, the preparation of fluorescent antibodies, and the visualization of specific determinants on cells are described in Chapter 13.

Production of monospecific (monoclonal) antibodies using cell fusion techniques (see Chapter 17) provides an important new approach for producing immunological reagents. While the initial investment is high, reagents prepared in this way will be much better defined and their production ultimately more economical than those produced by conventional immunization procedures. In the near future, many hybrid cell lines and/or antibodies produced by them will become available from commercial and noncommercial sources. As this occurs, individual laboratories will no longer need to produce many of the reagent antibodies required for cellular immunological studies.

Preparation and Testing of Antisera

11.1 HETEROLOGOUS ANTISERA TO MOUSE BRAIN

Stanley M. Shiigi and Maxwell Slomich

Heterologous antisera that will specifically lyse thymus-derived lymphocytes (T cells) in the presence of complement can be prepared in rabbits (or goats) (Golub 1971). This procedure takes advantage of the antigen that is shared between mouse brain cells and T cells but is absent on most other cells. After the antiserum is obtained, it is absorbed with mouse cells to remove the species-specific antibodies. Following absorption, rabbit anti–mouse brain serum (RAMB) must be tested to determine its effectiveness and specificity in the complement-mediated lysis of T cells. The specificity of antiserum intended for general use (see 2 under Comments) is determined by showing that the antiserum fails to kill significant numbers of other cell types, particularly B lymphocytes and accessory cells. Additional absorption may be required to render the antiserum sufficiently specific for other uses, such as in fluorescent labeling studies. The procedures described below are designed to produce antiserum of sufficient specificity for removing T cells from heterogeneous cell populations. The absorption protocols and specificity assays should be modified if the antiserum is to be employed for other purposes.

A. Preparation of Mouse Brain

MATERIALS AND REAGENTS

Mice, 1.5 brains/rabbit or goat to be injected
Balanced salt solution (BSS; Appendix A.3)
Complete Freund's adjuvant (CFA), 1.5 ml per rabbit or goat. Note:
  Freund's adjuvant is a potentially hazardous agent (see Appendix
  F).
Forceps and scissors for removing brains
Petri dishes
Centrifuge tubes
Equipment for preparing antigen-CFA emulsions (Appendix F)
Glass tissue homogenizer or electric blender

PROCEDURE

1. Bleed mice to deplete the brain of blood (peripheral blood contains
   B cells which can interfere with the specificity of the antiserum).
   Kill mice by cervical dislocation or CO_2 inhalation.
2. Make an incision at the base of the skull and reflect the skin. Open
   the skull to expose the brain. With forceps, remove the brain and
   place in a Petri dish containing BSS. Rinse brain to remove adherent blood.
3. Homogenize brains with an electric blender or a glass tissue homogenizer, using 1.5 brains in 1.5 ml BSS for each rabbit (or goat)
   to be injected. If using an electric blender, keep the antigen cold.
4. Prepare an emulsion of the homogenate with an equal volume of
   CFA by the procedure described in Appendix F.

B. Immunization of Rabbits and Collection of Antisera

The following protocol usually results in uniformly high-titer antisera.
Because an occasional rabbit may either produce antiserum of low titer or
become physically paralyzed by the formation of auto-antibodies, it is
best to immunize several rabbits and test the antiserum from each rabbit
prior to combining the antisera into a single pool.

MATERIALS AND REAGENTS

Rabbits (adult, either sex)
Antigen emulsified in CFA

Syringes, 3 ml, Luer-lock (1 per rabbit). Note: If Luer-lock syringes are not available, protective glasses should be worn (see Appendix F).

Needles, 22 gauge, 1 in.

PROCEDURE

1. Divide the emulsified antigen equally among the 3-ml syringes, one syringe for each rabbit.

2. Inject each rabbit intramuscularly, dividing the contents of one syringe between 4 sites (2 sites in each hind leg works well). In our experience, fewer animals develop paralysis if the injections are given intramuscularly rather than subcutaneously.

3. Repeat the immunization after 1 month and bleed the rabbits $2-2\frac{1}{2}$ weeks later. Repeat the boosting and bleeding cycle after a 3–4-week resting period. Alternatively, the rabbits may be bled 2 or 3 times after each booster injection. Bleed the rabbits on a weekly schedule, starting 10–12 days after the booster injection; then wait 3–4 weeks before repeating the cycle. Antisera obtained by either method should be separately absorbed to remove species-specific antibodies and then tested for cytolytic activity against T cells prior to pooling. Perform T cell cytolytic titrations and specificity tests on the pooled antiserum; carry out additional absorptions if necessary.

C. Absorption of Antisera

Antisera to be used for the complement-mediated lysis of T cells are absorbed with adult bone marrow, fetal liver, or peripheral blood cells (see comments 1 and 2). Prior to absorption, heat the antisera at 56°C for 30 minutes to inactivate the complement.

MATERIALS AND REAGENTS

Absorption with Bone Marrow or Fetal Liver Cells

Bone marrow cells (Section 1.8) or fetal liver cells from 15–21-day-old fetuses (one pregnant mouse frequently yields sufficient fetal liver cells to absorb approximately 1.5 ml of antiserum): Obtain cells from mice of the same strain as the brain donors.

Balanced salt solution (BSS; Appendix A.3)

Scissors and forceps

Glass tissue homogenizer

Plastic centrifuge tubes, graduated, conical
Centrifuge tube, 50 ml
Petri dishes
Rotator (Scientific Products, #R4193-1)

Absorption with Peripheral Blood Cells

Adult mice, same strain as brain donor
BSS or glucose-phosphate-buffered saline (G-PBS; Appendix A.11)
Alsever's solution (Appendix A.14)
Plastic centrifuge tubes, graduated, conical, with screw caps
Centrifuge tube, 50 ml
Rotator

PROCEDURE

Absorption with Bone Marrow or Fetal Liver Cells

1. Prepare bone marrow cells as described in Section 1.8. Prepare fetal liver cells as follows: Remove livers from 15–21-day-old fetuses. It is important to exclude gut fragments from the livers because enzymes from the gut might partially degrade the antiserum. Dissociate the livers into a single-cell suspension with forceps or a glass tissue homogenizer. Wash the cells in cold BSS at least 3 times ($200 \times g$, 10 min), executing the last wash in a graduated centrifuge tube to measure packed cell volume.

2. Add 1.0 ml of antiserum for each 0.1 ml packed cells. Resuspend the cells and rotate the antiserum-cell mixture for 45–60 minutes at 4°C. Remove the cells by centrifugation ($250 \times g$, 10 min). Finally, remove smaller debris by centrifugation at $12\,000 \times g$ for 20 minutes. Sterilize antiserum by membrane filtration (Appendix C.2). Distribute antiserum in aliquots and store at -70°C. Large amounts of antiserum can be stored precipitated in saturated ammonium sulfate (Section 11.9). Before use, dialyze, reconstitute to the original volume, and sterilize if necessary.

Absorption with Peripheral Blood Cells

1. Exsanguinate mice and collect blood in a tube containing a large volume of Alsever's solution (do not let the ratio of blood to Alsever's solution exceed 1 : 1). An adult mouse will yield approximately 1.5 ml of blood. (For bleeding techniques, see Garvey et al. 1977.)

2. Centrifuge the blood cells ($400 \times g$, 10 min) and wash cells 4 times with BSS or G-PBS, executing the last wash in a graduated centrifuge tube to measure packed cell volume.

3. Mix antiserum with $\frac{1}{3}$ volume of packed, washed peripheral blood cells. Rotate the antiserum-cell mixture for 45–60 minutes at 4°C. Remove cells by centrifugation (400 × g, 10 min).

4. Clarify (12 000 × g, 20 min) and store the antiserum as described above under 2 for Absorption with Bone Marrow or Fetal Liver Cells.

COMMENTS

1. If the antiserum is absorbed only with fetal liver cells, mouse red blood cell lysis (in addition to T cell lysis) may occur (Golub 1973). Apparently there is an antigen (or antigens) on circulating red blood cells that is (are) not present on red blood cells in the mouse fetal liver. We have observed no differences in the effectiveness of complement-mediated lysis of T cells between antisera absorbed with fetal liver and those absorbed with peripheral blood cells.

2. For functional tests, such as assays for primary anti-SRBC responses or for mitogen-induced proliferative responses, the absorption protocols described above are adequate. However, if the antiserum will be used for fluorescence studies, further absorption is usually required. Repeated absorption with bone marrow cells and B cell tumors generally yields highly specific T cell reagents. Specificity is confirmed by demonstrating that the RAMB and anti–mouse Ig sera bind to distinct cell populations by immunofluorescence (Chapter 13).

D. Titration of Cytolytic Activity

The cytolytic titer of the RAMB is determined by measuring the ability of doubling dilutions of antiserum to kill T cells in the presence of a nonlimiting amount of complement. The incidence of T cell death is measured by one of three methods: (1) the uptake of nigrosin in a microcytotoxicity test (Section 11.7); (2) the uptake of vital stains in a two-step cytotoxic test; (3) the release of ^{51}Cr. (Methods 2 and 3 are described below.) The results are graphically displayed by plotting the percent specific cytotoxicity against the antiserum dilution. Antisera of adequate potency should yield a plateau of maximum killing over a range of at least three dilutions. In the plateau region, 95–100% of the thymocytes, 35–50% of the spleen cells, and less than 10% of the bone marrow cells should be killed. For T cell removal, the antisera are used at a concentration of twice that with which a maximum of cells are killed.

MATERIALS AND REAGENTS

Uptake of Vital Stains

Lymphoid cell suspension (e.g., Sections 1.2, 1.5, and 1.8)

Guinea pig serum, absorbed with agarose (Appendix A.2), as a source of complement

Absorbed antiserum

Trypan blue (Section 1.11), eosin Y (Section 1.12), fluorescein diacetate (Section 1.14), or acridine orange-ethidium bromide (Section 1.15)

Balanced salt solution (BSS; Appendix A.3)

Plastic tubes, 12 × 75 mm (Falcon, #2054 or similar)

^{51}Cr Release

Lymphoid cell suspension

Guinea pig serum, absorbed with agarose (Appendix A.2), as a source of complement

Absorbed antiserum

Fetal calf serum (FCS), heat inactivated (56°C, 30 min)

$(Na)_2{}^{51}CrO_4$ 200–500 Ci/g, 1000 μCi/ml (New England Nuclear, #NEZ-030)

BSS

RPMI 1640 or Eagle's minimum essential medium (MEM), supplemented with sodium pyruvate, nonessential amino acids, L-glutamine, and 5% heat-inactivated FCS (as described in Section 2.2)

Plastic tubes, 12 × 75 mm (Falcon, #2054 or similar)

Glass tubes, disposable, 12 × 75 mm

Gamma counter

PROCEDURE

Uptake of Vital Stains

1. Suspend the washed cells in BSS to 1.5 × 10^7 viable cells/ml and distribute 0.5 ml (0.75 × 10^7 cells) to the appropriate number of 12 × 75-mm plastic tubes.

2. Pellet the cells (200 × g, 10 min), remove the supernatants, and add 0.5 ml of the appropriate dilution of antiserum in BSS (dilutions from 1:2 to 1:128 are adequate). Control tubes receive 0.5 ml BSS or 1:2 dilution of nontoxic normal rabbit serum in BSS. Resuspend the cells and incubate at room temperature for 30–45 minutes; avoid chilling the cells.

3. Centrifuge the cells (200 × g, 10 min) and discard the supernatants. Add 0.5 ml of diluted guinea pig complement (previously

titrated to contain a nonlimiting amount of complement activity). Resuspend the cells and incubate them at 37°C for 30–60 minutes.

4. Centrifuge the cells (200 × g, 10 min), resuspend in BSS, and determine total number of viable cells remaining in each tube by the procedure described in Section 1.11, 1.12, 1.14, or 1.15.

5. Calculate the % specific cytotoxicity by the following equation:

$$\% \text{ specific cytotoxicity} = \frac{x - y}{x} \times 100$$

where

x = number of viable cells in control tubes

y = number of viable cells in experimental tubes

^{51}Cr Release

Note: Established safety procedures must be followed when handling ^{51}Cr.

1. Label spleen cells and/or thymocytes by the procedure described in the part of Section 4.3 entitled "Radioactive Labeling of Target Cells." Incubate the cells with $(Na)_2{}^{51}CrO_4$ for 60 minutes. After the last wash, resuspend the labeled cells in BSS to a concentration of 1.5×10^7 cells/ml.

2. Distribute 0.5 ml of the labeled cells to the appropriate number of 12 × 75-mm plastic tubes (each experimental point should be done in triplicate). Pellet the cells (200 × g, 10 min.), remove the supernatant (discard in radioactive waste container), and add 0.5 ml of an appropriate dilution of antiserum in BSS (dilutions ranging from 1:2 to 1:128 are adequate). Add 0.5 ml of BSS or a 1:2 dilution of normal rabbit serum in BSS to triplicate tubes for both spontaneous release and maximum release controls.

3. Gently resuspend the cells and incubate them at room temperature for 30–45 minutes; avoid chilling the cells.

4. Pellet the cells and discard the supernatants. Add 0.5 ml of diluted guinea pig serum (previously titrated to contain a nonlimiting amount of complement activity). Resuspend the cells and incubate at 37°C for 30–60 minutes. Treat the maximum release control by freezing and thawing 3 times.*

---

* If Nonidet P40 (NP40) is used to lyse cells for maximum release controls (as described in Section 4.3), higher values are obtained than with the freeze-thaw method, because detergent lysis results in the release of both the ^{51}Cr incorporated into membrane proteins and that from cytoplasmic proteins. Too high a value for maximum release falsely reduces the calculated values of the percent specific cytotoxicity.

5. Centrifuge the cells (200 $\times$ g, 10 min) and carefully transfer 0.3 ml of the supernatants to 12 $\times$ 75-mm glass tubes. Determine the amount of ^{51}Cr released by measurement in a gamma counter.

$$\% \text{ specific cytotoxicity} = \frac{\text{experimental release} - \text{spontaneous release}}{\text{maximum release} - \text{spontaneous release}} \times 100$$

E. Specificity Tests

After the cytolytic titer of the antiserum has been established, its specificity is determined by functional criteria using the following methods (see comment 2).

1. Effects on Mitogen-Induced Proliferative Responses

Treatment of spleen cells with RAMB plus complement should eliminate T cell proliferation induced by concanavalin A (Con A) but not affect B cell proliferation induced by lipopolysaccharide (LPS). If the treatment reduces the proliferative response to LPS, the antiserum requires further absorption. Controls to assess the nonspecific toxicity of complement and RAMB must also be done. These controls should respond similarly to the untreated cells.

MATERIALS AND REAGENTS

As described in Section 6.2 with the following cell preparations:

Untreated cells
Cells treated with complement only (complement toxicity control)
Cells treated with RAMB only (RAMB toxicity control)
Cells treated with RAMB and complement (experimental)

PROCEDURE

Follow the procedures described in Sections 9.2 and 6.2.

2. Depletion of T Helper Activity from Normal Spleen Cells

Normal spleen cells treated with RAMB and complement should no longer generate an *in vitro* primary humoral response to sheep red blood cells

(SRBC) because of the loss of T helper cell activity. Furthermore, the addition of a source of T helper cells or factors with T cell-replacing activity should restore the primary humoral responses of the RAMB treated cells. Failure to restore indicates that the particular antiserum may also be cytotoxic to B cells or accessory cells.

MATERIALS AND REAGENTS

As described in Section 2.2 with the following additions:

Untreated spleen cells
Spleen cells treated with complement only
Spleen cells treated with RAMB only
Spleen cells treated with RAMB plus complement
One of the following as a source of T helper activity:
    Allogeneic-conditioned medium, pretitrated for maximal T cell-replacing activity (Appendix E)
    Thymus cells educated to SRBC (Section 1.6)
    Spleen cells primed to SRBC and irradiated with 1000–2700 R as described in Sections 2.5 and 2.6.

PROCEDURE

Follow the procedure as described in Sections 9.2 and 2.2 with the following modifications:

1. Set up the following cultures:
   a. Untreated spleen cells (positive control).
   b. Spleen cells treated with complement (toxicity control).
   c. Spleen cells treated with RAMB (toxicity control).
   d. Spleen cells treated with RAMB and complement (control for the effectiveness of the antiserum).
   e. Spleen cells treated with RAMB and complement, plus additional T helper cells or factors with T cell-replacing activity (cultures to test whether the responses of the treated cells can be restored). If educated thymocytes or irradiated primed spleen cells are used, these should be cultured alone (control to show that the T cell-restoring population cannot respond on its own). Add allogeneic-conditioned medium at a concentration previously determined to give a maximum of T cell-replacing activity. Add concentrations of educated thymus cells or irradiated, primed spleen cells equivalent to 100%, 50%, and 25% of the concentration of the cells treated with RAMB and complement.

   2. Feed the cultures daily and assay on day 5 for the number of direct anti-SRBC plaque-forming cells (Section 3.2).

3. Accessory Cell Specificity

To determine if RAMB has cytolytic activity against accessory cells, it is necessary to measure the effects of the antiserum on the activity of splenic accessory cells. Normal spleen cells are first depleted of accessory cells by Sephadex G-10 filtration (Section 7.2). The primary humoral responses of such a population depleted of accessory cells are low but can be restored by the addition of irradiated normal spleen cells (accessory cell function is usually radioresistant). Treatment of normal spleen cells with RAMB and complement (followed by irradiation) should not interfere with the subsequent ability of the cells to restore the response of G-10 filtered spleen cells, unless the antiserum contains antibodies against accessory cells.

Because 2-mercaptoethanol (2-ME) reduces dependency on accessory cells, it should not be included as a medium supplement in tests of accessory cell function. For these assays, cultures are established at the high cell densities indicated.

MATERIALS AND REAGENTS

As described in Sections 1.2, 2.2 (exclude 2-Me from the medium), and 7.2, with the following addition:

Irradiated (1500 R) normal spleen cells treated with RAMB and complement, as a source of accessory cells (Section 10.4)

PROCEDURE

Several controls (indicated below) are necessary to demonstrate that the test is a valid measurement of accessory cell function.

1. Prepare a normal spleen cell suspension as described in Section 1.2.

2. Prepare the following cell suspensions:

   a. Spleen cells filtered through Sephadex G-10 (Section 7.2).

   b. Irradiated spleen cells (1500 rad) (Section 10.4).

   c. Spleen cells treated with RAMB and complement.

   d. Irradiated normal spleen cells treated with RAMB and complement.

3. Set up the following cultures:
   a. Untreated spleen cells cultured at 1.5×10^7 cells/ml. This is the positive control for responding spleen cells.
   b. Sephadex G-10-filtered spleen cells cultured at 1.5×10^7 cells/ml. This is the negative control to demonstrate that filtration was adequate to remove accessory cell function.
   c. Irradiated spleen cells cultured at 1.5×10^7 cells/ml. This is a negative control to demonstrate that the accessory cell preparation does not develop antibody-forming cells.
   d. RAMB-and-complement-treated spleen cells cultured at 1.5×10^7 cells/ml. This is a negative control to demonstrate that T-depleted cells do not develop antibody-forming cells.
   e. Sephadex G-10-filtered spleen cells (1×10^7 cells/ml) plus irradiated spleen cells (5×10^6 cells/ml). This is a positive control to demonstrate that by replacing accessory cells, the filtered population can develop antibody-forming cells.
   f. Sephadex G-10-filtered cells (1×10^7 cells/ml) plus RAMB-and-complement treated, irradiated spleen cells (5×10^6 cells/ml). These are the experimental cultures to determine whether RAMB is inhibitory or cytolytic for accessory cells.

4. Feed daily and assay on day 5 for the number of direct anti-SRBC plaque-forming cells (Section 3.2).

REFERENCES

Garvey, J. S., N. E. Cremer, and D. H. Sussdorf. 1977. *Methods in Immunology*. W. A. Benjamin, Reading, MA. Chapter 3.

Golub, E. S. 1971. Brain associated θ antigen: Reactivity of rabbit anti–mouse brain with mouse lymphoid cells. *Cell. Immunol.* **2:**353.

Golub, E. S. 1973. Brain associated erythrocyte antigen: An antigen shared by brain and erythrocytes. *Exp. Hematol.* (Copenhagen) **1:**105.

11.2 MOUSE ALLOANTISERA TO LYMPHOCYTE ANTIGENS

Eva L. Chan, Robert I. Mishell, and Claudia Henry, with contributions from Susan L. Swain

Mouse alloantisera have been produced to a wide variety of cellular antigens, including determinants coded by the genes of the major histocompatibility complex (K, D, and I regions), minor histocompatibility antigens, allotypic markers on membrane immunoglobulins, and differentiation antigens of specific cell types such as Thy 1 and Ly. Some are readily raised (e.g., anti–H-2 sera) and others are raised with considerable difficulty (e.g., anti-Ly sera). The literature should be consulted regarding specific protocols that may be necessary for producing a particular alloantiserum (see References).

To illustrate the principles of alloimmunization, we describe a protocol for raising alloantiserum against the Thy 1 marker. Thy 1 is a differentiation antigen present on murine thymocytes, thymus-derived cells in peripheral lymphoid organs, and brain cells. Thy 1.1 is found in AKR mice, which carry the Thy 1^a allele, and Thy 1.2 is found in most other strains. Antiserum to Thy 1.2 is made by injecting C3H thymocytes into AKR mice. Since these two strains have a common H-2 haplotype ($H-2^k$), most of the antibodies obtained are against Thy 1.2. The antisera can be used for T cell removal without subjecting them to absorption, despite possible contamination with small amounts of antibodies specific for other non–H-2 alloantigens and endogenous viral antigens of C3H mice. For studies requiring the complete absence of contaminating antibodies, it is possible to prepare antisera using the congenic mice, AKR and AKR/Thy 1.2. However, the use of such congenic pairs may result in lower cytolytic titers.

MATERIALS AND REAGENTS

Mice
> Donor strain: C3H/HeJ, 4–6 weeks old, female
> Recipient strain: AKR/J, 12–20 weeks old, female (approximately two recipient mice per donor)

Saline, 0.85% (w/v) NaCl

Balanced salt solution (BSS; Appendix A.3)

Pelikan ink (Accurate Chemical & Scientific, #C11/1431A), diluted 1 : 5 in saline

Dissecting microscope

Scissors and forceps

Glass tissue homogenizer or stainless steel mesh

Centrifuge tubes, 12–15 ml

Needles, 25 gauge

Tuberculin syringes

Disposable Petri dishes

Equipment for bleeding mice from a tail vein or by puncture of the retro-orbital plexus (see Garvey et al. 1977)

PROCEDURE

1. Inject donor mice intraperitoneally with 0.05 ml of Pelikan ink diluted 1 : 5 in saline. This increases the visibility of the

parathymic lymph nodes, which are then easily dissected from the thymus under a dissecting microscope.

2. Thirty minutes after the injection, exsanguinate the mice and remove the thymuses (avoid cervical dislocation if bleeding is insufficient for death). Wash the thymuses free of any contaminating blood and tease away any blood vessels and black (ink) areas.

3. When the thymuses are clean and free of all visible blood and lymph nodes, prepare a single-cell suspension by teasing with forceps, pressing tissue through a mesh or by homogenizing with a glass tissue homogenizer. Wash once in BSS and resuspend to a concentration of $1-2 \times 10^8$ cells/ml.

4. With a 25-gauge needle and tuberculin syringe, inject 5×10^7 cells intraperitoneally into adult AKR/J mice. Depending on the concentration of the cells, the mice will receive 0.25–0.5 ml of the cell suspension.

5. Repeat the immunization weekly for 6 weeks. Bleed the mice 7 and 10 days after the last injection, from either the tail vein or the retro-orbital plexus. (For bleeding techniques, see Garvey et al. 1977.)

6. The mice can be boosted and bled repeatedly by resting them for 2 weeks, giving a further injection of 10^7 cells, and bleeding 7 and 10 days later.

7. Alloantisera against Thy 1.2 are characterized by the procedures used for examining rabbit anti–mouse brain sera (Section 11.1), although specificity tests to rule out activities against accessory cells are usually not done. Additional tests may be performed to demonstrate that the antisera are specific for T cells from mice of the appropriate genotype (Thy 1^b). Another method for characterizing anti–Thy 1.2 sera is to absorb its activity with brain tissue from mice carrying the Thy 1^b allele; contaminating antibodies against alloantigens not found on brain cells can be detected by this procedure.

COMMENTS

1. Each mouse yields about 20 drops (0.5 ml) of blood at each bleeding. Begin bleeding the mice close to the tip of the tail and move towards the base with successive bleedings.

2. If possible, avoid the use of male mice unless they can be prevented from fighting (Section 15.6). Scarring from fighting makes male mice unsuitable for tail bleeding.

3. It is important to bleed the mice at 7 and 10 days after injection; by 12 days the peak of antibody production has passed.

4. No clear advantage of any adjuvant has been established.

5. The anti–Thy 1.2 antisera obtained from the strain combination described above are of high titer but require absorption to yield reagents sufficiently specific for T cells in fluorescence studies.

6. The references at the end of this section describe some of the specific protocols used in raising antisera to other alloantigens.

REFERENCES

Chan, E. L., G. F. Mitchell, and R. I. Mishell. 1970. Cell interaction in an immune response *in vitro:* Requirement for theta-carrying cells. *Science* **170:**1215.

David, C. S., D. C. Shreffler, and J. A. Frelinger. 1973. New lymphocyte antigen system (Lna) controlled by the Ir region of the mouse H-2 complex. *Proc. Nat. Acad. Sci.* (USA) **70:**2509.

Garvey, J. S., N. E. Cremer, and D. H. Sussdorf. 1977. *Methods in Immunology.* W. A. Benjamin, Reading, MA. Chapter 3.

Hammerling, G. J., B. D. Deak, G. Mauve, U. Hammerling, and H. O. McDevitt. 1974. B lymphocyte alloantigens controlled by the I region of the major histocompatibility complex in mice. *Immunogenetics* **1:**68.

Shen, F.-W., E. A. Boyse, and H. Cantor. 1975. Preparation and use of Ly antisera. *Immunogenetics* **2:**596.

Shen, F.-W. 1977. Preparation of Lyt antisera. *Immunogenetics* **5:**291.

Reif, A. E., and J. M. Allen. 1966. Mouse thymic iso-antigens. *Nature* **209:**521.

11.3 ANTISERA TO HAPTENS

Claudia Henry and John Kimura

Rabbits are hyperimmunized with hapten-KLH conjugates to obtain high-titer anti-hapten sera. The same procedure can be used to raise antisera against a variety of azophenyl haptens such as lactoside, glucoside, benzoate, sulfonate, benzoylglutamate, and trimethylaniline. Antibodies obtained with these procedures have binding constants in the range of 10^5 to 10^6 M^{-1} and are suitable for the fluorescence and rosetting studies described in this book. The procedure to purify anti-hapten antibodies by affinity chromatography is described in Section 12.4.

MATERIALS AND REAGENTS

Rabbits, adult, either sex
Hapten-KLH conjugates: 2 mg/ml (see Section 16.2)

Complete Freund's adjuvant (CFA). Note: CFA is a potentially hazardous agent (see Appendix F).

Aluminum potassium sulfate (alum)

Syringe (Luer-lock), 3 ml, and needles, 22 gauge. Note: If Luer-lock syringes are not available, protective glasses should be worn (see Appendix F).

PROCEDURE

1. Emulsify the hapten-KLH conjugate with an equal volume of CFA, as described in Appendix F.

2. Immunize each rabbit with 4 intradermal injections on the back (0.1 ml/site) plus 0.1 ml into each hind footpad.

3. Repeat the 4 intradermal injections four weeks later. Do not repeat the footpad injections.

4. Two weeks later, boost the rabbits intravenously with 1.0 ml of alum-precipitated antigen at a final concentration of 1.0 mg/ml (see Section 2.5 for procedure to prepare alum-precipitated antigen).

5. Ear bleed 30–50 ml from the rabbits two and three weeks after the booster injection.

6. After a two-week rest, repeat the intravenous injection of alum-precipitated antigen and bleed the rabbits two and three weeks later. This cycle can be continued for months to produce a large amount of high-affinity anti-hapten IgG from each rabbit.

11.4   RABBIT ANTISERA AGAINST MOUSE IMMUNOGLOBULINS FOR DEVELOPING INDIRECT HEMOLYTIC PLAQUES

Claudia Henry and Anne H. Good

This procedure describes the use of ammonium sulfate-precipitated mouse immunoglobulins for the production of high-titer, polyspecific antisera directed primarily against the major isotypic determinants. Such antisera are relatively easy to prepare and are suitable for use as developing antisera in most studies of indirect hemolytic plaque-forming cells. Prior to use, it is necessary to determine the optimal concentration of each antiserum for developing indirect plaques. Because the optimal concentration of antiserum often inhibits direct (IgM) plaques, the antisera are also tested with spleen cells containing only IgM-producing cells so that the percentage of inhibition can be measured and a correction factor determined.

Antisera prepared by the procedure described below often contain antibodies against other serum components besides immunoglobulins. These antisera are therefore not suitable for studies based on radioimmunoprecipitation, fluorescent labeling, or cytotoxity, because such techniques require highly specific reagents. Methods for preparing sufficiently specific antisera against mouse immunoglobulins are described in Section 11.5.

A. Production of Antisera

MATERIALS AND REAGENTS

Rabbits
Mouse serum, 2 ml per rabbit to be immunized
Saline: 0.85% NaCl (w/v)
Complete Freund's adjuvant (CFA). Note: CFA is a potentially hazardous agent (see Appendix F).
Saturated ammonium sulfate (SAS; Section 12.2)
Dialysis tubing (Appendix D)
Syringe, Luer-lock, and 22-gauge, 1-in. needle. Note: If Luer-lock syringes are not available, protective glasses should be worn (see Appendix F).
UV spectrophotometer

PROCEDURE

1. Precipitate the mouse serum with 40% (v/v) SAS as described in Section 12.2. Place mixture on ice and stir it slowly for at least one hour.

2. Centrifuge the precipitate at 10 000 × g for 5 minutes.

3. Dissolve the precipitate in water, bring to original serum volume, and reprecipitate with 40% SAS. Centrifuge the precipitate at 10 000 × g for 5 minutes.

4. Dissolve the precipitate in a minimal amount of water (i.e., the smallest amount that will dissolve the precipitate) and remove the ammonium sulfate by dialysis against saline.

5. Centrifuge at 10 000 × g for 10 minutes to remove insoluble material and measure the absorbance at 280 nm. Adjust the protein concentration to about 4 mg/ml with saline, using an extinction coefficient of 1.45 for a 1 mg/ml solution.

6. Emulsify the protein in an equal volume of CFA as described in Appendix F.

7. Inject 2 ml of the emulsion (4 mg of protein), dividing it among 4 intramuscular sites on the back of each rabbit. Repeat the injections one month later.

8. Three to four weeks after the second immunization, obtain samples of sera from each rabbit and test for potency. If the results are satisfactory, bleed out the rabbit by cardiac puncture. If the titer is not satisfactory, boost the rabbit again and retest the serum after waiting another three to four weeks.

9. Heat inactivate the antisera at 56°C for 30 minutes and absorb with $\frac{1}{10}$ volume of packed SRBC (or other indicator red blood cells), if necessary. Freeze in small aliquots or precipitate with 40% SAS and store at 4°C (Section 11.9).

B. Titration of Antisera

MATERIALS AND REAGENTS

As described in Section 3.2 or 3.3, with the following additions:

Polyspecific rabbit anti–mouse Ig sera
One of the following cell populations, which contain predominantly IgG plaque-forming cells:
    Spleen cells from mice immunized intravenously 9–12 days previously with 0.2 ml of 10% SRBC (v/v) in BSS.
    Spleen cells from secondary cultures immunized with nitrophenyl or azophenyl hapten conjugates (Section 2.5 or 2.6).
The following cell population, which contains predominately IgM plaque-forming cells:
    Spleen cells from mice immunized intravenously 2–3 days previously with 0.2 ml of 10% SRBC (v/v) in BSS.

PROCEDURE

1. Prepare agar-red blood cell-lymphocyte suspensions for the measurement of the number of direct and indirect plaque-forming cells as described in Section 3.2 (slides), Section 3.3 (plates), or Section 3.8 (anti-hapten plaques). Prepare a separate set of slides or plates for the IgG- and IgM-producing populations.

2. Prepare 2-fold dilutions of antiserum from 1 : 50 to 1 : 1600 in BSS.

3. Treat the slides or plates containing the IgG-producing cells with

the various dilutions of antiserum and a predetermined concentration of guinea pig complement. Include a control with complement only to measure direct plaques.

4. Treat the slides or plates containing the IgM-producing cells with the various dilutions of antiserum and a predetermined concentration of guinea pig complement. Include a control with complement only to measure the total number of direct plaques.

5. Incubate the slides or plates at 37°C as described in Section 3.2 or 3.3, and count the number of hemolytic plaques.

COMMENTS

1. There is generally a range of dilutions of antiserum that is optimally effective in developing indirect plaques. When this optimal range is tested on cell populations containing only IgM plaque-forming cells, the number of plaques is usually 60–80% of the number obtained with complement alone. When calculating the number of IgG plaques, it is necessary to make corrections to account for the inhibition of IgM plaques:

Correction factor =
$$\frac{\text{IgM plaques measured with complement plus antiserum}}{\text{IgM plaques measured with complement only}}$$

IgG plaques = (total number of plaques obtained by indirect assay)
$-$ (number of direct plaques $\times$ correction factor)

2. Rare antisera completely inhibit IgM plaques at concentrations that promote the optimal development of IgG plaques. Such antisera are useful because the number of plaques obtained with them in the presence of complement gives the number of IgG plaques.

REFERENCE

Jerne, N. K., C. Henry, A. A. Nordin, H. Fuji, A. M. C. Koros, and I. Lefkovits. 1974. Plaque forming cells: Methodology and theory. *Transplant. Rev.* **18**:130.

11.5 SPECIFIC RABBIT ANTISERA AGAINST MOUSE IMMUNOGLOBULINS FOR USE IN STUDIES BASED ON HAPTEN ROSETTING, FLUORESCENT LABELING, AND RADIO-IMMUNOPRECIPITATION

Anne H. Good

Highly specific antisera directed against isotypic determinants of mouse immunoglobulins are required in procedures for hapten rosetting (Section 9.3), fluorescent labeling (Section 13.4), and radio-immunoprecipitation (Chapter 14). Such antisera are usually prepared by immunizing rabbits or goats with purified myeloma proteins or their Fc fragments and then rendering the antisera specific by the appropriate absorptions.

Myeloma proteins are used as antigens because they can be isolated in high yield and purity. Myeloma proteins are available commercially at various stages of purification. Circumstances will dictate whether it is most efficient (or economical) to obtain purified myeloma proteins, ascites fluid containing myeloma protein, or the myeloma tumors themselves. General procedures for propagating the tumors and purifying the antigens have been described by Dresser (1978). Detailed instructions for the individual techniques required are presented in Garvey et al. (1977) and Hudson and Hay (1976).

The following procedure describes the preparation of antisera in rabbits by immunization with purified myeloma proteins and absorption to render the antisera class or subclass specific. To obtain a preparation that recognizes multiple isotypic determinants on mouse immunoglobulins (e.g., in the fluorescent labeling of B cells), antisera raised against the appropriate individual myeloma proteins are combined. If immunofluorescence by the procedure described in Section 11.6 shows that the combined antiserum binds nonspecifically to mouse cells, the inappropriate antibodies can be removed by adsorption onto mouse liver cells.

MATERIALS AND REAGENTS

Production of Antisera

Rabbits
Purified myeloma proteins (Litton Bionetics) or their Fc fragments (Section 12.5)
Ascites fluid (Litton Bionetics)
Myeloma tumors (Cell Distribution Center, Salk Institute)
Complete Freund's adjuvant (CFA). Note: CFA is a potentially hazardous agent (see Appendix F).
Sodium alginate adjuvant

Saline: 0.85% NaCl (w/v)

Syringes, Luer-lock, and 22-gauge, 1-in. needles. (Note: If Luer-lock syringes are not available, protective glasses should be worn [see Appendix F]).

Absorption of Antisera

As described in Section 12.4, with the following modifications:

a. A 2–20 mg/ml solution of protein in 0.1 M $NaHCO_3$, pH 9, is used to couple protein to the CNBr-activated agarose.

b. Phosphate-buffered saline (PBS; Appendix A.8) or borate-buffered saline (BBS; Appendix A.9) may be used for the absorption.

c. Prepare a 1 M ethanolamine, pH 8.5 solution: Dissolve 61.1 g ethanolamine (liquid) in 750 ml distilled water. Slowly add 84 ml concentrated HCl. Adjust to pH 8.5 with additional HCl if necessary and bring volume to 1000 ml.

d. The eluting solution is 0.1 M acetic acid. This solution is neutralized after use with 1 M Tris-HCl, pH 8.0: Bring 121.1 g Trizma base (Sigma Chemical) and 44.2 ml concentrated HCl to a total volume of 1000 ml in water.

e. Myeloma protein precipitated with 40% saturated ammonium sulfate (SAS; see comment 1).

PROCEDURE

Production of Antisera

1. Emulsify a 1 mg/ml solution of protein in saline or PBS with an equal volume of CFA as described in Appendix F. Inject each rabbit with 0.1 ml of the emulsion in each rear footpad, plus an additional 0.3 ml divided among several subcutaneous sites on the back (0.5 ml total; 250 μg protein per rabbit).

2. Inject an additional 0.5 ml of the emulsion (freshly prepared) one month later, divided among several subcutaneous sites on the back. (Do not repeat the footpad injections.) Bleed the rabbits from the ear two to four weeks after the second injection. Rabbits can be boosted and bled in this way every three to four months for several years. It is not necessary to use CFA for the third and subsequent injections. Sodium alginate is a satisfactory adjuvant for the later injections (use a 1 : 1 mixture of sodium alginate and protein solution).

3. Store the serum as a 40% SAS slurry at 4°C (Section 11.9).

Absorption of Antisera

1. Reconstitute the antiserum from the SAS slurry and dialyze against PBS. Adjust to original serum volume.

2. Test the undiluted antiserum by immunodiffusion against 1 mg/ml solutions of purified myeloma proteins of each class and subclass to determine which immunoadsorbents are needed to remove unwanted specificities (see Garvey et al. 1977 for a description of immunodiffusion procedures).

3. Immunoadsorbents are most economically prepared using myeloma protein isolated from ascites fluid (see comment 2). Precipitate the myeloma protein from the ascites fluid with 40% SAS (Section 12.2). (Ascites fluid containing the IgM myeloma protein from MOPC 104E should be precipitated with 50% SAS to obtain an adequate yield.) Dialyze the precipitated protein against 0.1 M NaHCO$_3$, pH 9, and adjust protein concentration to about 20 mg/ml.

4. Activate 10 ml (or more) of agarose with CNBr by the procedure described in Section 12.4. Add the protein solution to the activated agarose (use 2–20 mg protein per ml of activated agarose). Stir or rotate the mixture gently for 24 hours at 4°C. Add sufficient 1 M ethanolamine, pH 8.5, to make the solution 0.05 M in ethanolamine. After a 5-minute incubation, wash immunoadsorbent as described in Section 12.4. Before use, wash the immunoadsorbent thoroughly with 0.1 M acetic acid until no protein can be detected in the eluate (OD$_{280}$ < 0.01). As soon as the eluate is free of protein, wash the adsorbent with PBS until the eluate is pH 7.2.

5. Perform a pilot absorption to determine the amount of immunoadsorbent needed to completely remove unwanted specificities. In most instances, satisfactory results are obtained with a 5:1 (v/v) serum to immunoadsorbent ratio, if at least two different immunoadsorbents are used. For example, 25 ml of anti-IgG2b serum are passed over a 5-ml IgG2a column connected in tandem to a 5-ml IgG1 column. After all of the serum has been applied to the first column, wash the sample through both columns with PBS. Collect all fractions that give visible turbidity when a drop of eluate is tested with 10% TCA. Concentrate the pooled fractions to $\frac{1}{4}$ the original serum volume or less.

6. Retest the antiserum for specificity by immunodiffusion and by immunoelectrophoresis against undiluted normal mouse serum. (If the antiserum is to be used for radio-immunoprecipitation or

fluorescent labeling studies, more sensitive tests must be used; see Section 11.6.) If the specificity tests are not satisfactory, repeat the absorption after regenerating the immunoadsorbent (see comment 2).

7. After obtaining satisfactory results from the pilot studies, absorb the remaining antiserum.

8. Store the absorbed antiserum frozen in small aliquots or as a 40% SAS slurry at 4°C (Section 11.9).

COMMENTS

1. Immunoadsorbents prepared from 40% SAS precipitates of ascites fluid are usually satisfactory and are often preferable for reasons of economy. However, purified myeloma proteins may be required in situations where high ratios of immunoadsorbents to serum are required to remove unwanted specificities. In such situations, the use of SAS-precipitated ascites fluid for preparation of the immunoadsorbent may result in unacceptable losses of specific antibody during the absorption process. The procedure to couple purified myeloma proteins to agarose is identical to that described above.

2. Regenerate the immunoadsorbent columns by eluting with 0.1 M acetic acid at room temperature until the absorbance of the eluate is less than 0.01 at 280 nm. Usually about 5 column volumes of acetic acid are needed. Immediately wash the columns with several volumes of PBS until the eluate is pH 7.2. Store columns at 4°C with 0.1% sodium azide as a preservative. The eluted antibodies can be recovered if the acetic acid is promptly neutralized with $\frac{1}{3}$ volume of 1 M Tris-HCl, pH 8.0, and the neutralized solution dialyzed against PBS prior to concentration.

3. When using class-specific antisera to detect immunoglobulins in mouse strains other than the strain in which the immunogen (the myeloma) originated, the ability of the antiserum to react with normal immunoglobulins of the strain being studied must be tested before the antiserum is used for quantitative work. Some "class-specific" heteroantisera recognize primarily allotypic determinants on the immunizing protein and are not suitable for general use as class-specific reagents (Epstein and Gottlieb 1977; Herzenberg and Herzenberg 1978).

REFERENCES

Dresser, D. W. 1978. Assays for immunoglobulin-secreting cells. In D. M. Weir (Ed.), *Handbook of Experimental Immunology,* third edition. Blackwell Scientific Publications, Oxford.

Epstein, S. L., and P. Gottlieb. 1977. Quantitative measurement of mouse
    IgG subclasses with the use of heteroantisera: The importance of al-
    lotypic considerations. *J. Immunol.* **118**:935.
Garvey, J. S., N. E. Cremer, and D. Sussdorf. 1977. *Methods in Immunology,*
    third edition. W. A. Benjamin, Reading, MA.
Herzenberg, L. A., and L. A. Herzenberg. 1978. Mouse immunoglobulin
    allotypes: Description and special methodology. In D. M. Weir (Ed.),
    Handbook of Experimental Immunology, third edition. Blackwell Scien-
    tific Publications, Oxford.
Hudson, L., and F. C. Hay. 1976. *Practical Immunology.* Blackwell Scientific
    Publications, Oxford.

11.6 RADIO-IMMUNOPRECIPITATION AND FLUORESCENT LABELING SPECIFICITY TESTS FOR ANTISERA AGAINST MOUSE IMMUNOGLOBULINS

Material for this section was provided by John North

Tests for specificity must have a sensitivity equal to or greater than that of
the experiments in which the antisera are used. Thus, the sensitivity of
precipitation in gel techniques is insufficient to assess the specificity of
antisera used in radio-immunoprecipitation and fluorescent labeling studies. Three highly sensitive specificity tests for antisera directed against
mouse immunoglobulins are described below. These tests are designed to
detect different types of nonspecific antibodies present in the antisera. The
radio-immunoprecipitation and fluorescent labeling tests will only detect
antibodies against unwanted class or subclass determinants, for example,
the presence of anti-κ chain antibodies in a preparation of anti-γ chain
antiserum. Neither test will detect antibodies against other serum components or against cell surface determinants (aside from immunoglobulins).
The double fluorescent labeling test will detect antibodies directed against
nonimmunoglobulin cell surface determinants present on a particular cell
type. The most commonly used test of this type is to determine whether
fluorescent-labeled anti-Ig sera bind to T cells.

A. Radio-Immunoprecipitation

In this procedure, radio-iodinated preparations of purified myeloma proteins (possessing determinants representing unwanted specificities) are
incubated separately with control antiserum, diluent, and the test antiserum. After incubation, any precipitate that forms is pelleted by high
speed centrifugation, and the radioactivity (i.e., the test antigen) remaining in the supernatant is measured. If the test antiserum is specific, the
amount of radioactivity remaining in the supernatant in its presence

should be equal to the radioactivity remaining in the presence of the diluent. This test is critically dependent on the purity of the myeloma proteins used as the test antigens.

MATERIALS AND REAGENTS

Test antibody at 1–5 mg/ml
Iodinated purified myeloma proteins as test antigens, containing determinants representing unwanted specificities (see Section 14.3 for general procedures for preparing radio-iodinated proteins)
Control antiserum, known to be class- or subclass-specific; one control antiserum for each test antigen
Bovine serum albumin (BSA)
Normal rabbit serum
Phosphate-buffered saline (PBS; Appendix A.8)
Tubes, 6 × 50 mm (Kimble, #45060 or similar)
Dilution buffer: 3% BSA in PBS or 10% normal rabbit serum diluted in PBS. (Select rabbit serum for its high level of C'1q complement.)

PROCEDURE

1. Dilute test antibody in dilution buffer (1 : 5, 1 : 10, and 1 : 20 of a 2.5 mg/ml stock).
2. Dilute iodinated myeloma protein antigens in dilution buffer to give approximately 10 000 cpm/50 μl.
3. Mix 50 μl of antibody dilution with 50 μl of iodinated antigen in duplicate tubes.
4. Set up positive controls for each test antigen with a known antiserum and negative controls with normal serum replacing the antiserum.
5. Incubate for 1½ hours at 37°C.
6. Incubate 30 minutes at 4°C.
7. Centrifuge at 45 000 × g for 20 minutes at 4°C.
8. Remove 50 μl of each supernate and measure the amount of radioactivity in the supernatant with a gamma counter.
9. Calculate the percentage of each antigen precipitated by each antiserum.

COMMENT

An alternate method using facilitating anti-antibody to precipitate the antigen-antibody complex is described in Section 14.3. In the alternate method, centrifugation at $4300 \times g$ is sufficient for the complete precipitation of the complex.

B. Fluorescent Labeling

In this procedure, several preparations of red blood cells, each coated with a different myeloma protein antigen of known purity, provide target cells for the binding of the test antibody. Visualization of antibody binding to the myeloma-coated red blood cells is achieved by immunofluorescence using either direct staining with fluorescent-labeled test antisera or indirect staining with fluorescent-labeled goat anti–rabbit Ig sera.

MATERIALS AND REAGENTS

Preparation of Myeloma Protein-Coated Sheep Red Blood Cells

Sheep red blood cells (SRBC)

Purified myeloma proteins: 5 mg/ml in saline (no phosphate), as test antigen containing determinants representing unwanted specificities

Saline: 0.85% NaCl (w/v) at pH 7.2

Phosphate-buffered saline (PBS; Appendix A.8)

$CrCl_3 \cdot 6H_2O$, $M_r = 266.5$

Sero-Fuge II (Clay Adams), optional

Polypropylene tube, 17×100 mm (Falcon, #2059), for use with Sero-Fuge II

Rotator (Scientific Products, #R4193-1)

Visualization of Antibody Binding

Reagents and buffers for fluorescent staining of immunoglobulin on cell membranes (Sections 13.3 and 13.4). A control antiserum specific for each test antigen is required as a positive control.

PROCEDURE

Preparation of Myeloma Protein-Coated SRBC

1. Wash SRBC 4 times in saline ($400 \times g$, 10 min; or, 2 min in Sero-Fuge).

2. Prepare a fresh solution of 2.5×10^{-4} M $CrCl_3 \cdot 6H_2O$ in saline. A simple procedure is to prepare a 6.7 mg/ml solution and dilute this 1 : 100 in saline.

3. For each myeloma protein antigen required in the fluorescence assay, prepare coated cells as follows (there must be no phosphate in the reaction mixture, since phosphate inhibits the coupling

reaction): To 0.2 ml packed SRBC, add 0.2 ml of myeloma protein at 5 mg/ml and mix. Add 2.0 ml of the 2.5×10^{-4} M solution of $CrCl_3 \cdot 6H_2O$ with continuous mixing.

4. Incubate with gentle agitation (e.g., in a rotator) for 1 hour at 30°C.
5. Wash in PBS 3 times.

Visualization of Antibody Binding

1. The binding of antibody to the myeloma protein-coated SRBC is visualized by the immunofluorescence methods described in Sections 13.3 and 13.4. Either direct or indirect procedures are applicable. Indirect procedures (Section 13.4B), using fluorescein-conjugated goat anti–rabbit Ig antibodies to detect the binding of rabbit anti–mouse Ig antibodies, are probably more efficient in studies requiring a large number of test antigens and control antisera. (If direct staining is used, all the control and test antisera must be fluorescent labeled).

2. Treat each test preparation of myeloma protein-coated SRBC with control antiserum, diluent, and test antiserum as described in Section 13.4B. Then stain with a second layer of fluorescein-conjugated goat anti–rabbit Ig antibodies.

3. Determine the percentage of labeled cells by fluorescence microscopy (Section 13.4E). If the test antiserum is highly specific, it should not stain inappropriate myeloma protein-coated SRBC.

C. Double Fluorescent Labeling

This procedure is used to detect antibodies in preparations of rabbit anti–mouse immunoglobulin sera that inappropriately bind to T cells. In the particular example given, the rabbit antibodies are conjugated with fluorescein and used to label spleen cell suspensions. This procedure will label B cells with fluorescein, but may also label T cells if anti–T cell antibodies are present in the antiserum. The T cells are then labeled with rhodamine-conjugated anti–T cell reagents. This is accomplished by a hapten-sandwich technique (Section 13.2): The spleen cell suspension is treated with a first layer of hapten-conjugated rabbit anti–mouse brain antisera, followed by a second layer of rhodamine-conjugated anti-hapten antibodies. Detection of cells labeled with both fluorescein and rhodamine indicates that anti–T cell antibodies are present in the anti–mouse immunoglobulin antisera.

MATERIALS AND REAGENTS

As listed in Sections 13.3 and 13.4, with the following additions:

Fluorescein-conjugated anti–mouse Ig sera (Sections 11.5 and 13.3)
Arsonate-conjugated rabbit anti–mouse brain sera (Sections 11.2 and 13.2)
Rhodamine-conjugated rabbit anti-arsonate antibodies (Sections 11.3, 12.4, and 13.3)

PROCEDURE

1. Prepare a spleen cell suspension as described in Section 1.2. Cell suspensions for fluorescent staining should be of high viability and essentially free of clumps and debris (see Chapter 1).

2. Double label the cell suspension with the fluorescein- and rhodamine-conjugated reagents as described in Section 13.4D.

3. Determine the percentage of T cells that are doubly labeled. If the anti-Ig serum is highly specific, there will be very few doubly labeled T cells.

11.7 MICROCYTOTOXICITY TEST

John North

The microcytotoxicity test provides a fast, economical, and accurate method for measuring the complement-mediated cytotoxic activity of antiserum. In this procedure, cells are treated with antiserum and complement in the wells of a microwell plate and the incidence of cell death is measured by nigrosin uptake (Section 1.13). The technique requires the expenditure of small volumes of antisera and small numbers of cells. Although it is preferable to perform the test in duplicate for accurate measurements of cytotoxic activities, single titrations are adequate for many purposes.

MATERIALS AND REAGENTS

Target cells at 5×10^5 cells/ml in medium-FCS: The initial cell viability should be about 95% (Sections 1.11–1.15). Tests are easier to read when red blood cells are removed (Sections 1.16–1.19). Select target cells to include a vulnerable cell type for measurement of activity and a specificity control (cells from a different organ or another strain of mice, which will not be killed).

Nontoxic fetal calf serum (FCS), prescreened

Rabbit serum as a source of complement, previously titrated and determined to be nontoxic for mouse lymphocytes (Appendix A.2 or Cedarlane Laboratories). (We have obtained nontoxic sera from rabbits 2–3 weeks old.)

RPMI 1640 or minimum essential medium, buffered with 0.025 M HEPES and containing 5% FCS (medium-FCS)

0.1% nigrosin in medium-FCS (Section 1.13)

Microtiter V plates (Cooke Laboratory Products, #220-25)

Microtest II plates (Falcon, #3034)

Inverted microscope

Micropipette to deliver 4 μl (Eppendorf or similar)

PROCEDURE

1. Prepare 2-fold dilutions of test serum in medium-FCS, starting at an initial dilution of 1 : 5. Since 4 μl of each serum dilution will be used for each test well, 10–20 μl of each dilution is enough for 2–4 tests. Dilutions are conveniently done in Cooke Microtiter V plates.

2. Dilute complement to twice the concentration previously determined by titration to be nonlimiting for antibody-dependent cytotoxicity. Keep diluted complement on ice.

3. The cytotoxic tests are done in Microtest II plates. For each target cell type, include two control wells that receive 4 μl of medium-FCS instead of antiserum. Starting with the most dilute antiserum, add 4 μl of antiserum to the experimental wells.

4. Add 4 μl of cell suspension (5×10^5 cells/ml) to each well, followed by 4 μl of diluted complement. Incubate plates in a humid chamber at 37°C for 45 minutes.

5. Place a pad of absorbent paper on a bench top. Invert the Microtest II plates 6–9 inches above the pad and forcefully tap the plates onto the pad to remove much of the fluid from the wells. Most of the cells will remain in the wells.

6. Using a finely drawn out Pasteur pipette, add 1 drop (~10 μl) of 0.1% nigrosin. Leave for 10 minutes at room temperature and repeat step 5.

7. Add one drop of medium-FCS to each well, and count dead (brown-black) and live (unstained) cells with the aid of an inverted microscope.

8. Determine the percent specific cytotoxicity using the following formula:

$$\% \text{ specific cytotoxicity} = \frac{(\% \text{ dead cells}_{experimental} - \% \text{ dead cells}_{control})}{100\% - \% \text{ dead cells}_{control}} \times 100$$

9. Plot the percent specific cytotoxicity against the serum dilution. The dilution of serum giving 50% of the maximum killing of a particular vulnerable target cell is conventionally taken as the titer. For a given serum this will vary with the different types of target cells used, because the display of antigen differs and/or cells differ in their susceptibility to killing by antibody and complement.

COMMENTS

1. If necessary, stained plates may be stored overnight at 4°C enclosed in a humid chamber. Longer storage may result in greater nonspecific cell death (which is detectable in the control wells).

2. Occasionally, a lower percentage of killing is observed at higher serum concentrations than at intermediate concentrations. This effect is due to anticomplementary components in the test serum and may sometimes be reduced by high speed centrifugation of the serum (30 000 $\times$ g for 30 min). Alternatively, a two-step procedure (described in Section 9.2) may be adopted.

3. A high rate of cell death in the controls is usually caused by toxic complement. However, it may also result from a lack of humidity during incubation, toxicity of the FCS, or dilution of the medium to hypotonicity.

11.8 SEMI-MICROPRECIPITATION TEST

This section is based on material provided by John Kimura

A simple qualitative microprecipitation test can serve as a preliminary assay for anti-hapten antibodies before purification. Though the example given here is for anti-Lac antibodies, the methods can be used for a variety of antibodies.

MATERIALS AND REAGENTS

Antigen (e.g., Lac-BGG): about 100 μg/ml (see Section 16.2 for general procedures for preparing Lac-modified proteins)

Antibody: 2–5 mg/ml (lower concentrations give weak precipitations that are difficult to read)

Capillary tubes, 1 × 30–50 mm

Modeling clay

PROCEDURE

1. Clarify the antigen and antibody solutions by centrifugation (10 000 × g, 5 min).

2. Allow 30–50 μl of antigen to penetrate into one tube by capillary action.

3. By a similar procedure, add 30–50 μl of antibody to another capillary tube.

4. Place the fluid-containing ends of the two tubes together while holding the capillary tubes horizontally.

5. Gently tilt the tubes vertically so that the tube containing antigen is on top. The antigen solution will flow into the tube containing the antiserum.

6. Seal the empty end of the capillary tube containing the antigen-antibody mixture with modeling clay and wipe tube.

7. Let the tube stand at room temperature in modeling clay. A milky precipitate indicates antibody activity. It may be necessary to further dilute the antigen solution to obtain a good precipitate.

11.9 STORAGE OF ANTISERA

Claudia Henry

Although most antibodies are stable at −70°C for prolonged periods, it is impractical to depend on freezing for routine storage. Freezers may be unreliable, and the space required for storage of large pools of antisera is prohibitive. As an alternative, sera can be precipitated in solutions of $(NH_4)_2SO_4$ and stored in this manner almost indefinitely without loss of activity.

A. Freezing

1. Fill labeled tubes to about $\frac{2}{3}$ capacity. Cap tightly and cover the cap with Parafilm to limit loss due to sublimation.

2. Quick freeze the sera in a dry ice-alcohol mixture. Store at $-70°C$ in a clearly labeled screw cap container.

B. Saturated $(NH_4)_2SO_4$

MATERIALS AND REAGENTS

Antiserum, clarified by centrifugation (10 000 $\times$ g, 5 min)
Saturated $(NH_4)_2SO_4$ (SAS), pH 7.4 (see Section 12.2)

PROCEDURE

1. With stirring, add SAS drop by drop to the antiserum to 40% saturation. Solutions containing <1 mg/ml should then be kept at 0°C (ice bucket in refrigerator) overnight. Store precipitated immunoglobulins at 0–4°C.

2. To reconstitute precipitated immunoglobulins, follow the procedure described in Section 12.2.

12

Purification of Immunoglobulins and Their Fragments

Material for this chapter was provided by Anne H. Good, Leon Wofsy, John Kimura, and Claudia Henry

12.1 INTRODUCTION

This chapter describes methods for the purification of immunoglobulins and their fragments, particularly as they apply to mouse immunoglobulins and to anti–azophenyl hapten antibodies. Current interest in alloantisera against cell surface differentiation antigens has stimulated the need for efficient procedures for purifying mouse immunoglobulins and their fragments. The anti–azophenyl hapten antibodies are used extensively in procedures for hapten rosetting (Section 9.3) and fluorescent double labeling (Chapter 13).

12.2 PRECIPITATION OF IMMUNOGLOBULINS BY AMMONIUM SULFATE

Immunoglobulins are precipitated in 40% saturated ammonium sulfate (SAS) either for preliminary fractionation prior to subsequent purification or for the storage of antisera (Section 11.9).

MATERIALS AND REAGENTS

Preparation of SAS (pH 7.4)

Ammonium sulfate
Ammonium hydroxide
Bunsen burner or hot plate
Flask or beaker, 4 liters
Buchner funnel, filter paper
Vacuum flask, 4 liters
pH meter

Precipitation of Immunoglobulins

Antiserum
SAS
High speed centrifuge
Magnetic stirrer and bar

Reconstitution of Precipitated Immunoglobulins

NaCl, $M_r = 58.4$
Appropriate buffer
Dialysis equipment

PROCEDURE

Preparation of SAS (pH 7.4)

1. Add about 900 g ammonium sulfate to 1.0 liter of water. Heat the mixture until the ammonium sulfate dissolves completely, and quickly filter the solution while it is hot. Let the solution cool to room temperature (crystals will form and should always be present in the bottle).

2. Adjust to pH 7.4 with ammonium hydroxide.

Precipitation of Immunoglobulins

1. Clarify antiserum by centrifugation (10 000 × g, 5 min).

2. To the antiserum, add SAS (slowly and with stirring) until 40% saturation is reached. Allow precipitate to form for some hours, preferably overnight at 0°C. Incubation in an ice bucket overnight is essential when precipitating immunoglobulins from dilute solutions (<1 mg/ml). The resulting precipitate can be stored in the 40% SAS at 0–4°C for a long time.

Reconstitution of Precipitated Immunoglobulins

1. Resuspend the 40% SAS slurry and centrifuge an aliquot at 10 000 × g for 5 minutes.

2. Dissolve the precipitate in a minimal amount of water and dialyze for at least 36 hours against 200 volumes of 0.15 M NaCl (or an appropriate buffer), changing the fluid 3 times.

3. If the ammonium ions must be completely removed from the immunoglobulin preparation, increase the length of time of the dialysis and the number of buffer changes. Alternatively, the reconstituted preparation can be passed through a Sephadex G-25 column.

COMMENTS

1. The solubility of ammonium sulfate is 103.4 g/100 g water at 100°C, and 70.6 g/100 g water at 0°C.

2. Adjustment of the reconstituted samples to a standard OD at 280 nm prior to titration of activity will eliminate the necessity of retitrating subsequently reconstituted samples.

3. Note that precipitation in 40–45% SAS is satisfactory either for storage (Section 11.9), as a preliminary step to further IgG purifications (e.g., DEAE chromatography; Section 12.3), or for concentrating purified solutions of IgG. See Heide and Schwick (1978) for the use of salts for the fractionation of immunoglobulins.

REFERENCE

Heide, K., and H. G. Schwick. 1978. Salt Fractionation of Immunoglobulins. In D. M. Weir, (Ed.), *Handbook of Experimental Immunology,* third edition. Blackwell Scientific Publications, Oxford.

12.3 DEAE CHROMATOGRAPHY

Some procedures require the use of highly purified IgG; for example, when antibodies are chemically modified for use in hapten-sandwich rosetting or fluorescent labeling. Purification of IgG free of contamination with other serum proteins or immunoglobulin classes can be accomplished with DEAE chromatography (Levy and Sober 1960). A procedure for the DEAE purification of rabbit IgG is described in detail in Chapter 26 of Garvey et al. (1977). The pH and ionic strength required to obtain IgG with a maximum of purity and the most satisfactory yield vary with the species: (1) for rabbit IgG: 0.0175 M phosphate, pH 6.3; (2) for mouse IgG: 0.04 M phosphate, 0.03 M NaCl, pH 8.0; (3) For goat IgG: 0.01 M phosphate, 0.05 M NaCl, pH 7.35. After chromatography, concentrate the pooled fractions by ultrafiltration. Dialyze the concentrated pool against an appropriate buffer and store frozen. Alternatively, precipitate the IgG with 40% SAS and reconstitute as needed (Sections 11.9 and 12.2).

REFERENCES

Garvey, J. S., N. E. Cremer, and D. H. Sussdorf. 1977. *Methods in Immunology.* W. A. Benjamin, Reading, MA. Chapter 26.

Levy, H. B., and H. A. Sober. 1960. A simple chromatographic method for preparation of gamma globulin. *Proc. Soc. Exp. Biol. Med.* **103**:250.

12.4 PURIFICATION OF ANTI-HAPTEN ANTIBODIES BY AFFINITY CHROMATOGRAPHY

The following procedure describes the use of hapten-modified agarose in purifying antibodies directed against the azophenylarsonate (Ars) and azophenyl-β-D-lactoside (Lac) haptens (Wofsy and Burr 1969). The titration method for activating agarose by CNBr is described. For a description of the buffer method of CNBr activation, see Chapter 30 in Garvey et al. (1977). Alternatively, CNBr-activated agarose can be purchased from Pharmacia Fine Chemicals.

MATERIALS AND REAGENTS

Coupling of Haptens to CNBr-Activated Agarose

Preswollen agarose (Agarose A1.5, Bio-Rad Laboratories or Sepharose 4B, Pharmacia Fine Chemicals)

Cyanogen bromide (CNBr; Eastman Kodak). Note: CNBr is extremely toxic and a potent lachrymator (tear gas). Store CNBr in a desiccator at $-20°C$ and handle only in a well-ventilated chemical hood.

4 M NaOH: 160 g/liter

0.1 M $NaHCO_3$, pH 9.0: Dissolve 67.2 g $NaHCO_3$ in 4 liters of distilled water. Adjust to pH 9.0 with about 18 ml 4 M NaOH. Bring to 8 liters with distilled water.

p-aminophenyl-β-D-lactoside, $M_r = 433$ or arsanilic acid, $M_r = 217.1$: Prepare a 4×10^{-2} M solution in 0.1 M $NaHCO_3$, pH 9.0 buffer. One milliliter of the solution will be used in the procedure described below.

pH meter

Balance

Magnetic stirrer and bar

Graduated cylinder, 25 ml
Beakers, 50 ml, 100 ml
Parafilm
Pasteur pipettes
Coarse, sintered glass funnel attached to 1000-ml vacuum flask
Ice bucket
Stainless steel spatulas

Purification of Antibodies

Antiserum
Phosphate-buffered saline (PBS; Appendix A.8) or borate-buffered
    saline (BBS; Appendix A.9). PBS is used during the purification of
    anti-Lac antibodies, whereas BBS is used during the purification of
    anti-Ars antibodies.
Trichloroacetic acid (TCA): 10% (w/v) in distilled water
Immunoadsorbent columns
Ringstand and clamps
Dialysis equipment
UV spectrophotometer
Ultrafiltration equipment
Dissociating solutions; maintain pH 7.5 to 8.6 with NaOH in order to
    dissolve:
        Benzenearsonic acid, $M_r = 202.0$: 0.3 M in BBS or in 0.34 M
            borate buffer, pH 8.6 (Section 16.2); for anti-Ars antibodies
        Solution of 0.5 M lactose, $M_r = 342.3$, and 0.01 M p-nitro-
            phenyl-β-D-lactoside, $M_r = 463$, in PBS; for anti-Lac anti-
            bodies

PROCEDURE

The procedure is designed to prepare 10 ml of hapten-modified
agarose. Larger amounts of agarose can be modified using this procedure as a guide.

Coupling of Hapten to CNBr-Activated Agarose

1. Place the balance, pH meter, magnetic stirrer, and sintered glass
   funnel with vacuum flask in a chemical hood.

2. Place 10 ml of preswollen agarose in a graduated cylinder. Pour
   the agarose onto the sintered glass funnel (under gentle suction)
   and wash with 200–300 ml of distilled water to remove preserva-
   tives. Transfer the agarose to a 50-ml beaker and add 10 ml of
   distilled water.

3. Weigh 1.0 g of CNBr into a 100-ml beaker and add 20 ml of distil-

led water. *Gently* stir with a magnetic stirrer. The CNBr will not completely dissolve at this stage.

4. Adjust the CNBr solution to pH 11 with the 4 M NaOH and immediately add the agarose to the CNBr solution. Continually monitor the pH and maintain it at 11–11.5 by addition of 4 M NaOH.

5. After an 8–10-minute reaction time, pour the mixture into the sintered glass funnel and wash the agarose with 200–300 ml of *ice cold* 0.1 M $NaHCO_3$, pH 9. Resuspend the washed agarose in a 50-ml beaker with 10 ml of cold 0.1 M $NaHCO_3$ buffer.

6. Add 1.0 ml of the hapten solution to the activated agarose. Cover the beaker with Parafilm and stir the mixture *gently* for 24 hours at 4°C. (Vigorous stirring will fracture the beads and result in poor flow rates during the purification step.)

7. Transfer the immunoadsorbent to a sintered glass funnel and wash extensively (but gently) with 1000 ml of ice cold distilled water followed by 1000 ml of ice cold 0.1 M $NaHCO_3$, pH 9.0 buffer. After the last wash, suspend the immunoadsorbent in the appropriate buffer (PBS or BBS).

Purification of Antibodies

1. Clarify the antiserum by centrifugation at $10\ 000 \times g$ for 10 minutes.

2. Place immunoadsorbent into a suitable column (the dimensions of the column are not critical; a syringe barrel is suitable). Wash adsorbent with the appropriate buffered saline.

3. Apply the antiserum slowly to the column and collect the eluate. Ten milliliters of immunoadsorbent will bind approximately 150–200 mg of anti-hapten antibody; however, aliquots of the eluate should be periodically tested to determine if the capacity of the column has been reached. (A simple precipitation test for anti-hapten antibodies is described in Section 11.8.)

4. Wash the column with the appropriate buffer until the eluate has an OD_{280} of less than 0.01.

5. Saturate the column with the appropriate dissociating solution. Clamp the column off and allow it to stand at room temperature for 15–30 minutes.

6. Pass several column volumes of dissociating solution through the column and collect the eluate until it no longer gives a visible turbidity with 10% TCA (1 drop of eluate into 0.5–1.0 ml 10% TCA).

7. Combine all TCA-positive fractions, dialyze against multiple

changes of buffered saline, and concentrate by ultrafiltration. The amount of antibody recovered can be determined from the absorbance at 280 nm, using an extinction coefficient of 1.46 for a 1.0 mg/ml solution of anti-hapten antibody.

COMMENTS

1. Immunoadsorbents prepared by CNBr-activation of agarose will "leak" small amounts of antigen during prolonged storage at 4°C. The immunoadsorbents should therefore be washed with several volumes of buffer before each use.

2. Columns can be reused. To remove any residual high-affinity antibody, wash column with 1 volume of 0.1 M acetic acid and re-equilibrate with large volumes of the buffer to be used in the subsequent purification. The immunoadsorbents must be stored at 4°C with 0.02% sodium azide as a preservative.

REFERENCES

Garvey, J. S., N. E. Cremer, and D. H. Sussdorf. 1977. *Methods in Immunology.* W. A. Benjamin, Reading, MA. Chapter 30.

Wofsy, L., and B. Burr. 1969. The use of affinity chromatography for the specific purification of antibodies and antigens. *J. Immunol.* **103**:380.

12.5   PREPARATION OF ACTIVE ANTIBODY FRAGMENTS

The optimal conditions for preparing active antibody fragments vary from species to species. Standard procedures and references for preparing Fab and (Fab')$_2$ fragments of rabbit IgG are described in Chapter 31 of Garvey et al. (1977). There is no satisfactory procedure for preparing mouse (Fab')$_2$ because mouse IgG tends to precipitate from solution at the acidic pH required for pepsin action. For preparation of mouse Fab by papain digestion, the following procedure based on the method of Dresser (1978) is advisable.

MATERIALS AND REAGENTS

Purified mouse immunoglobulin (Sections 11.5, 12.3): 3–30 mg/ml
Mercuripapain (Worthington Biochemical)
$Na_2HPO_4 \cdot 7H_2O$, $M_r = 268.09$
$NaH_2PO_4 \cdot H_2O$, $M_r = 137.99$
EDTA, $M_r = 292.24$

2-mercaptoethanol (2-ME), $M_r = 78.1$, specific gravity $= 1.114$
Iodoacetamide, $M_r = 185$
1 M Tris-HCl, pH 8 (Section 11.5)
Nitrogen tank and regulator
NaCl, $M_r = 58.4$
37°C water bath
Parafilm
Ice bucket
Dialysis equipment
DEAE-cellulose and equipment for ion-exchange chromatography
Solutions

    0.5 M sodium phosphate buffer (pH 7.5 when diluted to 0.1 M): Dissolve 112.6 g $Na_2HPO_4 \cdot 7H_2O$ and 11.0 g $NaH_2PO_4 \cdot H_2O$ in distilled water and bring to a final volume of 1.0 liter.

    0.1 M phosphate, 4×10^{-3} M EDTA buffer: Add 1.17 g EDTA to 200 ml of 0.5 M phosphate buffer and bring to 1.0 liter with distilled water. The pH of this buffer will be 7.2 after it has been made 0.01 M in 2-ME.

    1 M 2-ME: Mix 0.36 ml 2-ME with 4.64 ml 0.1 M phosphate, 4×10^{-3} M EDTA.

    Iodoacetamide: Prepare a 0.3 M solution (55.5 mg/ml) in 1 M Tris-HCl, pH 8, immediately before use. Make only the amount needed.

    0.005 M Tris-HCl, pH 8.0: Dilute 1 M Tris-HCl, pH 8.0, 1:200 with distilled water. Readjust to pH 8.0 if necessary.

    0.3 M NaCl, 0.005 M Tris-HCl, pH 8.0: Combine 17.5 g NaCl and 5.0 ml 1 M Tris-HCl, pH 8.0, and bring to a total volume of 1000 ml with distilled water. Readjust to pH 8.0 if necessary.

PROCEDURE

1. Dialyze the protein (mouse immunoglobulin) at a concentration of 3–30 mg/ml overnight against 0.1 M phosphate, 4×10^{-3} M EDTA buffer.

2. Immediately before addition of the papain, make the solution 0.01 M in 2-ME by adding 0.01 ml 1 M 2-ME per ml of protein solution. (Do not dialyze the protein against the 2-ME solution. Prolonged dialysis in the presence of a reducing agent is likely to cause irreversible precipitation of the protein.)

3. Add mercuripapain (2% of the weight of the protein) to the solution, flush the tube with nitrogen, cap securely, and place in a 37°C water bath. Mix thoroughly several times during the digestion period.

4. After 4 hours, terminate the reaction by adding 50 μl of 0.3 M iodoacetamide in 1 M Tris-HCl, pH 8.0, per ml of reaction mixture to bring the final concentration of iodoacetamide to 0.014 M, and place the mixture in an ice bath.

5. Hold on ice for 30 minutes, then dialyze against 0.005 M Tris-HCl, pH 8.0.

6. Apply the mixture to a column of DEAE-cellulose equilibrated with 0.005 M Tris-HCl buffer, pH 8.0. Elute column with a gradient of 0.005 M Tris-HCl, pH 8.0 to 0.3 M NaCl in 0.005 Tris-HCl, pH 8.0. Mouse Fab is isolated as the first eluted peak (Dresser 1978). Alternatively, mouse Fab can be purified by adsorption of undigested IgG and free Fc onto a staphylococcal protein A column (Goding 1978, also Section 17.9).

7. The absence of undigested IgG in the final preparation should be checked by electrophoresis in 7% SDS-acrylamide gels (Garvey et al. 1977; Weber and Osborne 1969).

REFERENCES

Askonas, B. A., and J. L. Fahey. 1962. Enzymatically produced subunits of proteins formed by plasma cells in mice. II. β_{2A}-Myeloma protein and Bence Jones protein. *J. Exp. Med.* **115:**641.

Dresser, D. W. 1978. Assays for immunoglobulin-secreting cells. In D. M. Weir (Ed.), *Handbook of Experimental Immunology,* third edition. Blackwell Scientific Publications, Oxford.

Garvey, J. S., N. C. Cremer, and D. H. Sussdorf. 1977. *Methods in Immunology.* W. A. Benjamin, Reading, MA.

Goding, J. W. 1978. Use of staphylococcal protein A as an immunological reagent. *J. Immunol. Meth.* **20:**241.

Weber, K., and M. Osborn. 1969. The reliability of molecular weight determinations by dodecyl sulfate-polyacrylamide gel electrophoresis. *J. Biol. Chem.* **244:**4406.

Modification and Use of Antibodies to Label Cell Surface Antigens

Material for this chapter was prepared on the basis of contributions from Leon Wofsy, Claudia Henry, John Kimura, and John North

13.1 INTRODUCTION

In general, antibodies are the most sensitive, specific, and versatile probes for the detection of cell surface antigens. By coupling the appropriate markers to antibodies, it is possible to prepare reagents that distinguish cells bearing characteristic antigens by fluorescence, electron microscopy, or radioactivity. These reagents can also target specific cell types for rosetting or isolation on immunoadsorbents.

In the following sections, we will outline or refer to well-established procedures for preparing fluorescent and other such detector-coupled antibodies. We will describe more fully the procedures for preparing hapten-conjugated antibodies for use in the hapten-sandwich labeling method. Although the latter technique only supplements conventional labeling methods, we emphasize it here because it is not fully described in other laboratory guides.

13.2 HAPTEN-SANDWICH LABELING

Hapten-sandwich labeling is an indirect procedure. The marker for detection of cell surface antigens is on a second-layer anti-hapten antibody which recognizes hapten groups that have been conjugated to the specific first-layer antibody. The conventional indirect (sandwich) antibody technique (Coons 1956) employs second-layer anti-immunoglobulin made in one species to label first-layer antibody made in another species. Sandwich procedures afford greater sensitivity by amplifying the number of detector antibodies focused on a given antigen.

The hapten-sandwich method is especially advantageous for studies of cell membrane alloantigens, where the antibody and antigen originate in the same species. Alloantisera, which are so important in distinguishing subpopulations of mouse lymphocytes, are usually of low titer and may be substantially inactivated when chemically modified to attach fluorescent or other markers. Attempts to use an anti-immunoglobulin sandwich to improve detection of cellular antigens that bind alloantibodies are, however, complicated by the fact that anti-Ig from another species will recognize both the specific first-layer antibody and all other cell surface immunoglobulins (e.g., those on B cells). With hapten-sandwich labeling, there is obviously no such problem because the second-layer antibody is specific for hapten and not immunoglobulin. Moreover, by selecting two non-cross-reactive haptens, the hapten-sandwich procedure can be applied in double-labeling studies to provide amplified detection of more than one antigen at a time.

The feasibility of the hapten-sandwich method depends on the availability of purified anti-hapten antibodies and simple procedures for conjugating haptens to antibodies without appreciable loss of antibody activity. The necessary anti-hapten antibodies are, of course, easy to prepare (Section 11.3) and can be readily purified by affinity chromatography (Section 12.4). However, most common procedures for the chemical modification of proteins are of limited value in preparing hapten-antibody conjugates. The requisite coupling reactions must yield covalent attachment of a reasonably large number of hapten groups without attacking "backbone" amino acid residues (e.g., tyrosine and histidine), without harsh conditions of pH or temperature, and without the use of denaturing solvents. To date, these requirements have been met most satisfactorily by the use of recently developed bifunctional amidinating reagents (Cammisuli and Wofsy 1976). The reagent of choice is methyl-p-hydroxybenzimidate hydrochloride (HB):

$$HO-\left\langle\!\!\!\bigcirc\!\!\!\right\rangle-\overset{\overset{\displaystyle NH_2^{\oplus}Cl^{\ominus}}{\|}}{C}-OCH_3$$

With HB, haptens are coupled to antibodies in a two-step procedure.

First, an aminophenyl hapten is converted to a diazonium reagent that is azo-coupled to the phenolic ring of HB. Second, the resulting hapten-azo-HB is reacted with antibody. The rationale for this procedure is that most of the imidate functions remain active after the azo-coupling is complete and, when the protein is added, can react with ϵ-amino groups of lysine to form amidine bonds.

A. Synthesis of Methyl-p-hydroxybenzimidate Hydrochloride (HB)

HB is available commercially (Pierce Chemical); however, it is easy and inexpensive to prepare.

MATERIALS AND REAGENTS

p-hydroxybenzonitrile, $M_r = 119$ (Aldrich Chemical)
HCl (gas), $M_r = 36.5$, lecture bottle
Methanol, absolute, $M_r = 32.0$; density = 0.79 g/ml
Ether, anhydrous
P_2O_5
Flask
Ice bucket
Sintered glass filter
Desiccator, vacuum
Drierite

PROCEDURE

This procedure is based on the Pinner synthesis as described by Hunter and Ludwig (1962).

1. Dissolve 50 mmol of p-hydroxybenzonitrile in 75 mmol of absolute methanol. Cool mixture to 0°C in an ice bath.

2. At 0°C, under strictly anhydrous conditions, pass HCl through the solution until it is saturated (75 mmol); at saturation, the bubbling of HCl to the surface becomes noticeably more vigorous.

3. About an hour after the flow of HCl has been stopped, the white HB crystals (which have turned the reaction mixture into a solid mass) should be taken up and thoroughly suspended in cold anhydrous ether, filtered on sintered glass, and washed with more cold ether.

4. Dry HB thoroughly over P_2O_5 under vacuum. HB melts with decomposition at 164°C. Store over Drierite at -20°C.

B. Preparation of Hapten-Antibody Conjugates

While many aminophenyl haptens may be used, we recommend arsanilic acid (Ars) because it is inexpensive and because Ars-HB-immunoglobulin conjugates have good solubility (conjugates with no charged groups on the hapten phenyl ring are less soluble). If two non-cross-reactive haptens are desired for double-labeling application, another good choice is either p-aminobenzoylglutamic acid or p-aminobenzoylglycine. Neither of these haptens cross-reacts with anti-Ars antibody, whereas benzenesulfonic acid and benzoic acid haptens do cross-react with anti-Ars in fluorescent double-labeling experiments.*

MATERIALS AND REAGENTS

Arsanilic acid, $M_r = 217.1$
p-aminobenzoylglutamic acid, $M_r = 266$ (Sigma Chemical)
p-aminobenzoylglycine, $M_r = 194$ (ICN Nutritional Biochemicals)
1 M HCl; 2 M HCl
5 M NaOH: 20 g/100 ml water
NaNO$_2$, $M_r = 69$
Phosphate-buffered saline (PBS; Appendix A.8), 5×
Borate buffer, 0.34 M, pH 8.6: Combine 128 g H$_3$BO$_3$ and 24 g NaOH and bring to 6 liters with deionized water.
Borate buffer, 0.017 M, pH 8.0: Dilute 0.34 M borate buffer 1:20 and adjust pH to 8.0.
HB, $M_r = 187$
Imidazole, $M_r = 68$
Bio-Gel, P-100 (Bio-Rad Laboratories); for hapten-HB-Ig conjugates
Bio-Gel P-60 (Bio-Rad Laboratories); for hapten-HB-Fab conjugates
DEAE-purified IgG, $M_r = 150\,000$
pH meter or pH-stat

PROCEDURE

Preparation of Diazonium Reagent

1. To prepare 12 ml of a 0.25 M diazonium solution, dissolve 3 mmol aminophenyl compound in 9 ml of 1 M HCl on ice.

2. At 0°C and with stirring, add 3 mmol NaNO$_2$ (0.21 g) in 3 ml water (react for 15–20 min). The resulting diazonium reagent may

---

* Since this chapter was prepared, we also have had occasion to use the biotin-avidin system (Heitzmann and Richards 1974) for cell surface labeling. This is an excellent hapten-sandwich variant. Moreover, it can be used in conjunction with any of the HB-hapten-antibody reagents for double labeling.

be reacted with HB or aliquoted, frozen, and stored for several months at $-20°C$.

Preparation of Hapten-Azo-HB

Diazonium reagent is reacted with HB in a molar ratio of $5:1$ to assure that no HB molecules lacking an azo-linked hapten group are present during the subsequent modification of antibody. It is important to carry out this procedure exactly as described.

1. To prepare a 20-ml stock solution of hapten-azo-HB (0.03 M HB, initial concentration), add 0.6 mmol HB (0.112 g) to 3 ml 0.34 M borate buffer adjusted to pH 9.8. (This prevents a dramatic drop in pH below the effective borate buffering range.)
2. On ice and with stirring, add (in portions) 12 ml of the 0.25 M diazonium solution to the HB solution, maintaining at pH 9.2 ± 0.2 with 5 M NaOH.
3. When the addition is complete (in about 20 min), allow the reaction to come to room temperature and continue for a total of 2 hours, maintaining at pH 9.2 ± 0.2 throughout.
4. Add 4 mmol solid imidazole (0.27 g) with stirring and allow mixture to stand for 1 hour to quench residual diazonium. (Most of the diazonium is exhausted after 2 to 3 hours at alkaline pH and room temperature.)
5. Adjust to pH 8.6 with 2 M HCl and dilute to a final volume of 20 ml with borate buffer. This 0.03 M hapten-azo-HB stock reagent may be aliquoted and stored at $-20°C$ for use over a two-week period, after which unused reagent should be discarded.

Modification of Antibody

1. Mix DEAE-purified immunoglobulin at 1.5–7.5 mg/ml (in 0.34 M borate, pH 8.6) with the hapten-azo-HB reagent to achieve a solution that is 0.02 M in the initial HB. This entails the addition of 1 part of immunoglobulin solution to 2 parts of the 0.03 M stock hapten-azo-HB reagent.
2. Allow this mixture to react for 15–20 hours at room temperature.
3. Pass the reddish black solution over the Bio-Gel P-100 column (for hapten-HB-Fab conjugates use P-60), using 0.017 M sodium borate, pH 8.0, as the column buffer. Collect the orange-colored conjugate at the front. (See comment 1.)
4. The conjugate may be aliquoted and frozen directly or precipitated in 45% SAS and stored at 4°C (Section 12.2).
5. Before using for cell labeling, adjust the hapten-antibody conju-

gates to physiological pH and ionic strength. (For samples in 0.017 M borate, add $\frac{1}{4}$ volume of 5× PBS; for preparations in 45% SAS, either dissolve precipitate in deionized water and dialyze against 0.017 M borate, pH 8.0, or dialyze directly against 1× PBS if no precipitate forms during dialysis. Ars-HB and Glut-HB conjugates are more soluble in PBS than Gly-HB conjugates.)

COMMENT

If the reaction volume is large and the protein concentration is greater than 1 mg/ml, the modified antibody can be concentrated after step 2 of Modification of Antibody by precipitation at 0°C in 45% SAS (as described in Section 12.2). This will permit the use of a smaller chromatography column in step 3 and thereby save time. After precipitation, centrifuge and dissolve the precipitate in a minimal volume of deionized water.

REFERENCES

Cammisuli, S., and L. Wofsy. 1976. Hapten-sandwich labeling. III. Bifunctional reagents for immunospecific labeling of cell surface antigens. *J. Immunol.* **117**:1685.

Coons, A. H. 1956. Histochemistry with labeled antibody. *Int. Rev. Cyt.* **5**:1.

Heitzmann, H., and F. M. Richards. 1974. Use of the avidin-biotin complex for specific staining of biological membranes in electron microscopy. *Proc. Nat. Acad. Sci.* (USA) **71**:3537.

Hunter, M. J., and M. L. Ludwig. 1962. The reaction of imidoesters with proteins and related small molecules. *J. Am. Chem. Soc.* **84**:3491.

Wallace, E. F., and L. Wofsy. 1979. Hapten-sandwich labeling. IV. Improved procedures and non-cross-reacting hapten reagents for double-labeling cell surface antigens. *J. Immunol. Meth.* **25**:283.

Wofsy, L., C. Henry, and S. Cammisuli. 1978. Hapten-sandwich labeling of cell surface antigens. In R. A. Reisfeld and F. P. Inman (Eds.), *Contemporary Topics in Molecular Immunology,* Vol. 7. Plenum Press, New York.

13.3 FLUORESCENT ANTIBODIES

In this "traditional" method of fluorochrome conjugation, immunoglobulin solutions are dialyzed against solutions of fluorochrome isothiocyanates. Techniques that make use of these fluorescent reagents are described in Section 13.4.

MATERIALS AND REAGENTS

Preparation of Solutions

$NaHCO_3$, $M_r = 84.0$
Na_2CO_3, anhydrous, $M_r = 106.0$
$NaH_2PO_4 \cdot H_2O$, $M_r = 137.0$
Na_2HPO_4, anhydrous, $M_r = 142.0$
$NaCl$, $M_r = 58.4$
6 M HCl
Fluorescein isothiocyanate (FITC; BBL)
Tetramethylrhodamine isothiocyanate (TRITC; BBL)
Dimethylsulfoxide

Coupling of Isothiocyanate Fluorochromes to Immunoglobulins

DEAE-purified IgG (10–20 mg/ml)
Dialysis tubing (Appendix D)

Purification of Fluorochrome-Conjugated Immunoglobulins

Sephadex G-25
DEAE-cellulose

Determination of Fluorochrome : Protein Ratio

UV Spectrophotometer

Evaluation of Staining

As described in Section 13.4

PROCEDURE

Preparation of Solutions

1. Prepare the following solutions:
   a. Stock 0.5 M bicarbonate-buffered saline, pH 9.2: Mix 10 ml of 0.5 M $NaHCO_3$ in 0.15 M NaCl and 5.8 ml of 0.5 M Na_2CO_3 in 0.15 M NaCl. Adjust to pH 9.2 with 6 M HCl.
   b. Stock 0.5 M bicarbonate-buffered saline, pH 8.5: Prepare as described in (a) but adjust to pH 8.5.
   c. 0.05 M bicarbonate-buffered saline, pH 8.5 and pH 9.2: Dilute the two stock solutions described in a. and b. 10-fold with 0.15 M NaCl.
   d. 0.02 M phosphate-buffered saline, pH 7.0.
   e. 0.02 M phosphate buffer, pH 7.5.
   f. 0.0175 M phosphate buffer, pH 6.5.
   g. Fluorochrome reagents: Dissolve fluorescein isothiocyanate in

0.5 M bicarbonate-buffered saline, pH 9.2, to a final concentration of 8–10 mg/ml. Dissolve tetramethylrhodamine in dimethylsulfoxide to a final concentration of 5 mg/ml.

Coupling of Isothiocyanate Fluorochromes to Immunoglobulins

1. Free IgG sample (10–20 mg/ml) of NH_4^+ ions by dialysis against 0.15 M NaCl (3 changes in two days). Then dialyze against 0.05 M bicarbonate-buffered saline, pH 8.5, for 4–5 hours, followed by 2 hours against 0.05 M bicarbonate-buffered saline, pH 9.2. All dialysis should be done at 4°C.

2. Couple the fluorochromes to the Ig by dialyzing the Ig solution against a solution of 100 µg fluorochrome/ml in 0.05 M bicarbonated-buffered saline, pH 9.2. The volume of fluorochrome-bicarbonate solution should be 10 times the sample volume in the dialysis bag. Dialyze at 4°C for 14–16 hours.

3. Stop the reaction by changing the dialysis buffer to 0.02 M phosphate-buffered saline, pH 7.0, at 4°C. Dialyze for 2–3 hours against this buffer.

Purification of Fluorochrome-Conjugated Immunoglobulins

1. Chromatograph conjugated samples on Sephadex G-25 in 0.02 M phosphate-buffered saline, pH 7.0, to remove free fluorochrome from the conjugates. Use a bed volume of about 10 times the sample volume.

2. Further purification of the fluorochrome conjugates is done by stepwise elution from DEAE columns. Procedures for FITC-conjugates and TRITC-conjugates differ.

   FITC-Conjugates

   a. Dialyze the sample against 0.0175 M phosphate buffer, pH 6.5.

   b. Centrifuge (10 000 × g, 10 min) to remove any precipitate and apply supernatant to a 10-cm DEAE column equilibrated with 0.0175 M phosphate buffer, pH 6.5.

   c. Elute fractions of increasingly modified immunoglobulins by steps of 0.1 M, 0.15 M, 0.2 M, and 0.25 M NaCl in 0.0175 M phosphate buffer, pH 6.5.

   d. Concentrate fractions with 50% SAS (Chapter 12.2), dialyze against the appropriate physiological solution, and test for fluorochrome:protein ratio and specificity of staining as described below.

TRITC-Conjugates

a. Dialyze sample against 0.02 M phosphate buffer, pH 7.5.

b. Centrifuge as described above and apply to a DEAE column equilibrated with 0.02 M phosphate buffer, pH 7.5.

c. Elute fractions with stepwise gradients of NaCl (in 0.02 M phosphate buffer, pH 7.5) as for fluorescein conjugates.

d. Concentrate fractions with 50% SAS, dialyze against the appropriate physiological solution, and test for fluorochrome : protein ratio as described below.

Determination of Fluorochrome : Protein Ratio

1. The ratios of fluorochrome to protein (F : P) in the FITC and TRITC conjugates are determined by spectrophotometric analysis. Measure the OD at 280 nm and 493 nm for FITC conjugates; and at 280 nm, 515 nm, and 555 nm for TRITC conjugates.

2. Estimates of F : P ratios for FITC conjugates are obtained by a formula and nomogram given in Goldman (1968):
   a. Concentration of FITC-protein (mg/ml) =
   $$\frac{OD_{280} - (0.36 \times OD_{493})}{1.4}.$$
   b. Use the nomogram in Figure 13.1 to calculate the F : P ratio.

3. Estimates of the F : P ratios for TRITC conjugates are obtained as described by Amante et al. (1972):
   a. Concentration of TRITC-protein (mg/ml) =
   $$\frac{OD_{280} - (0.56 \times OD_{515})}{1.4}.$$
   b. μg TRITC/mg protein $= \dfrac{OD_{555} \times 6.6}{\text{protein concentration (mg/ml)}}.$

4. A wider range of F : P ratios is satisfactory for FITC-conjugates than for TRITC-conjugates. For FITC conjugates, a molar F : P ratio of 2–3 : 1 is optimal for tissue sections, while a ratio of 5–6 : 1 is optimal for cell suspensions. TRITC-conjugates are generally unsatisfactory if the ratio of OD_{555} to OD_{280} is greater than 1 : 2. (For a detailed discussion of the problems of TRITC conjugation, see Goding 1976.)

Evaluation of Staining

Test each fraction of fluorochrome conjugate for sensitivity and specificity of staining, using a range of dilutions on the right and wrong target cells. Choose the dilution that gives maximal sensitivity on the right cells with minimal background on the wrong cells.

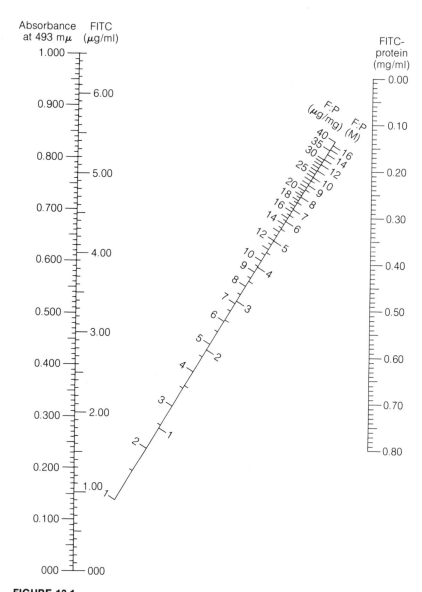

FIGURE 13.1
Nomogram for the calculation of the F : P ratios of FITC conjugates. (After Wells, A. F., C. E. Miller, and M. K. Nadel. 1966. Rapid fluorescein and protein assay method for fluorescent-antibody conjugates. *Appl. Microbiol.* **14**:271.)

COMMENT

An alternate method for conjugating fluorochrome to Ig is described by Goding (1976). He adds the fluorochromes directly to the Ig solutions in bicarbonate-buffered saline and allows the reaction mixture to stand at room temperature for 2 hours. This method has the advantage that the F:P ratios can be predicted.

REFERENCES

Amante, L. A., A. Ancona, and L. Forni. 1972. Conjugation of immunoglobulins with tetramethylrhodamine isothiocyanate. *J. Immunol. Meth.* **1**:289.

Goding, J. W. 1976. Conjugation of antibodies with fluorochromes: Modification to the standard methods. *J. Immunol. Meth.* **13**:215.

Goldman, M. 1968. Labeling agents and procedures of conjugations. In M. Goldman, *Fluorescence Antibody Methods.* Academic Press, New York.

13.4 FLUORESCENT LABELING AND VISUALIZATION

To minimize nonspecific fluorescent staining, it is essential to take care in the preparation of reagents and cell suspensions. Aggregates and complexes of immunoglobulins will bind to many lymphocytes both nonspecifically and via Fc receptors. Ultracentrifugation of reagents immediately prior to cell staining reduces these effects: The recommended speeds and times are $40\,000 \times g$ for 30 minutes or $100\,000 \times g$ for 12 minutes in a Beckman Airfuge. Fc receptor binding may be excluded by preparation of Fab or $(Fab')_2$ reagents (Section 12.5).

In addition to the desired binding activities, many antibody preparations contain activity directed towards other components of the cell membrane. These may be removed by absorption on cells that lack the determinants of interest. Because of the high sensitivity obtained with hapten-sandwich reagents, it is advisable to absorb them even though the original antiserum has already been absorbed for specificity. Two absorptions with an equal volume of packed cells (in the cold for 30 minutes, with gentle mixing) followed by centrifugation of $1000 \times g$ for 10 minutes will usually remove background staining. After absorption, reagents should be ultracentrifuged as described above to remove debris.

Nonspecific staining will, in general, increase with the concentration of the reagent. All antibody preparations are therefore titrated to find the optimal concentration giving minimal nonspecific binding but effective specific staining.

Cell suspensions for staining should be of high viability (Section 1.11, 1.12, 1.14 or 1.15) and essentially free of cell clumps and debris (Section 1.20, 1.21, or 1.22).

A. Direct Staining

MATERIALS AND REAGENTS

Nontoxic fetal calf serum (FCS)

Fluorescent antibody in PBS (or other physiological buffer), pretitrated to determine the optimal concentration for staining

MEM-FCS buffer: 5% FCS in minimum essential medium (MEM) plus 10 mM HEPES

Phosphate-buffered saline (PBS; Appendix A.8)

400-μl microsample tubes (Beckman Instruments) or 3-ml conical glass centrifuge tubes

Finely drawn out Pasteur pipettes

PROCEDURE

1. Load 5×10^5 target cells in MEM-FCS/400-μl tube or 2.5×10^6 target cells in MEM-FCS/3-ml tube.

2. Centrifuge at $300 \times g$ for 5–7 minutes to pellet. Decant supernatant using drawn-out Pasteur pipettes.

3. Add 20 μl fluorescent antibody/400-μl tube or 50–100 μl/3-ml tube. Carefully resuspend the cells, without forming bubbles, using drawn-out Pasteur pipettes. Incubate on ice for 15–20 minutes.

4. Fill 400-μl tube with FCS or add 1 ml FCS to 3-ml tube, and mix with cell suspension.

5. Centrifuge $400 \times g$ for 10 minutes, decant with drawn-out Pasteur pipettes. Resuspend pellet in MEM-FCS, fill tube, and centrifuge.

6. Repeat MEM-FCS wash as in 5.

7. Prepare sample for microscopy.

B. Indirect (Sandwich) Staining

1. The procedure described in A above is performed with the first-layer antibody. In indirect staining, the first-layer antibody is usually not itself fluorescent; it may be unmodified immunoglobulin or, for hapten-sandwich labeling, a hapten-antibody conjugate.

2. The entire procedure is repeated with a fluorescent second-layer antibody. This antibody may be anti-Ig (directed against the first-layer antibody) or anti-hapten (for hapten-sandwich labeling).

C. Distribution of Label

The distribution of labeled antibody on a cell membrane is influenced by several factors (Taylor et al. 1971; Loor et al. 1972). Cross-linking of membrane antigens causes the formation of aggregates or "patches" of label. If cross-linking is extensive enough and the temperature is not too low to prevent cellular metabolism, labeled antigen may be gathered into a "cap" over one portion of the cell surface. If Fab reagents are used for labeling, cross-linking does not occur and an even distribution of label is seen as "ring staining" under fluorescence microscopy. However, the capping of many cell surface antigens requires a second layer of cross-linking antibody. When membrane-bound Ig is the labeled antigen, the majority of labeled cells are capped with first-layer antibody if incubated at 37°C for 10–20 minutes; prolonged incubation at 37°C causes a loss of the labeled Ig through endocytosis or shedding. Since capping is dependent on metabolic activity, it may be inhibited by including 0.1% sodium azide in the buffers used in all steps of the labeling and visualization procedure. The considerations that may make capping desirable or not in any given situation depend on specific experimental objectives. They have no relevance if the object is simply to identify cells that bear a particular surface antigen.

D. Double Labeling

Two antigens on the same or different cells can be distinguished by immunospecific labeling with fluorescein and rhodamine markers. It is essential that the labeling reagents be highly specific. When either or both of the antigens require indirect detection, second-layer antibodies must combine exclusively with a single immunoglobulin in the labeling system. For double labeling with two hapten-sandwich combinations, Ars-HB and Glut-HB antibody conjugates (Section 13.2B) meet these requirements. The staining procedure is essentially as described in Section 13.4A and B. It is sometimes possible to get discrete hapten-sandwich double labeling without too extended a series of steps by adding the first-layer antibodies simultaneously and, subsequently, adding the FITC and TRITC anti-hapten antibodies together. Alternatively, each reagent may be added separately and each third wash (in MEM-FCS) may be omitted except for the final step after labeling with the second anti-hapten antibody.

E. Microscopy

1. Preparation of Slides

One can make wet mounts for immediate viewing or dry mounts for inspection at later times. Dry mounts will last for some months if they are refrigerated in the dark. However, we have found them less satisfactory when the intensity of staining is low.

MATERIALS AND REAGENTS

100% FCS
Phosphate-buffered saline (PBS; Appendix A.8)
PBS containing 5% heat-inactivated (56°C, 30 min) FCS
Glycerol-phosphate-buffered saline: 9 parts glycerol, 1 part PBS
95% ethanol
Pasteur pipettes
Slides
Cover slips (#1)
Permount (or colorless nail polish)
Stock solution of 4% paraformaldehyde (poison): Dissolve 4 g paraformaldehyde in 85 ml of 0.1 M phosphate buffer, pH 7.3, by heating the solution to 70°C with stirring. Add 5 ml of 0.001 M CaCl$_2$, cool, and filter the solution through Whatman #1 filter paper. Add 10 ml of 0.1 M phosphate buffer. The solution is stable for 1–2 weeks at 4°C. Just prior to use, dilute 1 : 4 in phosphate buffer to obtain 1% fresh paraformaldehyde.

PROCEDURE

Wet Mounts

1. Pellet stained cells and resuspend in a small volume of 100% FCS to a concentration of about 1–2 × 10^7 cells/ml. An ideal suspension should yield 20–30 cells/field at a magnification of 500×.

2. Place 1 small drop (5–10 μl) on a microscope slide, cover with a #1 cover slip, and seal with Permount or nail polish.

Dry Mounts

1. Pellet cells and resuspend in 100% FCS as above. Take up a small amount of the cell suspension into a Pasteur pipette by capillary action. Then streak 5–7 lines of the cell suspension onto a microscope slide.

2. Air dry *at least* 30 minutes at room temperature.

3. Fix for 20 seconds in 95% ethanol at room temperature. Air dry.

4. Add 1 small drop of glycerol-phosphate buffer, cover, and seal.

Fixation with Paraformaldehyde

An alternate method for fixing cells in dry mounts is by treatment with paraformaldehyde. This method of fixation can also be used to fix cells when staining two cell surface antigens to prevent movement of the first antigen during the staining of the second.

1. Wash cells free of serum.

2. Resuspend pellet in 2 ml ice cold 1% fresh paraformaldehyde. Fix for 30 minutes on ice.

3. Wash once in PBS without FCS, and once in PBS with 5% FCS.

4. Resuspend pellet in FCS, streak, fix with ethanol, and mount as described above.

2. Viewing

Discount all cells in aggregates and cells at the edge of the field. Use the fine focus adjustment when judging fluorescence.

3. Microscope Requirements

The following two systems of UV light source, filters, and objectives will provide incident-light excitation with a high yield and minimal quenching of fluorescence. They also permit visualization of specimens doubly stained with FITC and TRITC antibodies; the filter systems allow visualization of each fluorochrome while excluding the other.

Leitz System

UV Light Source:
    200 W ultra-high-pressure Hg lamp (Osram) with DC power supply

Leitz Ploem filter system for FITC:
    Excitation filters:
        4 mm BG 38 heat filter
        2× KP 490 or KP 500
    Suppression filters:
        TK 510 dichroic beam-splitting mirror

K 515
S 525 (type AL)
Leitz Filter system for TRITC:
Excitation filters:
4 mm BG 38
2 mm BG 36
KP 546
Suppression filters:
TK 580 dichroic beam-splitting mirror
K 580
K 610
Leitz Objective:
Phaco 3 40×/1.3 N. A.

Zeiss System

UV Light source:
50 W ultra-high-pressure Hg lamp (Osram) with 50 W DC power
supply
Filter system for FITC:
Excitation filters No. 42-79-02 with KP 490 plus KP 500 interfer-
ence filters
510 LP dichroic beam splitter No. 46-63-04
Barrier filter set No. 42-79-03 with KP 540 interference filter
Filter System for TRITC:
Excitation filter set No. 42-79-01 with two 546 BP interference
filters
580 LP dichroic beam splitter No. 46-63-05
Barrier filters No. 46-78-69 with LP 590 and LP 605 interference
filters plus BG 18 red-attenuating filter No. 48-79-92.
Zeiss Objective:
Planapochromat 63/1.4 N.A. oil phase

COMMENT

The properties of individual filters with a given designation vary such
that each system must be checked for satisfactory operation.

REFERENCES

Loor, F., L. Forni, and B. Pernis. 1972. The dynamic state of the lymphocyte
membrane. Factors affecting the distribution and turnover of surface
immunoglobulin. *Eur. J. Immunol.* 2:203.
Taylor, R. B., W. P. H. Duffus, M. C. Raff, and S. de Petris. 1971. Movement
of lymphocyte surface antigens and receptors. The fluid nature of the
lymphocyte plasma membrane and its immunological significance. *Nature, N. B.* **233**:225.

13.5 ANTIBODIES CONJUGATED TO OTHER MACROMOLECULES

For a variety of purposes, it may be desirable to conjugate antibodies to enzymes, to markers visible in the electron microscope, to beads, to cells, or to other surfaces. Procedures for conjugating antibodies to red cells for rosetting (Section 9.3) or to immunoadsorbents (Section 11.8) have been described. For electron microscopy, antibodies can be conjugated to electron-dense ferritin molecules (Singer 1959). A good procedure for preparing Fab-ferritin or IgG-ferritin conjugates with glutaraldehyde is described by Kishida et al. (1975).

Antibodies can be conjugated to keyhole limpet hemocyanin (a molecule readily identifiable in electron microscopy) by the following procedure based on work by Nicholson and Singer (1971).

MATERIALS AND REAGENTS

IgG (or Fab)
Keyhole limpet hemocyanin (KLH)
Glutaraldehyde, fresh, EM grade
0.1 M $(NH_4)_2CO_3$
Sepharose 2B
Phosphate buffers
    0.1 M, pH 6.8
    0.05 M, pH 7.5

PROCEDURE

1. Prepare a 1-ml solution containing 5 mg IgG and 25 mg KLH in 0.1 M phosphate buffer, pH 6.8.

2. Slowly add 0.1 ml of aqueous 0.5% glutaraldehyde (fresh) with stirring, at room temperature. Allow to react for 1 hour.

3. Terminate the reaction by dialysis against 0.1 M $(NH_4)_2CO_3$ for 3–4 hours at 5°C. Then dialyze overnight against 0.05 M phosphate buffer, pH 7.5.

4. Centrifuge at 10 000 rpm for 15 minutes to remove any precipitate.

5. Chromatograph on a Sepharose 2B column (1 × 40 cm) in 0.05 M phosphate, pH 7.5. Collect the first peak, which includes the IgG (or Fab)-KLH conjugates. Samples may be concentrated if necessary and stored in 0.1% azide at 4°C.

REFERENCES

Kishida, Y., B. R. Olsen, R. A. Berg, and D. J. Prockop. 1975. Two improved methods for preparing ferritin-protein conjugates for electron microscopy. *J. Cell. Biol.* **64**:331.

Nicholson, G. L., and S. J. Singer. 1971. Ferritin-conjugated plant agglutinins as specific saccharide stains for electron microscopy: Application to saccharides bound to cell membranes. *Proc. Natl. Acad. Sci.* (USA) **68**:942.

Singer, S. J. 1959. Preparation of electron-dense antibody conjugates. *Nature* **183**:1523.

IV

ADDITIONAL METHODS

Several procedures used for cellular immunological research and in the application of immunological methods to other areas of biological investigation are described in Part IV.

Methods for producing monoclonal antibodies based on cell hybridization techniques are radically transforming the use of immunological reagents in biological research. Such antibodies can be produced in abundance and by their nature represent a degree of purity far greater than that obtained with conventionally prepared reagents. The method presented in Chapter 17 is a modification of that originally described by Köhler and Milstein (1975) and has been employed with much success both in the laboratory of the authors and elsewhere.

Radioimmune assays are widely employed for accurately measuring small amounts of antigen or antibody, even when they are present as part of a complex mixture. Two approaches, using conventional liquid-phase precipitation and solid-phase binding, are described. The solid-phase method has been particularly useful in the selection of appropriate clones during the preparation of hybrid cell lines.

Protein antigens modified with various haptens are used primarily for producing hapten specific antisera and for research in the response of hapten-specific B cells. Hapten modification is also used as a convenient way to mark proteins so that they can be identified with labeled hapten-specific antibodies.

The methods required for conducting single- and two-dimensional polyacrylamide gel electrophoresis studies are presented in Chapter 19. These techniques combine the use of immunological reagents and sophisticated physical separation procedures, and provide elegant tools for analyzing the macromolecular constituents of the membranes of lymphocytes and other cell types. The techniques will become even more useful for such analytic studies as better immunological reagents become available through the application of the monoclonal antibody preparative technique.

Also included are several procedures for the surgical manipulation of laboratory animals. These techniques are used for the preparation of cell populations with particular biological properties.

14

Double Antibody Radioimmunoassay for the Quantitation of Cellular Proteins

Elizabeth L. Mather

14.1 INTRODUCTION

The radioimmunoassay (RIA) is a specific, sensitive, and rapid technique for quantitating proteins, hormones, or other molecules that are or can be made immunogenic (Yalow and Berson 1960; Hunter 1978). It takes advantage of the specificity associated with antibodies and the sensitivity obtainable with radiolabeled molecules. Because it is not necessary to purify the substance from the biological fluids being assayed, quantitation is rapid and simple. However, it is necessary to use highly purified reagents as standards and indicators. In addition, a high-affinity antibody is necessary if the assay is to be sensitive and is to be carried out in the presence of detergents.

The RIA procedures described below have been used in the quantitation of immunoglobulin and J chain in lymphoid cells.

REFERENCES

Hunter, W. M. 1978. Radioimmunoassay. In D. M. Weir (Ed.), *Handbook of Experimental Immunology,* third edition, Vol. 1. Blackwell Scientific Publications, Oxford.
Yalow, R. S., and S. A. Berson. 1960. Immunoassay of endogenous plasma insulin in man. *J. Clin. Invest.* **39**:1157.

14.2 SAFETY PRECAUTIONS FOR WORKING WITH SODIUM ^{125}IODIDE AND IODINATED MATERIAL

Two types of hazards must be considered when working with radioactive iodine: (a) external exposure to gamma radiation, and (b) internal exposure. Although the energy level of ^{125}I is relatively low, care must be taken to minimize short-range exposure, especially when handling quantities of one or more millicuries. Internal exposure to radioactive iodine is a greater hazard than external exposure because iodine is concentrated in the thyroid when ingested or inhaled. Precautions must be taken at all times to prevent self-contamination and contamination of general laboratory glassware and equipment.

General Procedures

The following is a list of recommended procedures taken in part from *Radioisotope Safety Procedures,* U. C. Berkeley Office of Environmental Health, December 19, 1977. We suggest you consult your institution's radiation safety manual for additional or alternate procedures.

1. Areas for radioactive work must be covered with absorbent paper backed with an impervious material for easy and rapid clean up in case of spillage.

2. Work areas designated for radioactive work must be clearly marked "For Radioactive Work Only" and *used* for radioactive work only.

3. Waste containers (a plastic bag in a metal container) should be placed conveniently near the work area. Waste containers on work benches should be used for wastes that contain minimal amounts of radioactivity. Wastes containing substantial amounts of radioactivity or dry protein precipitates should be stored in a fume hood behind lead shielding.

4. Radioactive wastes should be removed from the laboratory on a regular basis by the appropriate agency. Large amounts of radioactivity should not be allowed to accumulate.

5. Gloves and laboratory coats should be worn when working with ^{125}I or ^{125}I-labeled material. Extra gloves should be readily available. Gloves used for radioactive work should be removed before touching common laboratory items and should be disposed of in radioactive wastes.

6. Na^{125}I and iodinated material should be stored in lead containers.

7. Dosimeter badges and rings should be worn when working with radioactivity.

8. Free iodine may be released from iodinated protein. This has been observed in assays that used small volumes and relatively little protein (Bogdanove and Strash 1975). We routinely cover immune precipitates with a protein solution to minimize the release of iodine into the air.

9. Accidents and spills should be reported to the appropriate agency.

10. Never mouth pipet radioactive material.

Additional Recommended Safety Procedures for Iodinations

Because larger amounts of radiation are handled during iodinations, it is essential to take a number of special precautions.

1. Iodinations and other operations involving a millicurie or more of ^{125}I must be performed in a functioning fume hood.

2. A lead apron should be worn during iodinations.

3. The stock solution of $Na^{125}I$ should be kept basic to minimize the release of free iodine.

4. All necessary items should be assembled before an iodination to minimize movement throughout the laboratory during the iodination.

5. A Geiger counter should be used during the iodination procedure to detect relatively large quantities of radiation. To monitor clean up of small spills, swipe the contaminated areas with a moist swab and count the swab in the gamma counter.

6. Once the container of $Na^{125}I$ has been opened in any way, it should be treated as if it were a contaminated container. Change gloves after handling.

REFERENCE

Bogdanove, E. M., and A. M. Strash. 1975. Radioiodine escape is an unexpected source of radioimmunoassay error and chronic low level environmental contamination. *Nature* 257:427.

14.3 RADIO-IODINATION OF PROTEINS

The development of methods to label proteins and hormones to a high specific activity was critical to the development of the radioimmunoassay (RIA) (Yalow and Berson 1960). Since radioactive iodine has a high specific activity, it is commonly used for RIAs. ^{125}I (or ^{131}I) can be covalently linked to the molecule of interest by a number of different methods (Hunter 1978). One of the more gentle means of introducing iodine is by enzyme catalysis; lactoperoxidase, an enzyme isolated from milk, catalyzes the substitution of iodine onto tyrosine rings (Morrison and Hultquist 1963; Marchalonis 1969). The advantage of this method of labeling is that a relatively high specific activity (2–8 μCi/μg) is obtained with little loss of antigenic determinants.

A. Purification of Lactoperoxidase

The purity of lactoperoxidase is determined by examining the ratio of absorbance at 412 nm to the absorbance at 280 nm; extensively purified enzyme has a ratio of 0.93 (Hubbard and Cohn 1976). Because we have found commercial preparations to have ratios of between 0.4 and 0.5, we further purify the commercial enzyme by carboxymethyl (CM) cellulose ion-exchange chromatography as described by Morrison and Hultquist (1963).

MATERIALS AND REAGENTS

Preparation of Carboxymethyl (CM) Cellulose

CM cellulose (Cellex CM, Bio-Rad Laboratories)
NaCl, $M_r = 58.4$
$CH_3COONa\cdot3H_2O$ (sodium acetate), $M_r = 136.1$
Acetic acid, glacial
0.5 M HCl
Beaker, 1 liter
Sintered glass funnel
pH meter
Chromatography column, 1 × 11 cm
Buffers
    0.5 M sodium acetate, pH 5.7: Dissolve 68.04 g $CH_3COONa\cdot$
    $3H_2O$ in 800 ml distilled water. Adjust to pH 5.7 with glacial
    acetic acid and dilute to 1000 ml with water.
    0.01 M sodium acetate, pH 5.7: Dissolve 1.36 g $CH_3COONa\cdot$
    $3H_2O$ in 800 ml distilled water. Adjust to pH 5.7 with glacial
    acetic acid and dilute to 1000 ml with water.

CM Cellulose Chromatography of Lactoperoxidase

Lactoperoxidase, $M_r = 78\,000$ (Sigma Chemical); $\epsilon_{412}^{0.1\%} = 1.39$

NaCl, $M_r = 58.4$
$CH_3COONa \cdot 3H_2O$, $M_r = 136.1$
Acetic acid, glacial
$NaH_2PO_4 \cdot H_2O$, $M_r = 138.0$
Na_2HPO_4, $M_r = 142.0$
Tris base, $M_r = 121.1$ (Sigma Chemical)
HCl, concentrated
Guaiacol (Sigma Chemical)
H_2O_2: 30% solution
CM column of washed and equilibrated CM cellulose, 1×11 cm
Dialysis tubing
Magnetic stirrer and bar
Spectrophotometer
High speed centrifuge
Gradient maker or two flasks (or bottles) connected by a tube
Fraction collector, test tubes
Ultrafiltration equipment
Buffers

    0.01 M sodium acetate, pH 5.7: Prepared as described above.

    0.05 M sodium acetate, pH 5.7: Dissolve 0.68 g $CH_3COONa \cdot 3H_2O$ in 80 ml water. Adjust to pH 5.7 with acetic acid and dilute to 100 ml.

    0.05 M sodium acetate, 0.5 M NaCl, pH 5.7: Dissolve 0.68 g $CH_3COONa \cdot 3H_2O$ and 2.92 g NaCl in 80 ml water. Adjust to pH 5.7 with acetic acid and dilute to 100 ml.

    0.01 M phosphate buffer, pH 7.0: Dissolve 0.538 g $NaH_2PO_4 \cdot H_2O$ and 0.866 g Na_2HPO_4 in 100 ml water.

    0.02 M Tris, 0.15 M NaCl, pH 7.4: Dissolve 2.42 g Tris base and 8.5 g NaCl in 800 ml water. Adjust to pH 7.4 with HCl and dilute to 1000 ml.

PROCEDURE

Preparation of Carboxymethyl (CM) Cellulose

1. Stir approximately 6 g CM cellulose into 600 ml 0.5 M HCl. Allow it to stir for 30 minutes, then transfer the resin to a sintered glass funnel. Wash 4–5 times using 500 ml of distilled water for each wash. Return the resin to a beaker and add 500 ml 0.5 M sodium acetate, pH 5.7. Allow the resin to stand for several hours or overnight, then measure the pH of the buffer.

    a. If the pH is near 5.7, remove the 0.5 M sodium acetate and replace with 0.01 M sodium acetate, pH 5.7.

    b. If the pH is less than 5.5, remove the buffer and add more

0.5 M sodium acetate, pH 5.7. Allow to stand for several hours. Remove the buffer and replace with 0.01 M sodium acetate, pH 5.7.

2. Wash the resin several times with 0.01 M sodium acetate, pH 5.7. This is also a good time to remove the fines. Stir the resin for 5 minutes, let it settle for 30 minutes, and remove the fines and supernatant fluid. Replace with fresh 0.01 M sodium acetate, pH 5.7 buffer. Repeat as often as necessary until the pH is 5.7 and the fines are removed. The last washes may be carried out at 4°C; alternatively, the resin may be stored overnight at 4°C.

3. Pour a 1 × 11-cm column at 4°C. Run at least 2 column volumes of 0.01 M sodium acetate through the column. Check the pH of the effluent and run more buffer through if necessary to obtain a pH of 5.7.

CM Cellulose Chromatography of Lactoperoxidase

This procedure should be carried out at 4°C.

1. Dissolve 6 mg of lactoperoxidase in 1 ml 0.01 M sodium acetate, pH 5.7, and dialyze against 500 ml of the same buffer overnight at 4°C.

2. Centrifuge at $17\,000 \times g$ for 20 minutes to remove large aggregates. Record the volume and the absorbance at 280 nm and 412 nm.

3. Apply the sample to the equilibrated CM cellulose column. Wash the column with 20 ml of 0.01 M sodium acetate, pH 5.7. Elute the lactoperoxidase by applying a linear gradient of NaCl in 0.05 M sodium acetate, pH 5.7. To make the gradient, use a siphon to connect two flasks of the same size and shape containing: (a) 50 ml 0.05 M sodium acetate, pH 5.7, and (b) 50 ml 0.05 M sodium acetate, 0.5 M NaCl, pH 5.7. Connect the flask containing 0.05 M sodium acetate, pH 5.7, to the column and start the gradient. The flask connected to the column must be stirred vigorously to insure good mixing.

4. Collect 1-ml fractions and read the absorbance of the fractions at 280 nm and 412 nm (Figure 14.1). Pool those fractions that have a 412 nm to 280 nm ratio of 0.8 or greater and concentrate to approximately 3 ml by ultrafiltration. Read the absorbance at 280 nm and 412 nm and calculate the ratio and the yield. Dialyze against 0.02 M Tris, 0.15 M NaCl, pH 7.4. Make 4–5-μg aliquots and store at $-20°C$ to $-70°C$. The enzyme is stable for at least a year at $-70°C$. Three to four micrograms are used per radio-iodination.

5. The activity of the enzyme may be assayed as described by

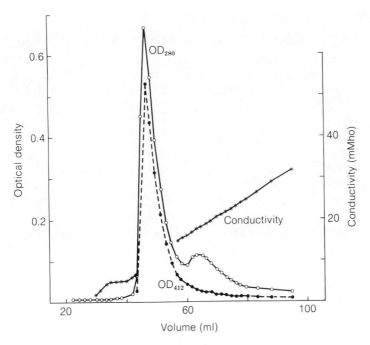

FIGURE 14.1
Carboxymethyl (CM) cellulose purification of lactoperoxidase. Six
milligrams of lactoperoxidase in 0.01 M sodium acetate was layered
onto a 1 ×11-cm column of CM cellulose equilibrated in 0.01 M sodium
acetate, pH 5.7. The sample was washed into the resin with 0.01 M
sodium acetate, pH 5.7, and eluted with a salt gradient of 50 mM
sodium acetate to 50 mM sodium acetate, 0.5 M NaCl, pH 5.7. (From
Ewan, V. A., A role for J chain in the activation of B lymphocytes, Ph.D.
dissertation, 1978, University of California, Berkeley.)

Maehly and Chance (1954). Mix 2.0 ml of 0.020 M guaiacol (0.22
ml guaiacol in 10 ml water) and 4.0 ml of 0.010 M phosphate
buffer, pH 7.0. To 3.0 ml of this mixture, add 0.005 ml of the
enzyme. Start the reaction by adding 0.02 ml of 0.01 M H_2O_2 (11.3
μl H_2O_2 in 10 ml water). Record the change of absorbance at 470
nm as a function of time, reading against the guaiacol-phosphate
mixture. We find that 1 μg of purified enzyme changes the absorbance 0.12–0.20 units every 20 seconds.

B. Radio-Iodination

The iodination procedure of Marchalonis (1969) as modified by John C.
Brown (unpublished notes) is described below.

MATERIALS AND REAGENTS

1.0 mCi Na^{125}I, carrier free, in 0.02 ml 0.1 M NaOH (New England Nuclear; specify a V-vial when ordering). Note: A 0.05 ml Hamilton syringe is used to remove the Na^{125}I from the vial. Do not remove the serum stopper from the vial. The syringe should be used for this purpose only and should be stored in the fume hood properly labeled.

80–500 μg of the protein to be iodinated: Dialyze against 0.1 M Tris, 0.15 M NaCl, pH 7.4 (see buffers and solutions below). Note: Azide inhibits the lactoperoxidase catalyzed reaction and thus must be removed.

Sephadex G-25 (Pharmacia Fine Chemicals): Hydrate Sephadex G-25 for 3 hours in 0.1 M Tris, 0.15 M NaCl, pH 7.4 (see buffers and solutions below). De-fine and pour a column in a 10-ml disposable pipette. Shortly before using, precoat the column with protein to prevent nonspecific losses; 0.3–0.5 ml of 3% bovine serum albumin solution is adequate.

CM cellulose-purified lactoperoxidase

0.1 M NaOH: Make a fresh preparation of 1.0 M NaOH (4.0 g/100 ml) and dilute 1:10.

Tris base, M_r = 121.1 (Sigma Chemical, #T-1503)

NaCl, M_r = 58.4

KI, M_r = 166.0

H$_2$O$_2$: 30% solution

2-mercaptoethanol (2-ME), M_r = 78.1 (Sigma Chemical)

1.0 M HCl

Bovine serum albumin (BSA)

Dialysis tubing and a disposable jar for dialysis (preferably with a tight-fitting lid)

Disposable gloves

pH paper (range 6.0–8.0)

Pasteur pipettes

Disposable micropipettes and test tubes

Gamma counter

Buffers and solutions

1.0 M Tris, pH 7.4: Dissolve 121.2 g Tris base in 900 ml water. Adjust to pH 7.4 with approximately 50 ml of concentrated HCl and dilute to 1000 ml.

0.1 M Tris, 0.15 M NaCl, pH 7.4: Dissolve 8.5 g NaCl in 100 ml 1.0 M Tris, pH 7.4, and dilute to 1000 ml.

1.0 M KI in 0.1 M Tris, 0.15 M NaCl, pH 7.4: Dissolve 83.5 mg of KI in 0.5 ml of 0.1 M Tris, 0.15 M NaCl, pH 7.4.

0.010 M H_2O_2 in 0.1 M Tris, 0.15 M NaCl, pH 7.4: Add 0.010 ml 30% H_2O_2 to 8.8 ml 0.1 M Tris, 0.15 M NaCl, pH 7.4. This dilution should be made immediately before addition to the iodination mixture.

0.10 M 2-ME in 0.1 M Tris, 0.15 M NaCl, pH 7.4: Add 0.010 ml 2-ME to 1.43 ml 0.1 M Tris, 0.15 M NaCl, pH 7.4. This dilution should be made immediately prior to use.

20% BSA: Dissolve 100 mg BSA in 0.5 ml 0.1 M Tris, 0.15 M NaCl, pH 7.4.

PROCEDURE

Keep the reaction volume at less than 0.5 ml and maintain the pH at 7.3–7.4.

1. Neutralization of Na^{125}I solution: To a disposable test tube in a lead pig, add 0.18 ml 0.1 M NaOH, 0.02 ml 1.0 M Tris (pH 7.4), 0.02 ml 1.0 M HCl, and 0.02 ml Na^{125}I in 0.1 M NaOH. Check the pH with pH paper and adjust to 7.3–7.4 if necessary. Dispose of the pH paper in the radioactive waste container. Note: The volume of 0.1 M NaOH is arbitrary and may be changed to fit the situation. If it is changed, the volumes of 1.0 M HCl and 1.0 M Tris must also be adjusted so that the final pH is 7.3–7.4 and the final Tris concentration is 0.1 M.

2. To the neutralized ^{125}I, add 80–500 μg of the protein in a volume of 0.24 ml or less. Add 3–4 μg of purified lactoperoxidase and 0.002 ml of 10 mM H_2O_2. React for 15 minutes at room temperature, mixing frequently.

3. Terminate the iodination by adding 0.010 ml of 0.1 M 2-ME and 0.005 ml 1 M KI. Incubate 15 minutes.

4. After adding 0.04 ml of 20% BSA as carrier protein, separate the protein from the free iodine by passing the mixture through a 10-ml Sephadex G-25 column. Collect 0.5-ml fractions and count the fractions or small aliquots of the fractions in a gamma counter. Pool the void volume fractions containing radioactivity and dialyze against 0.02 M Tris, 0.15 M NaCl, 0.02% sodium azide, pH 7.4. Additional BSA may be added before dialysis to help prevent nonspecific loss of the sample. Dialyze for 3–6 days, changing dialysis buffer daily. The progress of the dialysis may be monitored by counting aliquots of the dialysate. The dialysate, G-25 column, dialysis jar, and test tubes should be disposed of as radioactive wastes.

5. After dialysis, measure the total volume of the iodinated sample with a disposable pipette, count a 0.005–0.010 ml aliquot, and calculate the specific activity (cpm/μg or ng). We usually assume a 90% recovery of the sample.

6. Store the iodinated material at 4°C in a lead pig.

COMMENTS

1. We use a Tris buffer system for the iodination, but it is also possible to use phosphate buffers; they are actually better buffers at pH 7.4. Marchalonis (1969) uses 0.05 M sodium phosphate, 0.15 M NaCl, pH 7.3.

2. For proteins whose antigenic determinants are not destroyed by trichloroacetic acid (TCA), TCA precipitation is a faster way to separate protein from free iodide. Follow the protocol outlined above through step 3; then add 0.020 ml 20% BSA. Calculate the total volume of the reaction mixture and add $\frac{1}{4}$ to $\frac{1}{3}$ volume of 50% TCA. Let sit for 2 hours at 4°C, then centrifuge at 10 000 $\times$ g for 15 minutes in a refrigerated centrifuge. Wash 2× with 0.5 ml of 10% TCA and 3× with cold (-20°C) acetone. Dissolve the pellet in 1.0 ml of 3% BSA in phosphate-buffered saline containing 0.02% azide and 10^{-4} M phenylmethylsulfonylfluoride (see Materials and Reagents, Section 14.4). Count a 0.005-ml aliquot to determine the specific activity.

3. In an attempt to increase the specific activity of certain proteins, we make a second addition of 0.01 M H_2O_2 after the first 15 minutes of incubation. We incubate the reaction mixture for another 10 minutes before terminating the reaction.

REFERENCES

Bogdanove, E. M., and A. M. Strash. 1975. Radioiodine escape is an unexpected source of radioimmunoassay error and chronic low level environmental contamination. *Nature* **257**:427.

Ewan, V. A. 1978. A role for J chain in the activation of B lymphocytes. Ph.D. Dissertation, University of California, Berkeley.

Hubbard, A. L., and Z. A. Cohn. 1976. Specific labels for cell surfaces. In E. H. Maddy, (Ed.), *Biochemical Analysis of Membranes*. Wiley, New York.

Hunter, W. M. 1978. Radioimmunoassay. In D. M. Weir (Ed.), *Handbook of Experimental Immunology*, third edition, Vol. 1. Blackwell Scientific Publications, Oxford.

Maehly, A. C., and B. Chance. 1954. The assay of catalases and peroxidases. *Meth. Biochem. Anal.* **1**:357.

Marchalonis, J. J. 1969. An enzymatic method for the trace iodination of immunoglobulin and other proteins. *Biochem. J.* **113**:299.

Morrison, M., and D. E. Hultquist. 1963. Lactoperoxidase. II. Isolation. *J. Biol. Chem.* **238**:2847.

Yalow, R. S., and S. A. Berson. 1960. Immunoassay of endogenous plasma insulin in man. *J. Clin. Invest.* **13**:1157.

14.4 ASSAY

The basic radioimmunoassay (RIA) protocol is as follows: Labeled antigen is incubated with a limited amount of antibody, usually that amount of antibody which binds 50% of the radiolabeled antigen. Known amounts of unlabeled standard antigen or cellular lysate are added and allowed to inhibit the binding of radiolabeled antigen to antibody. After the removal of free radiolabeled antigen, the amount of radiolabeled antigen bound to antibody is determined. The amount of standard required for 50% inhibition is used to calculate the amount of antigen in the quantity of cellular lysate giving the same amount of inhibition.

In preparing cellular lysates for the RIA, the objective is to maximize the amount of antigen recovered while minimizing changes in the immunological properties of the antigen. A common way of lysing cells is to treat them with detergent, either ionic or nonionic. Although detergents have been shown to inhibit antigen-antibody binding (Crumpton and Parkhouse 1972), it is often possible to select a concentration of detergent that allows recovery of a large percentage of antigen but does not appreciably inhibit the antigen-antibody reaction. We routinely lyse cells with the nonionic detergent Nonidet P40 at a concentration of 1% and then dilute to a concentration of 0.4% during the RIA. The procedure described below was developed to measure nanogram quantities of IgG in rabbit spleen cell lysates. A sample protocol is given in Table 14.1.

MATERIALS AND REAGENTS

Bovine serum albumin (BSA), crystalline (Reheis Chemical)
Purified rabbit IgG
Goat anti–rabbit γ Ig, ammonium sulfate precipitated and DEAE purified (Sections 12.2 and 12.3) (anti-γ Ig is specific for γ chain)
^{125}I-labeled rabbit IgG, specific activity of 1000–10 000 cpm/ng
Normal goat IgG, ammonium sulfate precipitated and DEAE purified
Guinea pig anti–goat IgG serum or immunoglobulin
KH_2PO_4, $M_r = 136.1$
Na_2HPO_4, $M_r = 142.0$

TABLE 14.1
Sample Protocol for IgG RIA on Spleen Lysate

Reagents	Abbreviated Protocol
Rabbit IgG standard: Dilute to 1.0 μg/ml in 0.44% NP40, 1% BSA in PBS Goat anti–rabbit γ Ig: Dilute to a concentration that binds 50% of ^{125}I IgG ^{125}I-labeled rabbit IgG: Dilute so that 0.02 ml contains 4 ng ^{125}I IgG Goat IgG: 1 mg/ml Guinea pig anti–goat IgG serum: 0.04 ml quantitatively precipitates 12 μg IgG Rabbit spleen lysate: 5×10^7 cells/ml Buffer: 0.44% NP40, 1% BSA in PBS	1. Make serial dilutions of rabbit IgG standard and cell lysate. Add buffer and goat anti–rabbit γ Ig. Incubate for 4 hours at 37°C (Step 1). 2. Add ^{125}I-labeled rabbit IgG and incubate 4 hours at 37°C (Step 2). 3. Add goat IgG and guinea pig anti-goat IgG. Incubate overnight at 4°C (Step 3). 4. Determine total number of cpm/tube. 5. Centrifuge and wash the precipitate. 6. Determine the cpm/tube and calculate the percent inhibition.

		Step 1			Step 2		Step 3	
Tube No.	Buffer (ml)	Rabbit IgG Standard (ml)	Buffer (ml)	Goat Anti-Rabbit γ Ig (ml)	^{125}I Rabbit IgG (ml)	Goat IgG (ml)	Guinea Pig Anti-Goat IgG (ml)	Amount of Inhibitor† (ng)
1	—	0.02	0.46	—	0.020	0.012	0.04	—
2	—	—	0.46	0.020	0.020	0.012	0.04	—
3	—	—	0.46	0.020	0.020	0.012	0.04	—
4	—	0.02	0.44	0.020	0.020	0.012	0.04	20.0
5	0.02	0.02*	0.44	0.020	0.020	0.012	0.04	10.0
6	0.02	0.02	0.44	0.020	0.020	0.012	0.04	5.0
7	0.02	0.02	0.44	0.020	0.020	0.012	0.04	2.5
8	0.02	0.02	0.44	0.020	0.020	0.012	0.04	1.3
9	0.02	0.02	0.44	0.020	0.020	0.012	0.04	0.6
10	0.02	0.02 Discard	0.44	0.020	0.020	0.012	0.04	0.3

		Cell Lysate (ml)						Number of Cells‡
11	—	0.02	0.44	0.020	0.020	0.012	0.04	1.0×10^6
12	0.02	0.02*	0.44	0.020	0.020	0.012	0.04	5.0×10^5
13	0.02	0.02	0.44	0.020	0.020	0.012	0.04	2.5×10^5
14	0.02	0.02	0.44	0.020	0.020	0.012	0.04	1.3×10^5
15	0.02	0.02	0.44	0.020	0.020	0.012	0.04	6.3×10^4
16	0.02	0.02	0.44	0.020	0.020	0.012	0.04	3.1×10^4
17	0.02	0.02 Discard	0.44	0.020	0.020	0.012	0.04	1.6×10^4

TABLE 14.1 (continued)

		Step 1			Step 2		Step 3	
Tube No.	Buffer (ml)	Cell Lysate (ml)	Buffer (ml)	Goat Anti-Rabbit γ Ig (ml)	^{125}I Rabbit IgG (ml)	Goat IgG (ml)	Guinea Pig Anti-Goat IgG (ml)	Number of Cells‡
18	—	0.02	0.46	—	0.020	0.012	0.04	1.0×10^6
19	0.02	0.02*	0.46	—	0.020	0.012	0.04	5.0×10^5
20	0.02	0.02	0.46	—	0.020	0.012	0.04	2.5×10^5
21	0.02	0.02	0.46	—	0.020	0.012	0.04	1.3×10^5
22	0.02	0.02	0.46	—	0.020	0.012	0.04	6.3×10^4
23	0.02	0.02	0.46	—	0.020	0.012	0.04	3.1×10^4
24	0.02	0.02 ⟶ Discard	0.46	—	0.020	0.012	0.04	1.6×10^4

* Denotes serial dilutions of rabbit IgG standard or cell lysate.
† Denotes ng of rabbit IgG standard added to the tubes.
‡ Denotes the equivalent number of cells added to the tubes as cell lysate.

NaCl, $M_r = 58.4$

Nonidet P40 (NP40; Particle Data Laboratories)

Phenylmethylsulfonylfluoride (PMSF; Sigma Chemical). Note: Do not breathe in PMSF or get it on your skin.

Ethanol, 95%

NaN$_3$: 0.2% (w/v) in water. Caution: Sodium azide is extremely toxic.

Iodoacetamide, $M_r = 184.9$

Disposable test tubes (Falcon, #2038)

Parafilm

Hamilton syringe, 50 μl (Hamilton)

Pipettes

Disposable gloves

Refrigerated centrifuge

Gamma counter

Volumetric test tube, 1 ml

Buffers and solutions

    0.075 M phosphate, 0.075 M NaCl, pH 7.2: Dissolve 2.45 g KH$_2$PO$_4$, 8.09 g Na$_2$HPO$_4$, and 4.25 g NaCl in 900 ml water. Adjust to pH 7.2 and bring volume to 1000 ml. Note: This buffer is referred to as "PBS" in the following procedure. It is *not the same* as the buffer described in Appendix A.8.

1% NP40 in PBS: Dispense 1 g of NP40 into a 100-ml volumetric flask. Dilute to 100 ml with PBS.

3% BSA, 10^{-4} M PMSF, 0.02% NaN_3 in PBS: Dissolve 1.5 g BSA in 40 ml PBS. Dissolve 1.85 mg PMSF in 0.2 ml 95% ethanol. Add 0.1 ml of the PMSF solution to the BSA solution. Add 0.5 ml 2% NaN_3 (w/v) in water to the BSA solution. Adjust volume of BSA solution to 50 ml with PBS. Note: Do not breathe in PMSF or get it on your skin.

1% NP40, 0.1 M iodoacetamide in PBS: Dissolve 18.5 mg iodoacetamide in 1 ml 1% NP40 immediately before use.

0.42% NP40, 1% BSA in PBS: Mix 4.2 ml 1% NP40, 3.3 ml 3% BSA, and 2.5 ml PBS.

0.44% NP40, 1% BSA in PBS: Mix 4.4 ml 1% NP40, 3.3 ml 3% BSA and 2.3 ml PBS.

PROCEDURE

Titrating the Primary Antibody

The antibody is titrated to determine the amount required to bind 50% of the labeled antigen.

1. Make an appropriate dilution of the goat anti–rabbit γ Ig in 0.42% NP40, 1% BSA. The dilution will depend upon the concentration and affinity of the antibody. For the initial titration, dilute the goat anti–rabbit γ Ig to approximately 0.2 mg/ml.

2. To a series of disposable test tubes, add 0.020 ml 0.42% NP40, 1% BSA in PBS, with a 50-μl Hamilton syringe.

3. Serially dilute 0.020 ml of the goat anti–rabbit γ Ig in the 0.020 ml buffer, again using the Hamilton syringe. Titers vary considerably with different antisera so a large number of dilutions (10–14) should be done in the initial titration. Include controls to which no antiserum is added.

4. Adjust the volume of each tube to 0.48 ml with 0.42% NP40, 1% BSA.

5. Make a dilution of the stock ^{125}I-labeled rabbit IgG in 3.0% BSA such that 0.020 ml contains 4 ng of ^{125}I-IgG.

6. Add 0.020 ml of the ^{125}I-labeled rabbit IgG dilution to each titration tube (total volume is 0.5 ml). Cover the tubes with Parafilm and incubate for 4 hours at 37°C.

7. Separate the free and bound ^{125}I-labeled rabbit IgG by immune precipitation: Add normal goat IgG to each tube so that the total amount of goat IgG (normal goat IgG + goat anti–rabbit γ Ig)

equals 0.012 mg. Add sufficient guinea pig anti–goat IgG to precipitate the goat IgG quantitatively. (This amount is determined in advance by adding varying amounts of guinea pig anti–goat IgG to 0.012 mg normal goat IgG. The amount of guinea pig anti–goat IgG giving the maximum of precipitation is selected.)

8. Determine the total counts added per tube.

9. Incubate overnight at 4°C.

10. Centrifuge at 4300 × g for 15 minutes in a refrigerated centrifuge.

11. Remove the supernatant and discard in radioactive waste container. Add 0.5 ml cold PBS to the pellet and vortex.

12. Centrifuge at 4300 × g for 15 minutes. Remove the supernatant, add 0.3–0.4 ml of 0.5% BSA, and determine the radioactivity in the pellets.

13. Calculate the percentage of counts bound (cpm in pellet/total cpm in tube) and plot versus the antibody dilution. At the lowest dilutions, the curve should plateau with 85–100% of the counts bound. If it does not, there are several possible explanations:

    a. Free ^{125}I may not have been adequately removed from the radiolabeled antigen.

    b. Antigen determinants may have been destroyed during the iodination.

    c. The ^{125}I-labeled antigen is not as pure as the immunizing antigen.

14. Determine the dilution of goat antibody that binds 50% of the ^{125}I-labeled rabbit IgG.

RIA Standard Curve

1. Dilute the purified rabbit IgG that is to be used as a standard to 1.0–2.0 μg/ml in 0.44% NP40, 1% BSA.

2. Add 0.02 ml 0.44% NP40, 1% BSA with a Hamilton syringe to a series of disposable test tubes in which serial dilutions of the rabbit IgG standard are to be performed (tubes 5–10 in Table 14.1).

3. Add 0.02 ml of the standard rabbit IgG solution to tube 4. Add 0.02 ml of the standard rabbit IgG solution to tube 5; mix and transfer 0.02 ml to tube 6. Continue the serial dilutions through tube 10, discarding the final 0.02 ml transfer from tube 10. (A suitable range might be 40–0.5 ng of rabbit IgG per tube.)

4. Set up duplicate uninhibited tubes to which no unlabeled rabbit IgG standard is added (tubes 2 and 3).

5. Set up nonspecific precipitation controls that contain rabbit IgG standard but no antiserum (tube 1).

6. Adjust the volume of tube 1 to 0.48 ml and those of tubes 2–10 to 0.46 ml with 0.44% NP40, 1% BSA.

7. Add 0.02 ml of the dilution of goat anti–rabbit γ Ig that bound 50% of the ^{125}I-labeled rabbit IgG to all tubes except the nonspecific precipitation control (tube 1).

8. Incubate for 4 hours at 37°C.

9. Add 4 ng of ^{125}I-labeled rabbit IgG in 0.020 ml to each tube.

10. Incubate for 4 hours at 37°C.

11. Count, immune precipitate, and wash the pellets as described in steps 7–13 of the titration procedure.

12. Calculate the percent inhibition as follows:

$$\% \text{ inhibition} = \frac{\% \text{ bound in uninhibited control pellet} - \% \text{ bound in sample pellet}}{\% \text{ bound in uninhibited control pellet}} \times 100$$

13. Plot the percent inhibition as a function of the unlabeled rabbit IgG added. The amount required for 50% inhibition is often used for comparison purposes.

Lysing Spleen Cells

1. Wash and pellet 5×10^7 spleen cells in a test tube that will withstand $43\,000 \times g$ centrifugation.

2. To the cell pellet, add 0.45 ml 1% NP40, 0.1 M iodoacetamide. Mix and let stand on ice for 20 minutes.

3. Centrifuge at $43\,000 \times g$ for 30 minutes. Remove the supernatant and place in a 1-ml volumetric test tube. Adjust volume to 1.0 ml with PBS.

RIA-Cellular Lysates

1. The procedure is identical to the standard curve protocol except that varying amounts of cellular lysate are used to inhibit the binding of ^{125}I-labeled rabbit IgG. For the IgG assay, start with 0.020 ml of cell lysate prepared as described, and serially dilute. Tubes 11–17 (Table 14.1) are the experimental lines; tubes 18–24 are controls that do not receive goat anti–rabbit γ Ig.

2. Run a standard curve with each assay (tubes 1–10).

COMMENTS

1. Incubation times are selected to give the desired sensitivity; more or less time may be required with different antibody preparations. Although the labeled antigen may be added at the same time, it has been found that the sensitivity is greater if the unlabeled antigen is incubated with the antibody before the addition of the radio-labeled antigen.

2. The titer of the antibody required to bind 50% of ^{125}I IgG will decrease with time after labeling presumably because of the destruction of the iodinated material. The length of time an iodinated preparation can be used seems to vary. The titer of some preparations drops dramatically in several weeks; the titer of others remains fairly constant for months. If trouble develops (e.g., low percent binding, flat slopes), it is usually the iodinated material that needs to be replaced.

3. In some of our assays, we have had trouble with high nonspecific backgrounds. In most of the IgG and J chain assays, the nonspecific background is 1% of the counts or less. However, in the IgM assays backgrounds of 10–30% have appeared. We have reduced these high backgrounds to 2–5% by decreasing the time between immune precipitation and the washing of the pellet. For example, after the addition of goat IgG and guinea pig anti–goat IgG, the tubes are incubated for 30 minutes at 37°C and for 1 hour at 4°C; they are then centrifuged and washed.

4. Care should be taken in handling the radioactive pellet since escape of radioactive iodine from radiolabeled proteins has been reported (Bogdanove and Strash 1975). We routinely add 0.3–0.4 ml 0.5% BSA to the pellets to prevent the release of the radioactivity into the air.

5. The use of BSA as a carrier protein may not be suitable in all assays.

REFERENCES

Bogdanove, E. M., and A. M. Strash. 1975. Radioiodine escape is an unexpected source of radioimmunoassay error and chronic low level environmental contamination. *Nature* **257**:427.

Brown, J. C., and M. E. Koshland. 1977. Evidence for a long-range conformational change induced by antigen binding to IgM antibody. *Proc. Nat. Acad. Sci.* (USA.) **94**:5682.

Crumpton, M. J., and R. M. E. Parkhouse. 1972. Comparison of the effects of various detergents on antigen–antibody interaction. *FEBS Letters* **22:**210.

Patrick, J. W. 1977. Radiation Safety in the Performance of the Radioimmunoassay. In Guy E. Abraham (Ed.), *Handbook of Radioimmunoassay*. Marcel Dekker, New York.

Selected Surgical Procedures

Jirayr Roubinian

15.1 INTRODUCTION

The ontogeny of the lymphoid system is characterized by an intricate interaction between its component tissues. This interdependency involves tissue interactions within each developing rudiment as well as interactions between separate organs such as the thymus and spleen, the bone marrow, and peripheral lymphoid tissues.

The surgical procedures contained in this chapter can be used to change the cellular composition or alter the function of immune tissues in experimental animals. Thymectomy and skin grafting are two surgical procedures commonly used in immunological studies. Thymectomy has traditionally served as a way of obtaining sources of T depleted lymphoid tissues. In recent years it has been used more frequently to study experimental manipulations of T cells and T cell precursors. Skin grafting has frequently been used both to assess T cell functions and to sensitize donors to histocompatibility antigens. In addition to descriptions of these two procedures, this chapter outlines techniques for splenectomy, castration, and ablation of olfactory function (i.e., anosmia). Splenectomy can be used to study immune regulation and the traffic of lymphocyte populations because the spleen is the major lymphoid organ receiving immunologically active cells. Castration has major effects on the subsequent behavior of immune cells *in vitro,* illustrating the intimate and complex relationships of the immune system to other physiological components of the organism. Anosmia, among other effects, greatly reduces the aggressiveness of male mice and is therefore helpful when such mice are used to raise alloantisera.

15.2 THYMECTOMY

A. Neonatal Thymectomy

MATERIALS AND REAGENTS

Preparation for Thymectomy

Pasteur pipettes
Glass cutter
Bunsen burner
Suction tubing
Plastic tuberculin syringe barrel cut to a length of 5 cm
Beaker, 50 ml
Corkboard, 4 × 5 in., $\frac{1}{4}$ in. thick
Adhesive tape (one-sided masking tape is good)
Flask, 500 ml

Anesthesia

Pan containing crushed ice

Thymectomy

70% ethanol
Parlodion-gentian violet solution (Appendix A.16)
Silver nitrate applicators, 75% silver nitrate, 25% potassium nitrate
   (Arzol Chemical)
Dissecting microscope and light source
Scissors, fine-tipped, straight-edged
Forceps, fine-tipped, ophthalmic
Prepared Pasteur pipettes and suction apparatus
6-0 silk sutures
Suture needle holder, small
Cotton-tip applicator

Post-thymectomy

Lamp to warm mice

PROCEDURE

Preparation for Thymectomy

1. Select wide-bored Pasteur pipettes. Cut off the distal half inch of each pipette (the remaining tip should be approximately 8 mm long with a 1–1.5-mm diameter bore). Bend the remaining narrow portion to 45° by gently heating on the burner. Carefully fire polish the tip without sealing the pipette. Prepare at least 5 pipettes and place them in a cotton-lined box.

2. Attach the pipette to the suction apparatus. To achieve adequate control of suction intensity, make a 3-mm hole in a 5-cm plastic tuberculin syringe barrel and place the barrel between the pipette and the tubing leading to the vacuum. Control the suction by appropriate placement of a finger over the hole. Suction intensity, which should be low, can be tested by dipping the tip in a beaker full of water. The water should gently bubble in the pipette.

3. Place two strips of tape on the corkboard, with gummed side facing up, and fasten their ends to the underside of the corkboard with more tape.

4. Allow neonates to nurse prior to the planned surgery. Milk is usually visible in the stomach after nursing.

Anesthesia

1. Anesthetize the neonates by covering them up to the neck with finely crushed ice (1 min/day of age, up to 3 minutes). The anesthesia will last for approximately 3 minutes. After cooling, dry the animal and place it on the taped board, with its back on the tape. Spread the limbs and fasten them to the tape.

Thymectomy

1. Set the dissecting microscope magnification at 1.6X. Swab the neck and upper chest area of the neonate with ethanol. Make a midline incision extending from the chin to the xyphoid process and reflect the skin to expose the thoracic cage (Figure 15.1). Move the submandibular glands laterally. Remaining on the left border of the sternum, gently cut into the sixth intercostal space. Keeping the tip of the scissors in an upward direction (the heart is directly underneath), extend the incision upward to separate the bony thorax. Extend the incision further to separate the neck muscles. Dissect the connective tissue that forms the superior mediastinal border.

2. The thymic lobes should be visible as two flat, flask-shaped structures occupying the superior mediastinum on either side of the

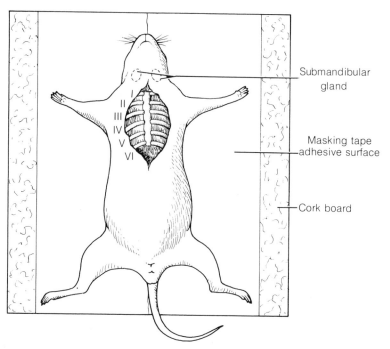

FIGURE 15.1
Exposure of the thoracic cage.

median plane (Figure 15.2). To appreciate the position occupied
by the lobes, separate the borders of the transected bony thorax.
The lobes lie behind the sternum and are covered superiorly by
the converging pleura. They lie anterior to the great vessels at the
base of the heart and extend down halfway over the heart.

3. With gentle suction on the pipette, engage each thymic lobe at the
lower pole and gently tease it off. The removal process must be
deliberate, steady, and entirely visualized under the microscope.
Since the aortic arch and its branches, as well as the major veins,
are situated behind the thymic lobes (Figure 15.3), excessive pressure on the pipette tip should be avoided. At times, sudden and
significant bleeding develops, filling the mediastinal cavity. This is
commonly caused by either an excessively forceful suction that
disrupts a major artery or a chipped Pasteur pipette. Inspect the
tip of the pipette under a microscope to rule out this latter
possibility.

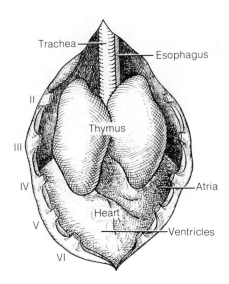

FIGURE 15.2
Contents of the superior mediastinum.

4. After removing the thymic lobes, carefully inspect the mediastinal cavity for remnants. If there are large remnants, discard the animal and start anew. If there are small remnants, an attempt may be made to remove them.

5. Release the upper limbs of the animal from the tape. Using 6-0 silk suture material, approximate the skin edges together. Three or four *interrupted* stitches will be necessary to adequately close the incision. At times, nursing mothers will bite and cut a suture and if the suturing has been continuous, the incision will open. However, with interrupted suturing, a break in one stitch will not result in the complete exposure of the incision.

6. Cover the incision with Parlodion-gentian violet solution. Parlodion forms a protective gelatin covering over the wound, while the gentian violet is for antisepsis.

7. Experimental animals can be distinguished from sham-operated ones by tail or ear clipping. Stop bleeding that results from the clipping by chemical cautery with silver nitrate.

Post-thymectomy

1. After surgery, warm the mice under a lamp and allow them to regain their normal respiratory activity and pink color. They

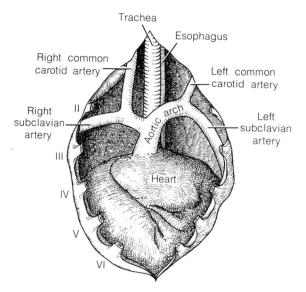

FIGURE 15.3
The aortic arch and its branches
(veins, located next to the arteries,
are not shown).

should react briskly to very gentle tactile stimuli. An irregular breathing pattern with visible thoracic contractions may be
a sign of surgical laceration of the trachea. This could result from
pointing the tip of the scissors downward while incising the chest
wall. If tracheal damage is present, the animal will not survive.

2. The nursing mother should be in a familiar cage. Since mice recognize and assess their environment through pheromones, it is
best *not* to change the cage. Placing a nursing mother with surgi-
cally treated suckling mice in a new cage can delay nursing and
increase the likelihood of cannibalization. If a new cage must be
used, transfer some of the wood shavings from the old cage to the
new one.

3. Stimulate the neonates to activate them and observe for bleeding.
Cover dried or fresh blood on the skin with Parlodion-gentian
violet solution to prevent cannibalization. Liberally apply Parlodion-gentian violet solution to the nostrils of the nursing mother
to prevent her from smelling blood and foreign odors. The nostrils
will not become obstructed because the animal begins to expel the
solution immediately.

4. Arrange the neonates in a group at the side of the cage, away from
the tip of the water bottle and cover them with wood shavings.

Place the cage in a dark and quiet environment for 24 to 48 hours, before transferring it back to the colony. Briefly examine the cage 3 to 6 hours later. If the mother has scattered the neonates and appears disinterested in nursing, gather and cover them again.

5. If a nursing mother cannibalizes the entire litter, one of the following should be considered: (a) The mother may have been agitated (noisy environment, bright lighting); or (b) blood from one mouse may have smeared onto other mice as a result of delayed postoperative bleeding. A nursing mother will not tolerate the smell of blood on the neonates. It is of utmost importance that there is no bleeding around the stitches of the neonates prior to their return to the mother.

COMMENTS

It is important to determine that the thymectomy results in complete removal of the gland. Two steps can be taken to confirm the operator's technique:

1. Perform the thymectomy procedure on at least 20 neonates. Starting with postoperative day 5, perform a complete autopsy on one animal each day to determine if any thymic remnants are present. The examination should not be confined to the mediastinal cavity. A common, yet unsuspected, site is the posterior aspect of the thoracic cavity. Since opening the mediastinal cavity invariably results in bilateral collapse of the lungs, thymic remnants left behind tend to fall by gravity into the posterior aspect of the chest cavity. Upon closure of the incision, the lungs expand and cover them. If subsequent examination is confined to the mediastinum, such remnants will be missed. Suspicious tissues must be examined histologically.

2. T cell depletion must be assessed by performing a histological evaluation of secondary lymphoid organs (spleen, lymph nodes) and by assessing small lymphocyte depletion in the so-called thymus-dependent areas. In addition, T cell depletion can be assessed by functional tests, such as the humoral response to sheep erythrocytes, or by fluorescent staining with T specific antisera.

B. Perinatal and Adult Thymectomy

MATERIALS AND REAGENTS

Nembutal, 50 mg/ml (Wellcome Reagents Division): Dilute to 6.7 mg/ml in water for injection.

70% ethanol
Parlodion-gentian violet (Appendix A.16)
Corkboard
Tape
Fine-tipped, straight-edged scissors
Blunt-edged forceps, 2
Surgical metal clips
Metal clipper
Tuberculin syringe, 1 ml, glass
25- or 26-gauge needle
Cotton balls
Lamp to warm mice

PROCEDURE

1. Swab the abdominal wall of the mouse with 70% ethanol.

2. Anesthetize the mouse by intraperitoneal injection of diluted Nembutal. Weigh the mouse to calculate an accurate dose of anesthetic. For mice older than 4 weeks, the dose is 0.01 ml/g of body weight. For mice between 2–4 weeks old, a lower dose of 0.005–0.007 ml/g of body weight is best. (If the procedure is of short duration it is safer to inject a smaller dose than that calculated.) Use a *glass* tuberculin syringe for the injection since it is much easier to control than a plastic one. Insert the needle over the lower third of the abdomen along the midline and point the needle towards the upper quadrant to avoid the liver, which is situated in the upper right quadrant. The mouse is usually asleep within 2–5 minutes. (When working with nursing mice, it is advisable to perform the surgical procedures early in the day to allow the mice to recover fully from Nembutal anesthesia before they are returned to their mothers. If the mice are transferred in a somnolent state, the likelihood of cannibalization increases.)

3. Place the mouse on its back on the corkboard and immobilize it by taping its stretched limbs to the board.

4. Swab the neck region with ethanol. Using the scissors, make an incision extending from the xyphoid process to the submandibular region. Reflect the skin edges laterally (Figure 15.1).

5. Remaining as close to the midline as possible, enter the 5th intercostal space and start the thoracic incision. Always point the edge of the scissors upward (even if the chest wall must be lifted). Extend the incision toward the manubrium and beyond it to sepa-

rate the upper cervical muscles. The process of making the surgical incision should not result in bleeding or collapse of the lungs.

6. Gently separate the edges of the incision. The upper and lower
poles of the thymic lobes should be visible under the fine
mediastinal-pleural covering (Figure 15.2).

7. With the forceps in one hand, separate the edges of the incised
chest wall. This will expose the lower poles of the thymic lobes.
Using the second pair of forceps in the other hand, gently grasp
the thymic lobes at the lower pole and lift. As the lobes are lifted
with the forceps in one hand, they are kept retracted with the
forceps in the other hand. The process of lifting the lobes pro-
ceeds from the lower pole towards the upper pole.

8. One has 15–30 seconds to remove the thymic lobes because the
lungs will invariably collapse with the initial attempts to lift them.
However, although speed is required, the procedure must be
performed very gently to prevent disruption of a major blood
vessel.

9. After removing the thymic lobes, separate the edges of the incision and take a quick glance to make sure there are no thymic
remnants.

10. Immediately grasp the skin edges of the incision and compress
them tightly to seal the opening of the thoracic cavity. As the
animal gasps for air and expands its lungs, negative intrathoracic
pressure is re-established.

11. Hold the skin edges compressed together for at least 2 minutes,
during which time the animal should resume a normal respiratory
rhythm and rate. Breathing should not be labored.

12. Clip the skin edges together with metallic surgical clips, covering
the entire surgical wound. Apply Parlodion-gentian violet solution to the incision.

13. Place the animal on its left side, under a lamp. Full recovery from
the anesthesia and surgery takes approximately 60 minutes.

14. Return nursing mice to their mothers by the procedure described
in Section 15.2A.

REFERENCES

Miller, J. F. A. P. 1964. The thymus and the development of immunulogic
responsiveness. *Science* **144**:1544.
Miller, J. F. A. P. 1965. Effects of thymectomy in adult mice on immunological responsiveness. *Nature* **208**:1337.

15.3 SKIN GRAFTING

MATERIALS AND REAGENTS

Preparation of Skin to be Grafted

70% ethanol
Electric hair cutter
Cotton balls
Scissors, straight-edged
Forceps, straight-tipped
Corkboard and pins
Dulled round-edged knife or scalpel
Whatman #1 filter paper
Cork borer, No. 8 (sharp-edged)
Petri dish, large, filled with cold, sterile saline (0.85% NaCl, w/v)
Crushed ice

Grafting Procedure

Nembutal, 50 mg/ml (Wellcome Reagents Division): Dilute to 6.7
    mg/ml in water for injection.
Neosporin ophthalmic solution
70% ethanol
Electric hair cutter
Masking tape
Curved scissors with serrated edges
Curved forceps
Blunt-nosed scissors
Sterile gauze squares, 2 × 2 in.
Ventilated tape (Johnson and Johnson, Air Vent Tape, 1 × 150 in.)
Owen's cloth (Davis-Geck Division)
Telfa nonadhesive pads
Tuberculin syringe, 1 ml, glass
25- or 26-gauge needle

PROCEDURE

Preparation of Skin to be Grafted

1. Kill donor mouse by cervical dislocation.
2. Shave hair of donor animal as completely as possible, without
   nicking the skin. Wet a cotton ball with 70% ethanol and swab the
   donor to remove loose hair.
3. Make a cylindrical, cufflike incision around the extremities and

neck followed by a dorso-ventral incision. Remove the skin from the body.

4. Place the skin, with its hair surface down, on a cork dissecting board and pin it in place. Scrape the undersurface to remove the fatty layer and the panniculus carnosus, using a dulled, round-edged knife or scalpel.

5. Place the skin onto a piece of Whatman #1 filter paper, with the hair surface up, gently spreading and pressing it so it adheres firmly to the paper.

6. With a No. 8 cork borer and a firm, circular motion, punch out uniform circles of skin and their filter paper backing. Place the punched, circular grafts in a large Petri dish filled with cold, sterile saline solution so that they float with their hair surface up.

Grafting Procedure

1. Swab the abdomen of the recipient with 70% ethanol and anesthetize the mouse by the procedure described in Section 15.2B.

2. Shave the recipient from its axillae to halfway down its back and swab it thoroughly with 70% ethanol to remove loose hair.

3. Tape the recipient, abdomen down, on a clean corkboard, stretching its limbs before taping them down, to ensure a taut skin surface. Turn the corkboard so that the animal's head faces the hand of the operator that will be used for cutting the graft bed.

4. Press the animal's rib cage forward (to make the skin firm) with one hand and snip through the superficial dermis and epidermis with the other hand. Curved scissors with serrated edges must be used. The diameter of the graft bed should be 1–3 mm larger than the graft.

5. Remove the prepared graft from the saline and filter paper with the curved forceps, and place it on the prepared bed. If the edges of the graft curl, flatten and spread it evenly.

6. Using a sterile 2 × 2-in. gauze pad, gently press the graft on its bed to remove the excess saline. This enables the graft to adhere to the bed firmly.

7. Place two drops of Neosporin ophthalmic solution on the graft.

8. Cover the exposed graft with a 2 × 2-cm piece of Owen's cloth. Onto the Owen's cloth, place a 2 × 2-cm square of Telfa non-adhesive pad.

9. Tear off approximately 3 in. of ventilated tape. Hold the top and

the bottom of the tape in the tips of the thumb and forefinger of the left and right hand respectively. Place the bottom of the tape in contact with the Owen's cloth-Telfa pad and press it in place. Carry the tape completely around the animal's body. Apply tension to compress the rib cage slightly and fasten the free edge of the tape to the other tape edge by direct pressure. Avoid blocking the air vents to the graft. The graft thus receives a dirt-proof, aerated cover.

10. Nine days later, remove the bandages by anesthetizing the recipient and cutting the tape on the ventral side with a blunt-nosed scissors. Pull the tape away by applying tension posteriorly (any other way will tear the animal's skin under the forelimbs). Wet the Telfa pad-Owen's cloth with 2–3 drops of sterile saline prior to removing them, to avoid disrupting the graft.

11. Analyze the grafted skin for the following characteristics: the size that it occupies on the bed; the presence of erythema, crusting, and purulent discharge; and the status of the hair on the grafted skin. Using a toothpick, apply gentle pressure on the grafted skin. If the pressure produces a "soft" sensation, it is a sign of a healthy "take"; a firm, boardlike sensation may mean an early rejection of the graft. Examine the grafted skin daily. If there is any open area around the graft bed, the graft should be covered as before. The grafted skin may be devoured by the other mice if a number of animals are housed in the same cage.

15.4 SPLENECTOMY

MATERIALS AND REAGENTS

Corkboard
Tape
Scissors, fine-tipped, straight-edged
6-0 silk suture material
Small suture needle holder
Cotton swabs
70% ethanol
Cotton balls
Electrocautery, with fine tip
Pan filled with finely crushed ice
Nembutal, 50 mg/ml (Wellcome Reagents Division): Dilute to 6.7 mg/ml in water for injection.

Tuberculin syringe, 1 ml, glass
Needle, 25 or 26 gauge
Parlodion-gentian violet (Appendix A.16)

PROCEDURE

1. The procedure, with minor variations, is applicable to neonates as well as adults. Anesthetize the neonates by placing them in ice as described in Section 15.2A. Anesthetize mice older than 7 days by intraperitoneal injection of diluted Nembutal as described in Section 15.2B.

2. After anesthesia, place the animal on its right side. Immobilize neonates by placing them on the taped corkboard and adults by taping the tips of their limbs to the corkboard.

3. Both right limbs should be perpendicular to the long axis of the body. The left foreleg should be taped after it is stretched toward the head; the left hind leg should be taped after it is stretched toward the tail. This maneuver exposes the left upper quadrant of the abdomen. Swab the abdomen with 70% ethanol.

4. Make the abdominal incision right above the iliac crest. Always determine the border of the left costal (chest) margin before making the incision. To avoid the development of pneumothorax (collapsed lungs), do not make the incision close to the costal margin.

5. After the skin incision, reflect the edges laterally to expose the abdominal wall. Remaining close to the iliac crest, incise the muscle layers. The incision should extend from the midline of the anterior abdominal wall towards the left costovertebral angle.

6. In neonates, the spleen appears as reddish, flat tissue overlying the stomach, which should be filled with milk and thus appear white. (Neonates should always be allowed to nurse prior to surgery.) In adults, the spleen is a sizeable structure, reddish in color, that overlies the left kidney and borders the greater curvature of the stomach.

7. Remove the spleen of neonates with electrocautery. The intensity of the heat in the tip should be moderate (scale of 3 over 6). Care should be taken not to traumatize the stomach. Gently lift the spleen at its lower pole and cauterize the inferior vascular bundle. This allows further mobilization of the organ. Cauterize the superior vascular bundle next. This frees the spleen, which can then be removed intact. Initially, it is helpful to remove the spleen with the aid of a dissecting microscope. However, with experience, magnification becomes unnecessary.

8. With adult mice, gently exteriorize the spleen at its inferior pole to expose the inferior vascular bundles. It is more efficacious and safer to tie the blood vessels than to cauterize them. Cauterization is possible but one must expose the vessels to the heat for 30–60 seconds in order to obtain an adequate hemostasis. After sectioning the vessels that supply the lower pole of the spleen, move the organ to expose the blood vessels of the upper pole. Tie the vascular bundle with silk suture, transect the organ, and remove the spleen. There should be no bleeding in the surgical wound.

9. Suture the abdominal wall with a continuous suture. Approximate the skin edges with interrupted sutures. Treat the incision with Parlodion-gentian violet.

10. Return nursing mice to their mothers by the procedure described in Section 15.2A.

REFERENCE

Battisto, J. R., and J. W. Streilein, Eds. 1976. *Immuno-aspects of the Spleen.* Elsevier/North Holland, Amsterdam.

15.5 CASTRATION

Sex hormones influence many immunological responses in both normal and abnormal strains of mice. Females manifest heightened immune responsiveness when compared to males. This is observed in enhanced antibody or serum levels of IgA, IgM, and IgG, enhanced antibody formation both in primary and secondary immune responses, and enhanced mixed-lymphocyte reactions. It is also easier to induce immunological tolerance in males than females. Both androgens and estrogens produce lymphoid atrophy. Conversely, castration of males and females has been associated with lymphoid hyperplasia.

Sex hormones also appear to play an important role in autoimmunity. For example, NZB/NZW mice, a laboratory model for systemic lupus erythematosus, are greatly influenced by the administration of sex hormones. All female B/W mice spontaneously develop, after 4 months of age, a lupus-like disorder characterized by the formation of antibodies to nucleic acids and the development of immune complex nephritis; death occurs between 8 and 12 months of age. Males develop a similar disease later in life. Androgens appear to suppress autoimmunity in B/W mice, while estrogens appear to worsen the disease process.

MATERIALS AND REAGENTS

Nembutal, 50 mg/ml (Wellcome Reagents Division): Dilute to 6.7 mg/ml in water for injection.

Parlodian-gentian violet (Appendix A.16)

70% ethanol

Scissors, straight-tipped

Forceps, fine, surgical

6-0 silk sutures

Small suture needle holder

Electrocautery with fine tip

Corkboard

Tape

Cotton balls

Tuberculin syringe, 1 ml, glass

Needle, 25 or 26 gauge

Surgical metal clips

Metal clipper

Cotton-tip applicators

PROCEDURE

Castration can be performed on 5–7-day-old mice with the aid of a microscope and on mice older than 2 weeks without a microscope. If mice are 2 weeks or younger, perform the surgical procedure early in the day, since recovery from the anesthetic can take 2–3 hours. Follow the procedure described in Section 15.2A when returning suckling mice to their mothers.

Castration of Males (Orchiectomy)

1. Swab the abdomen with 70% ethanol. Anesthetize 5–7-day-old mice in ice as described in Section 15.2A and older mice by Nembutal injection as described in Section 15.2B.

2. When fully anesthetized, place each mouse on its back and tape its limbs to the corkboard. The testicles and/or the scrotal sac can be identified above the tail and anal opening. If the testes cannot be palpated or visualized, gentle pressure over the abdomen will force the testes to emerge in the scrotal sac. Cleanse scrotal area with 70% ethanol.

3. Using fine surgical scissors, make an incision over the scrotal sac. The incision must be situated halfway between the anal opening and the penis. It must be a straight incision, not an irregular one.

4. Dissect the scrotal sac bluntly with the scissor tips and make a

small incision over the tunica vaginalis (the sac covering the testis). Gentle pressure over the abdomen will deliver the testis out of the tunica vaginalis.

5. Identify the spermatic cord that contains the vas deferens and the spermatic vessels. With electrocautery, transect the spermatic cord distal to the epididymis, so that the testes, epididymis, and gubernaculum are removed.

6. Approximate the edges of the scrotal sac using the 6-0 silk sutures. Treat the incision with Parlodion-gentian violet.

Castration of Females (Oophorectomy)

1. Swab the abdomen with 70% ethanol and anesthetize the mouse as described in 15.2A or 15.2B.

2. Place the mouse on the corkboard, *on its abdomen,* so that its back faces the operator and tape its limbs to the corkboard.

3. With fine surgical scissors, make the incision over the midline, and extend it from the midback downward toward the tail. By blunt dissection, separate the skin from the abdominal wall on the back.

4. Identify the kidneys on both sides. The ovaries are situated over the lower poles of the kidneys. They appear as pinkish, punctate masses. Incise the abdominal wall over the ovaries.

5. Using a fine opthalmic forceps, gently hold each ovary separately, and deliver it out of the abdominal cavity. Identify the uterine horn to which the ovary is attached. Using the electrocautery, transect the uterine horn distal to the ovary and remove the ovary with periovarian fat.

6. After removing both ovaries, close the skin with surgical steel clips. Cover the area with Parlodion-gentian violet.

REFERENCES

Eidinger, D., and T. J. Garret. 1972. Studies of the regulatory effects of the sex hormones on antibody formation and stem cell differentiation. *J. Exp. Med.* **136:**1098.

Castro, J. E. 1974. Orchidectomy and the immune response. *Proc. R. Soc. Lond. B.* **185:**425.

Roubinian, J. R., N. Talal, J. S. Greenspan, J. R. Goodman, and P. K. Siiteri. 1978. Effect of castration and sex hormone treatment on survival, anti–nucleic acid antibodies, and glomerulonephritis in NZB/NZW F_1 mice. *J. Exp. Med.* **147:**1568.

15.6 INDUCTION OF ANOSMIA

Olfactory stimuli control some aspects of animal behavior. Complete elimination of olfactory sensation can be achieved by either surgical ablation of the olfactory bulbs or chemical destruction of the olfactory nerve endings. Induction of anosmia causes disruption of sexual, maternal, territorial, and aggressive activities in various species. It is very useful as a method to prevent male mice from behaving aggressively when caged together. Elimination of olfaction prevents them from fighting with each other, thereby removing a main cause of infected skin lesions and debilitation.

MATERIALS AND REAGENTS

Chemical Anosmia

Saline: 0.85% NaCl (w/v)
$ZnSO_4$: 7.6% (w/v) in saline

Olfactory Bulbectomy

Nembutal, 50 mg/ml (Wellcome Reagents Division): Dilute to 6.7 mg/ml in water for injection.
70% ethanol
Tuberculin syringe, 1 ml, glass
Needle, 25 or 26 gauge
Scissors, fine, straight-tipped
6-0 silk suture
Small suture needle holder
Electrocautery with fine tip
Corkboard
Tape (masking tape is suitable)

PROCEDURE

Chemical Anosmia

1. Hold the mouse firmly in one hand with the head completely immobilized.
2. Instill 3–5 drops of $ZnSO_4$ solution into each nostril, drop by drop.
3. Perform 3 intranasal treatments with zinc sulfate, spaced 5 days apart. This will cause most strains to become permanently anosmic. However, some strains (e.g., SJL) may require additional treatments on a weekly or biweekly basis, if aggressive behavior appears.

Olfactory Bulbectomy

1. Swab the abdominal wall of the mice with 70% ethanol and anesthetize them by intraperitoneal injection of Nembutal as described in Section 15.2B. Place each mouse on a corkboard with its abdominal surface down and immobilize it by taping its limbs to the board.

2. Make a midline incision extending from the tip of the nose towards the top of the mouse's forehead (to the line that forms between the ears) and dissect the skin from the cranium. Identify two cranial humps superior and medial to the eyes. The olfactory bulbs are located under the calvarium.

3. Using a sharp scissors, make a hole in the calvarium over the humps. Slight bleeding is no cause for alarm. Place the electrocautery tip in the hole made in the humps and cauterize to a depth of 1–2 mm.

4. Suture the skin edges with 6-0 silk.

REFERENCES

Schoots, A. F. 1978. Zinc-induced peripheral anosmia and exploratory behavior in two mouse strains. *Physiol. Behav.* **21:**779.

Slotnick, B. M. 1977. Evaluation of intranasal zinc sulfate treatment on olfactory discrimination in rats. *J. Comp. Physiol. Psychol.* **91:**942.

Preparation of Hapten-Modified
Protein Antigens

Material for this chapter was prepared on the basis of contributions from
Anne H. Good, Leon Wofsy, Claudia Henry, and John Kimura

16.1 INTRODUCTION

Hapten-modified antigens are commonly used both in immunochemistry and cellular immunology because of the many advantages of working with antigens that have known chemical groups as major antigenic determinants (see also Sections 2.5 and 2.6). This chapter contains a number of procedures for the hapten modification of protein antigens. The degree of modification achieved in a given case can be controlled (within limits) by appropriate selection of the conditions used for modification. However, if a particular degree of haptenation is desired, it may be necessary to determine the exact conditions experimentally using the following representative procedures as guides. The methods used for the hapten modification of antigens are less stringent than those used for the hapten modification of antibodies (Section 13.2) because the preservation of active sites is usually not relevant when modifying antigens.

16.2 MODIFICATION OF KEYHOLE LIMPET
HEMOCYANIN WITH AZOPHENYL HAPTENS

The following procedures describe the modification of keyhole limpet hemocyanin (KLH) with *p*-azophenyl-β-D-lactoside (Lac), *p*-azophenyl-

343

β-D-glucoside (Glu), or p-azophenyl-arsonate (Ars). The reaction conditions are designed to couple approximately 40 mol of hapten groups per 100 000 g of KLH. (The molecular weight of KLH is 8×10^6.)

MATERIALS AND REAGENTS

Keyhole limpet hemocyanin (KLH): Prepare by the method described in Garvey et al. (1977) or obtain commercially (Calbiochem); $\epsilon_{280}^{0.1\%} = 2.02$

p-aminophenyl-β-D-lactoside, $M_r = 433$, *or*
p-aminophenyl-β-D-glucoside, $M_r = 271$, *or*
arsanilic acid, recrystallized, $M_r = 217$
NaNO$_2$, $M_r = 69.0$
1 M HCl
NaOH, $M_r = 40.0$: 0.1 M, 1.0 M, and 5 M solutions
H$_3$BO$_3$, $M_r = 61.8$
Test tubes and flat-bottom vials
pH paper
Dialysis tubing
Sephadex G-25 column, $\sim 1.5 \times 35$ cm (Pharmacia Fine Chemicals)
Ice bucket
Magnetic stirrer with flea bar
Buffers
  0.5 M borate buffer, pH 8.6: Dissolve 30.9 g H$_3$BO$_3$ and 6 g NaOH in 900 ml water. Adjust to pH 8.6 with 1 M NaOH. Bring volume to 1000 ml.
  0.3 M, 0.05 M and 0.01 M borate buffers, pH 8.6: Dilute the 0.5 M borate buffer, pH 8.6, to the appropriate concentration. Readjust to pH 8.6 if required.

PROCEDURE

1. Dialyze KLH ($\sim$ 50 mg/ml) against 0.5 M borate, pH 8.6.

2. Prepare diazonium reagent: Dissolve 0.14 mmol p-aminophenyl-β-D-lactoside (60 mg), or p-aminophenyl-β-D-glucoside (38 mg), or arsanilic acid (30 mg) in 0.35 ml *ice cold* 1 M HCl. Keep solution on ice. Add 10 mg NaNO$_2$ dissolved in 0.65 ml ice cold water. Let mixture react for 15–20 minutes on ice.

3. Place 2 ml of KLH solution (100 mg) in a flat-bottom vial with a magnetic flea bar and stir solution on ice. Slowly add 0.9 ml of diazonium reagent drop by drop to the KLH solution. Check pH with pH paper and maintain between pH 8.5 and pH 9.0 with 5 M

NaOH. After 1–2 hours of stirring, allow reaction mixture to stand overnight at 4°C.

4. Place reaction mixture on a Sephadex G-25 column equilibrated with 0.05 M borate buffer, pH 8.0. Elute and pool the colored front material. Store at 4°C. Membrane filter preparation if required (Appendix C.2).

16.3 MODIFICATION OF KEYHOLE LIMPET HEMOCYANIN WITH TRINITROPHENYL HAPTEN

When sodium trinitrobenzene sulfonate (TNBS) is used for the haptenation reaction, modification of keyhole limpet hemocyanin (KLH) occurs exclusively at free amino groups. The procedure described below normally yields a protein substituted with 7–8 mol of trinitrophenyl haptens (TNP) per 100 000 g of KLH. The degree of haptenation can be varied by varying the ratio of TNBS to protein, the reaction time, the temperature, or the pH. The exact conditions needed to obtain a desired degree of modification must be determined experimentally.

MATERIALS AND REAGENTS

Keyhole limpet hemocyanin (KLH): Prepare by the methods described in Garvey et al. (1977) or obtain commercially (Calbiochem); $\epsilon_{280}^{0.1\%} = 2.02$

2,4,6-trinitrobenzene sulfonic acid (TNBS; Sigma Chemical): trihydrate, $M_r = 347$; anhydrous, $M_r = 293$

H_3BO_3, $M_r = 61.8$

$NaH_2PO_4 \cdot H_2O$, $M_r = 138.0$

$Na_2HPO_4 \cdot 7H_2O$, $M_r = 268.1$

NaCl, $M_r = 58.4$

0.15 M NaOH (6 g/liter)

AG1-X8 resin (Bio-Rad Laboratories)

Dialysis tubing

Magnetic stirrer and bar

Aluminum foil

UV spectrophotometer

Buffers

Borate-buffered saline (BBS; Appendix A.9)

0.001 M phosphate buffer, pH 7.4: Dilute the 0.15 M phosphate buffer described in Appendix A.12 150-fold with water. Readjust to pH 7.4 if required.

PROCEDURE

1. Dialyze about 100 mg of KLH against BBS overnight. Readjust protein concentration to about 20 mg/ml. Centrifuge the KLH solution at 13 000 × g for 20 minutes to remove insoluble material. Dilute an aliquot of the KLH solution to 0.1–0.2 mg/ml in BBS and measure its absorbance at 280 nm to determine the protein concentration.

2. Prepare a 15 mg/ml TNBS solution in BBS. Add 38 μg TNBS per mg of KLH (drop by drop and with stirring) to the KLH solution. Wrap the container with aluminum foil to shield the reaction mixture from light and stir the mixture gently at room temperature for 2 hours.

3. Terminate the reaction by passing the reaction mixture over a column of AG1-X8 resin equilibrated with BBS. Use about 5 ml of resin per 100 mg KLH.

4. Combine all protein fractions and dialyze against 0.001 M phosphate buffer, pH 7.4, for two days at 4°C (change diluent 2–3 times a day). Centrifuge the protein solution at 13 000 × g for 20 minutes to remove insoluble material.

5. Dilute an aliquot of the KLH solution to approximately 0.1–0.2 mg/ml in phosphate buffer and measure absorbance at 280 nm and 340 nm. Determine the protein concentration and number of TNP groups by the following calculations:

    a. Extinction coefficients:

    KLH* (per 100 000 g) $\epsilon_{280} = 2.02 \times 10^5$;

    $\epsilon_{340} = 0.257 \times \epsilon_{280}^{KLH}$

    TNP (as mono-ϵ-TNP-lysine; $\epsilon_{280} = 0.337 \times \epsilon_{340}^{TNP}$

    molar extinction) $\epsilon_{340} = 1.25 \times 10^4$.

    b. Equations for contributions of protein and TNP-lysine residues to the absorbance of TNP-KLH at 280 nm and 340 nm:

    $$OD_{280} = [KLH](2.02 \times 10^5) + [TNP](.337)(1.25 \times 10^4);$$

    $$OD_{340} = [KLH](.257)(2.02 \times 10^5) + [TNP](1.25 \times 10^4).$$

---

* KLH dissociates reversibly into subunits. Therefore, to avoid ambiguity, the degree of haptenation is expressed in moles of hapten per 100 000 g of KLH rather than in moles of hapten per mole of KLH.

Solve equations for concentration of KLH (in 100 000 g units per liter) and TNP (in moles per liter):

$$[KLH] = \frac{(OD_{280}) - (.337)(OD_{340})}{1.85 \times 10^5} \, ;$$

$$[TNP] = \frac{(OD_{340}) - (.257)(OD_{280})}{1.14 \times 10^4} \, .$$

  c. The number of moles of TNP per 100 000 g KLH is obtained by dividing the TNP concentration by the KLH concentration. The concentration of the protein in g/liter or mg/ml is obtained by multiplying the KLH concentration (in 100 000 g units per liter) by 100 000.

6. Sterilize TNP-KLH solution by membrane filtration, aliquot into tubes, and store at $-20°C$. Wrap the tubes with aluminum foil to block out light.

COMMENT

The degree of substitution achieved can be varied by changing the amount of TNBS. If 140 μg TNBS per mg KLH is used, about 19 mol of TNP per 100 000 g KLH are coupled; and if 14 μg TNBS per mg KLH are used, about 2 mol of TNP are coupled.

16.4 MODIFICATION OF BOVINE GAMMA GLOBULIN WITH DINITROPHENYL HAPTEN

Dinitrophenylated bovine gamma globulin (DNP-BGG) is simple to prepare and elicits antibodies of high affinity. DNP-BGG can also be used to generate a population of B cells primed to DNP, which can then be used in conjunction with T cells primed to another carrier (e.g., KLH). When sodium dinitrobenzene sulfonate (DNBS) is used for haptenation, modification of the protein occurs almost exclusively at the free amino groups of lysine residues. High pH is essential for efficient conjugation since protonation of the amino groups will interfere with the reaction. For heavily haptenated conjugates, a 10-fold molar excess of DNBS over moles of lysine residues in the protein is usually satisfactory. The procedure outlined below normally yields a product containing 30–50 dinitrophenyl (DNP) groups per molecule of BGG. The degree of modification can be varied by varying the conditions of the coupling reaction.

MATERIALS AND REAGENTS

2,4-dinitrobenzene sodium sulfonate (DNBS), recrystallized, $M_r = 270.2$ (Eastman Kodak)

K_2CO_3, reagent grade, $M_r = 138.2$

$NaH_2PO_4 \cdot H_2O$, $M_r = 138.0$

$Na_2HPO_4 \cdot 7H_2O$, $M_r = 268.1$

Bovine gamma globulin (BGG; Miles Research Products or Calbiochem)

UV spectrophotometer

Aluminum foil

Test tube or Erlenmeyer flask, 20 ml

Magnetic stirrer and bar

Dialysis tubing

Buffer

> 0.001 M phosphate buffer, pH 7.4: Dilute the 0.15 M phosphate buffer described in Appendix A.12 150-fold with water. Readjust to pH 7.4 if required.

PROCEDURE

1. In a test tube or flask, dissolve 100 mg K_2CO_3 in 5 ml of distilled water (0.15 M solution). Add 100 mg of BGG and stir gently with a magnetic stirrer until protein is dissolved.

2. Dissolve 100 mg DNBS in 1.0 ml of warm distilled water and add drop by drop (with stirring) to the protein solution. Cover reaction mixture with foil to protect it from light and allow the mixture to stir overnight at room temperature.

3. Dialyze against 0.001 M phosphate buffer for 5–7 days, with 2–3 changes of buffer per day. Remove a sample of the dialysate before each change of buffer and measure absorbance at 360 nm. When the OD is less than 0.005 for 3 successive buffer changes, the dialysis can be stopped.

4. Centrifuge the mixture at 13 000 × g for 20 minutes to remove insoluble material. Dilute an aliquot to 0.1–0.2 mg/ml in the 0.001 M phosphate buffer and measure absorbance at 280 nm and 360 nm. Determine the protein concentration and number of DNP groups by the following calculations:

   a. Molar extinction coefficients:

   BGG $\quad\quad\quad\quad\quad\quad\quad\quad$ $\epsilon_{280} = 2.34 \times 10^5$ (calculated from $M_r = 160\ 000$ and $\epsilon = 1.46$ for a 1 mg/ml solution);

$\epsilon_{360} = 0.01 \times \epsilon_{280}^{BGG}$ (determined by absorbance readings on suitable dilutions of the protein).

DNP (as ϵ-DNP-L-lysine) $\epsilon_{280} = 0.316 \times \epsilon_{360}^{DNP}$ (measured at pH 7.4);

$$\epsilon_{360} = 1.74 \times 10^4.$$

b. Equations for contributions of protein and DNP-lysine to the absorbance of DNP-BGG at 280 nm and 360 nm:

$$OD_{280} = [BGG](2.34 \times 10^5) + [DNP](0.316)(1.74 \times 10^4);$$

$$OD_{360} = [BGG](0.01)(2.34 \times 10^5) + [DNP](1.74 \times 10^4).$$

Solving for concentration of BGG and of DNP groups in mol/liter:

$$[BGG] = \frac{(OD_{280}) - (.316)(OD_{360})}{2.33 \times 10^5};$$

$$[DNP] = \frac{(OD_{360}) - (0.01)(OD_{280})}{1.73 \times 10^4}.$$

c. The average number of DNP groups per BGG molecule is obtained by dividing the DNP concentration by the BGG concentration. The protein concentration in g/liter or mg/ml is obtained by multiplying the molar concentration of BGG by the molecular weight (160 000).

5. Sterilize the DNP-BGG by membrane filtration, aliquot into tubes, and store at $-20°C$ wrapped in foil. It can be kept for several years at $-20°C$ and thawed samples can be kept at least 2 weeks at 4°C.

COMMENTS

1. The number of DNP groups per molecule of BGG will vary from batch to batch and should always be determined experimentally.

2. It is essential to remove all free hapten before making absorbance readings to determine the concentration and degree of substitution with DNP.

3. DNP-BGG is soluble in water and in very dilute buffers above neutral pH, but is not soluble at concentrations above 0.1–0.2 mg/ml in isotonic buffers or PBS. (When these proteins are used in any type of precipitation assay, great care should be used to in-

clude adequate controls for detection of nonspecific precipitation of the DNP-conjugated protein.)

4. Since the absorbance of many proteins at 360 nm is negligible ($\sim 1\%$ of reading at 280 nm), it is common practice to calculate the DNP concentration directly from the absorbance at 360 nm without correcting for the contribution of the protein. The equation then reduces to:

$$DNP = \frac{OD_{360}}{1.74 \times 10^4}.$$

It is only necessary to correct the absorbance reading at 280 nm for the DNP contribution before calculating the protein concentration. This simplification can be used for gamma globulins and albumins, but not for KLH because its absorbance at 360 nm is 21% of its absorbance at 280 nm.

REFERENCES

Corneil, I., and L. Wofsy. 1967. Specific purification of equine anti-SII antibodies by precipitation with a hemocyanin-glucuronide conjugate. *Immunochemistry* **4**:183.

Eisen, H. N. 1964. Preparation of purified anti–2,4-dinitrophenyl antibodies. *Meth. Med. Res.* **10**:94.

Eisen, H. N., S. Belman, and M. E. Carsten. 1953. The reaction of 2,4-dinitrobenzenesulfonic acid with free amino groups of proteins. *J. Am. Chem. Soc.* **75**:4583.

Garvey, J. S., N. E. Cremer, and D. H. Sussdorf. 1977. *Methods in Immunology*, W. A. Benjamin, Reading, MA.

Nisonoff, A. 1967. Coupling of diazonium compounds to proteins. In, C. A. Williams and M. W. Chase (Eds.), *Methods in Immunology and Immunochemistry*. Academic Press, New York and London.

17

Immunoglobulin-Producing Hybrid Cell Lines

Vernon T. Oi and Leonard A. Herzenberg

17.1 INTRODUCTION

The problems of producing and characterizing antisera were radically altered when Köhler and Milstein (1975) demonstrated that antibody-producing hybrid cell lines could be generated by somatic cell hybridization. Within three years, antibodies of defined specificity produced by continuous cultures of monoclonal cell lines became routine laboratory reagents providing exquisite serological and biochemical probes (Oi et al. 1978). This chapter describes a modified version of the technique described by Galfre et al. (1977) to fuse murine spleen cells with the 8-azaguanine-resistant, nonsecreting mouse myeloma cell line NS-1 (a derivative of MOPC-21 (P3)). In this procedure polyethylene glycol is used as the fusion agent (Pontecorvo 1976) and Littlefield's hypoxanthine-aminopterin-thymidine (HAT) medium (Littlefield 1964) is used for selecting stable, monoclonal antibody-producing hybrid cell lines.

From the start (immunizing mice and growing the myeloma cell parent) to the end (when stable, cloned cell lines have become established), this method requires three to four months of continuous bench work. In addition, the generation of monoclonal antibody-producing cell lines demands constant attention and should not be undertaken unless one can afford

351

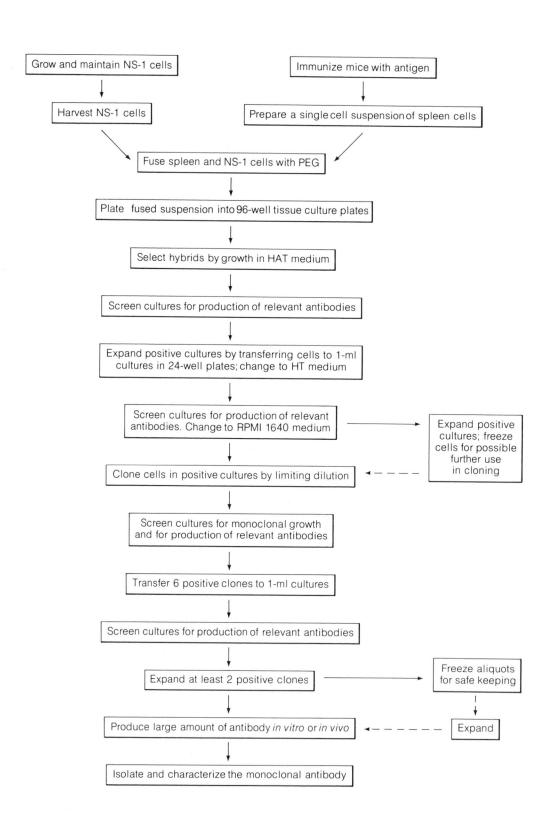

both the time and the effort. Moreover, it is necessary to establish the antibody detection system to analyze the products of the hybrid cell lines before beginning hybridization because there may not be sufficient time to work out technical problems after hybrid cells begin to grow.

Tissue culture facilities for generating antibody-producing hybrid cell lines minimally require the following equipment and supplies:

1. Tissue culture hood
2. Humidified incubator with a CO_2-in-air atmosphere
3. Bench top centrifuge
4. Inverted phase contrast microscope
5. Bright field microscope
6. Tissue culture supplies
7. Liquid nitrogen storage containers

In addition, investigators using these methods will require the laboratory equipment necessary for producing antibody in usable amounts, analyzing antibody activity, and characterizing the antibody molecules produced by the hybrids. The exact equipment and materials required for each of these operations will depend on the nature of the antibodies being produced and the scale to which production is carried out.

The procedure we describe for the development and use of antibody-producing hybrid cell lines (Figure 17.1) includes growing the parental myeloma cell line, immunizing mice to provide immune donor spleen cells, conducting the cell fusion, and selecting the resulting hybrids with HAT medium. Supernates of the surviving hybrid cell cultures are then tested for antibody activity. An aliquot of cells from the antibody-producing cultures is grown and prepared for freezing while another aliquot is employed in cloning the hybrids. To derive cloned cell lines, the cells are grown at limiting dilutions. Clones that secrete the desired antibody are expanded, and several aliquots of these clones are frozen while others are used for the large-scale production of antibody. The resulting antibodies are purified and characterized.

FIGURE 17.1
Flow chart indicating steps in the production of hybrid cell lines secreting monoclonal antibody.

17.2   PREPARATION OF THE FUSION PARTNERS

A.   NS-1 Myeloma Parent Cell Line*

NS-1, abbreviated from P3-NS1-1, is a cell line derived from MOPC-21, a BALB/c myeloma cell line. NS-1 does not produce the MOPC-21 γ_1 heavy chain; it synthesizes the original MOPC-21 κ chain but internally degrades it. This line is 8-azaguanine resistant and therefore susceptible to HAT selection (see Section 17.4). The advantage in using NS-1 as the fusion myeloma parent cell line, rather than other myeloma cell lines (such as P3-X63Ag8), is its inability to produce a heavy chain. Antibody-producing hybrid cell lines derived with this fusion partner will produce mixed molecules with only the MOPC-21 κ light chain; the molecules will not have both light and heavy chains derived from the myeloma cell (see Section 17.10).

Not all NS-1 cell lines are equivalent. Some sublines of NS-1 have been reported not to give rise to antibody-producing hybrid cell lines. Therefore, care should be taken when recloning NS-1. Recloning is necessary to maintain a homogeneous cell line; long-term maintenance of NS-1 (or any other cell line) in tissue culture gives rise to spontaneous genetic drift of the cell population. Such drift affects many characteristics, for example, continued resistance to 8-azaguanine. Upon recloning NS-1, testing of the new NS-1 clone for the ability to fuse with immune spleen cells and yield antibody-producing hybrid cell lines is recommended. This is a tedious procedure. If a particular cell line is a good fusion partner, establishing frozen stocks of the cells as a continual source of the original cell line is the best way of assuring continued success in generating antibody-producing hybrid cell lines.

---

* Three new cell lines have been developed for somatic cell hybridization with immune spleen cells to generate antibody-producing hybrid cell lines. The two mouse lines Sp2/0-Ag14 (Shulman et al. 1978) and P3X63-Ag8.653 (Kearney et al.; in press, *J. Immunol.*) are total nonsecretors. They do not synthesize either light or heavy chains, and hybrid cells derived with these parental cell lines will only produce antibody of the spleen cell parent. The third cell line is a rat myeloma cell line, Y3-Ag1.2.3 (Galfre et al. 1979), which secretes κ light chains. Antibody-producing hybrid cell lines derived from rat spleen cells fused with a mouse myeloma cell line are difficult to grow as tumors in either mice or rats. The development of this myeloma cell line permits the production of hybridomas using rat cells for both fusion partners. The resulting hybrids can be adoptively transferred for growth and antibody production in rats because these cells present no xenogeneic antigens to the host.

1. Maintaining NS-1

MATERIALS AND REAGENTS

NS-1 myeloma cell line (P3-NS1-1; Cell Distribution Center, Salk
   Institute)
Culture medium:
   RPMI 1640
   L-glutamine
   Sodium pyruvate
   Penicillin
   Streptomycin
   Fetal calf serum (FCS), screened (see comment 1)
CO_2 incubator, humidified
7% CO_2-in-air gas mixture
Stationary T flasks, roller bottles, or Spinner flasks

PROCEDURE

1. Culture NS-1 cells in RPMI 1640 supplemented with 2 mM
   L-glutamine, 1 mM sodium pyruvate, 50 units/ml penicillin, 50
   μg/ml streptomycin, and 15% FCS in a humidified 7% CO_2-in-air
   atmosphere at 37°C.

2. NS-1 can be grown either in stationary T flasks, roller bottles, or
   Spinner flasks. In any of these containers, NS-1 and hybrid cell
   lines derived from NS-1 grow to a maximum density of 2–5 × 10^5
   cells/ml with a doubling time of 12–24 hours. When this density is
   reached, there is a precipitous fall in cell viability. Generally NS-1
   cultures must be split (i.e., diluted either by removing the contents
   of the old flask and adding fresh medium or by addition to a new
   flask with medium) every 3–4 days. A 1-in-10 or 1-in-20 split,
   depending on the condition of the cells, is recommended. Cultures
   with cell densities lower than 10^4 cells/ml grow poorly.

COMMENTS

1. The FCS should be a screened lot known to support the clonal
   growth of at least the parental myeloma cell line NS-1. To test this
   capacity, clone NS-1 with batches of FCS by limiting dilution (see
   Section 17.7) without feeder cells. A good serum lot will support
   100% cloning efficiencies of NS-1, but sera yielding 70–80% cloning efficiencies are satisfactory. Generally, 10–20% of the serum
   lots tested are suitable. Most commercial suppliers of FCS will

reserve serum lots for three weeks while one is determining whether the lot is usable. Obviously, only serum lots with adequate quantities in reserve should be tested.

2. The 7% CO_2-in-air atmosphere assures a slightly acidic medium pH. NS-1 and hybrid cell lines derived from NS-1 grow better under such conditions. These cells are somewhat intolerant of basic pH medium. (Adequate buffering of RPMI 1640 medium is provided by 5–10% CO_2-in-air atmospheres.)

3. Should one find that an NS-1 cell culture has overgrown and is dying, it is better to start again from frozen stock than to attempt to salvage the culture. Selective forces in the dying cultures might result in the growth of cells with altered phenotypes that make them unsuitable fusion partners.

2. Preparation of NS-1 for Fusion

A total of 1.5×10^8 NS-1 cells is generally used for fusion. These cells should be in log-phase growth. To insure that the cells are in log-phase growth, they should be at a density of about 10^5 cells/ml. Thus, 1–2 liters of NS-1 cells are grown in preparation for fusion. Cell viability at the time of collecting the cells should be greater than 95%. Because cell viability determinations with trypan blue are influenced by the presence of serum albumin, either the albumin must be washed away before cell counts are made or another method of determining viabilities must be used. A convenient method using acridine orange-and-ethidium bromide and fluorescence microscopy is described in Section 1.15.

B. Immune Spleen Cells

Mice are generally immunized with limited immunization protocols to provide the immune spleen cells used for fusion. In most cases, hyperimmunization is not necessary.

GUIDELINES FOR IMMUNIZATION PROCEDURE

1. If the antigen is soluble, prime mice intraperitoneally with 100 μg of antigen precipitated in alum, mixed with 2×10^9 killed *Bordetella pertussis* organisms. (See Section 2.5 for sources of reagents and procedures for alum precipitation of antigen.) Boost mice (intraperitoneally or intravenously) 1–3 weeks later with 10 μg aqueous antigen without *B. pertussis*. Use the spleen cells

for fusion 3 days after the boost. Best results have been obtained using this immunization protocol. Alternatively, fusion can be done 3–4 days after the priming dose, or 3 days after a second boost.

2. If the antigen consists of cells, prime and boost mice intraperitoneally with 2×10^7 cells or less. The critical parameter to remember is that fusion should be done 3 days after the last antigen boost.

3. If hyperimmune mice are used as the spleen cell donor, the mice should be rested (generally 3–4 weeks) before receiving the final antigen boost prior to fusion.

17.3 FUSION OF NS-1 WITH IMMUNE SPLEEN CELLS

The immediate event in somatic cell hybridization is the fusion of cell membranes, generating multinucleated (generally binucleated) cells or heterokaryons in which the cell membranes of the fusion partners surround a common cytoplasm with two or more nuclei. In a matter of days, synkaryons form when the nuclei fuse and are capable of synchronous mitosis; in the process, a variable number of chromosomes of both fusion partners are lost. With subsequent cell divisions, more chromosomes are lost, but the hybrid cell line eventually stabilizes.

MATERIALS AND REAGENTS

NS-1 myeloma cells and immune spleen cells (see Section 17.2)
Medium (see Section 17.2A): with FCS (30 ml); without FCS (approximately 100 ml)
37°C water bath
Glass beakers for preparing a makeshift water bath for use in a tissue culture hood
Centrifuge tube, 50 ml, plastic (Corning Glass Works, #25330)
Bench top centrifuge
Pipettes, 1 ml and 10 ml
Stopwatch (optional)
96-well cluster dish (Costar, #3596; see comment 2)
50% solution of polyethylene glycol (PEG) 1500 (BDH Chemicals): PEG 1500 comes as large waxy chunks. It should be odorless and white. Cut away and discard any discolored material. Prepare 50% PEG by the following procedure: Weigh 20–50 g of PEG 1500 in a 100-ml glass reagent bottle and steam autoclave for 20 minutes at

121–132°C. As the PEG cools but before it solidifies, add a volume of RPMI 1640 (20–50 ml) equal to the number of grams of PEG autoclaved. Mix the solution thoroughly. Store the reagent at room temperature. During storage, the 50% PEG solution becomes very alkaline; however, this does not seem to affect the PEG as a fusion agent and nothing should be done to alter the pH.

PROCEDURE

The following description of the fusion procedure takes into account several characteristics of the 50% PEG solution: (1) The PEG solution is hypotonic; (2) proteins precipitate in 50% PEG; and (3) cells are damaged by PEG treatment. The entire procedure takes 6–7 minutes.

1. Warm 30 ml of medium with FCS and 20 ml of serum-free medium to 37°C. Also, warm the 50% PEG solution to 37°C.

2. Make a 37°C water bath using two glass beakers. Place one beaker of water within a larger beaker, also filled with water. Keep this at 37°C until needed.

3. Harvest the NS-1 cells and wash once with serum-free medium at room temperature. Remove spleens from primed mice, as described in Section 1.2. Prepare a cell suspension and wash 3 times in serum-free medium at room temperature.

4. Mix together 1.5×10^8 NS-1 cells and 1.5×10^8 immune spleen cells in a 50-ml centrifuge tube and centrifuge the mixture at $400 \times g$ for 10 minutes at room temperature to form a tight pellet.

5. Remove all supernate from the pellet and keep the tube at 37°C for further manipulations in the makeshift water bath.

6. Using a 1-ml pipette, add 1 ml of warm 50% PEG over a one-minute period. Gently *stir* the cell pellet with the tip of the pipette as the PEG is being added. Do not pipet the cell suspension. (A stopwatch is helpful to keep track of time.)

7. Continue to *stir* the cell pellet for an additional minute. The goal is to expose the cells to the PEG while maintaining as much cell contact as possible. The cell suspension should look like homogeneous clumps of cells.

8. With the same 1-ml pipette, take one minute to stir in 1 ml of serum-free medium that has been warmed to 37°C. Slow addition of warm medium serves to gradually dilute the PEG without lysing the cells.

9. Repeat step 8.

10. Finally, with a 10-ml pipette, stir in 7 ml of 37°C serum-free medium over 2–3 minutes. Continuous stirring motions should be used. (Pipetting the cell suspension must be avoided as this disrupts the cells.)

11. Centrifuge the suspension at $400 \times g$ for 10 minutes at room temperature and remove the supernate.

12. Fill a 10-ml pipette with 37°C medium with FCS and aim the tip of the pipette at the cell pellet. By releasing the medium directly at the cell pellet and stirring with the pipette, a suspension of fine cell clumps is obtained.

13. Add an additional 20 ml of warm medium with FCS and swirl the tube to suspend the contents.

14. Avoiding excessive pipetting, plate 0.1 ml of this suspension (10^6 total cells) into each well of three 96-well tissue culture plates. These plates are referred to as the master plates.

15. Place plates into the 7% CO_2-in-air incubator at 37°C.

COMMENTS

1. The ratio of NS-1 to immune spleen cells in the above protocol is $1:1$; however, a ratio of $1:4$ (e.g., 4×10^7 NS-1 cells mixed with 1.6×10^8 immune spleen cells plated into two 96-well tissue culture plates) has been successfully used. A ratio of $1:10$ can also be used. Whichever ratio and however many total cells are used in the fusion, the critical parameter is to maintain the initial culture density at 10^6 total cells per 0.1-ml culture well. The day of fusion is referred to as day 0.

2. Individual cultures in Costar plates are more isolated from each other than they are in similar plates from other suppliers. Costar plates, because of their design, provide the least opportunity for contamination and the best opportunity for eliminating it should it occur. If a plate develops mold contamination, the surest way to prevent its spread to other plates is to discard the contaminated plate. However, if the contamination occurs in one or two wells of a plate that contains valuable cultures, an attempt can be made to salvage the remaining cultures in the plate by rinsing the contaminated well 3 times with 5 M NaOH. To avoid contaminating other plates in the CO_2 incubator, isolate the contaminated plate either in a separate incubator or in a humidified culture chamber (Bellco Glass, #7741-10005) until it is clear that the mold has been eliminated.

17.4   SELECTION OF HYBRID CELLS (HAT SELECTION)

Cell fusion is a random process and necessitates a means of selecting the desired hybrid cells. Fusion of a population of NS-1 and immune spleen cells results in a mixture of fusion events (NS-1 : NS-1, NS-1 : spleen, and spleen : spleen cells). Selection of NS-1 : spleen cell hybrids is accomplished by culturing the fusion mixture in hypoxanthine-aminopterin-thymidine (HAT) medium. The mechanism of this selection is as follows:

1. Aminopterin (an analog of folic acid) blocks the *de novo* biosynthesis of purines and pyrimidines. To survive in the presence of aminopterin (as in HAT medium), cells must be able to synthesize these nucleotides by utilizing an exogenous source of hypoxanthine and thymidine (provided in HAT medium). They do this via alternate nucleotide biosynthetic pathways aptly called the salvage pathways. (Aminopterin also blocks glycine synthesis, but RPMI 1640 medium supplies enough exogenous glycine to meet this requirement.)

2. NS-1 cells are 8-azaguanine resistant and hence lack an enzyme, hypoxanthine-guanine-phosphoribosyltransferase (HGPRTase), that is required in one of the salvage pathways of nucleotide biosynthesis. NS-1 and NS-1 : NS-1 fused cells are therefore not capable of growing when *de novo* nucleotide synthesis is blocked with HAT medium.

3. Should NS-1 fuse with a normal, albeit antibody-producing spleen cell, the normal cell provides the fused partners with the required enzyme, HGPRTase. This allows the hybrid cell to utilize exogenous hypoxanthine and to grow in HAT medium.

4. There is no positive selection against the growth of infused normal spleen cells and spleen-spleen cell fusions in this scheme; hence it is called half-selection. Passive selection takes place because normal spleen cells have a limited growth potential in culture. By two weeks in culture most spleen cells have died.

5. As a result of this half-selection, the desired NS-1 : spleen cell hybrids are selectively grown.

MATERIALS AND REAGENTS

Preparation of 50× HT and HAT Stock Solutions and 1× HT and HAT Media

Supplemented culture medium (see Section 17.2)
Thymidine
Hypoxanthine

Aminopterin
   Note: All of the above reagents are available from a number of
   commercial firms (e.g., Sigma Chemical). Each new batch of
   reagents should be tested for toxicity before routine use in tissue
   culture. This is easily done by testing whether the reagent is
   toxic to a HAT-resistant cell line (e.g., hybridoma cell line developed by HAT selection).
NaOH: 0.1 M (4 g/liter)

HAT Selection

1× HAT medium
1× HT medium
Needle, 1½ in., 21 or 23 gauge, attached to tubing that is connected to
   an aspirator
Pasteur pipettes and bulb

PROCEDURE

Preparation of 50× HT and HAT Stock Solutions and 1× HT and HAT Media

1. *100× and 50× HT Stock Solutions*
   Prepare a 100× HT solution by dissolving 0.1361 g hypoxanthine
   and 0.0388 g thymidine in 100 ml double-distilled water warmed to
   70–80°C. The 100× HT stock solution is used in preparing the 50×
   HAT stock solution (see below). To prepare 50× HT stock solution, dilute the 100× solution to 50× with double-distilled water.
   Sterilize by membrane filtration (Appendix C.2) and store in
   aliquots at −20°C. (Four-ml aliquots are prepared in our laboratory for addition to 200-ml medium bottles.)

2. *1000× Aminopterin Stock Solution*
   Dissolve 17.6 mg aminopterin in 80 ml double-distilled water. If
   the aminopterin does not dissolve readily, add several ml of 0.1 M
   NaOH. Bring volume up to 100 ml with double-distilled water.
   Store the 1000× aminopterin stock in 10-ml aliquots at −20°C.

3. *50× HAT Stock Solution*
   Combine 100 ml of 100× HT stock, 10 ml of 1000× aminopterin
   stock, and 90 ml double-distilled water. Sterilize the solution by
   membrane filtration (Appendix C.2) and store in aliquots at
   −20°C.

4. *1× HT and 1× HAT Media*
   Add the 50× stock to an appropriate amount of supplemented
   culture medium. When thawing the aliquots of 50× stock, some
   material may come out of solution. However, this material quickly
   dissolves when the 50× stocks are added to the culture medium.

HAT Selection

The following procedure describes a progressive HAT selection scheme. Two objectives are accomplished with this protocol: (a) selection for the growth of hybrid cells; and (b) dilution of immunoglobulin produced by spleen cells. The dilution eliminates some false positive test results in the subsequent assessment of antibody production by hybrid cells.

1. On day 1 (i.e., the day after the fusion), add 0.1 ml of 1× HAT medium to each well. This is done with sufficient accuracy by adding 2 drops of HAT medium with a Pasteur pipette.

2. On days 2, 3, 5, 8, and 11, aspirate off half of the medium from each well and add two drops of fresh HAT medium. After day 11, continue to exchange half of the culture fluid with fresh HAT medium every 3–4 days.

   Aspirating half of the medium from the wells is done visually. The procedure is made easier by placing one edge of the microwell plate onto the edge of another plate thereby having the plate resting at a slight angle. The aspiration needle can then be applied along the upper side of the well to withdraw half of the volume of the culture medium.

COMMENTS

1. On days 1, 2, and 3 the culture medium will appear quite acidic; thereafter, HAT selection will drastically deplete the cell numbers and the cultures will appear dead. With the aid of an inverted phase-contrast microscope, cells approximately the size of the NS-1 parent can usually be observed growing as colonies among the cellular debris by days 6 to 14 (sometimes, they are not apparent until day 21). Live, growing cells have a distinct appearance with phase-contrast microscopy: bright and translucent. Dead or dying cells appear dark (brown) and opaque. These qualities are not evident without phase-contrast optics.

2. At some point, cells that have grown in HAT medium are transferred to normal medium (RPMI 1640). However, before making this switch, it is necessary for them to grow in HT medium for about one week in order to dilute any remaining intracellular aminopterin. The transfer from HAT medium can be done as early as day 14 but to avoid keeping track of which plates have HAT, HT, and normal media, cells are generally kept in HAT medium until they are transferred from the 96-well plates into 1-ml cultures.

3. As long as the cultures are fed regularly (i.e., with half the medium replaced every 3 days) and not disturbed (i.e., not resuspended), the hybrid cells can remain in the 96-well plates for up to 4 weeks, sometimes even 6 weeks. Successful hybridization will yield growing colonies in every well of the culture plate.

17.5   INITIAL SCREENING TO IDENTIFY CULTURES PRODUCING RELEVANT ANTIBODIES

Between two and four weeks after cell fusion (allowing three to four days after the last medium change for antibody to accumulate), the supernates of cultures are harvested using individual pipettes for each culture plate well. The supernates can be tested undiluted or diluted (e.g., 1:5 or 1:10). Dilution of supernates reduces the likelihood of selecting weakly positive wells that may represent marginal antibody production or simply a high assay background. The type of assay used for antibody detection will depend on the goal of the investigator. It is possible to use cytotoxicity or lytic assays; however, these will only detect complement-fixing antibodies and will miss non-complement-fixing antibodies. Solid-phase antibody-binding or cell-binding assays such as those described in Chapter 18 are recommended. When solid-phase antibody-binding or cell-binding assays are used, it is necessary to control for the detection of nonspecific antibody binding (i.e., antibodies that seemingly bind to plastic). Controls for auto-antibodies should be included in work involving alloantigens.

Multiple assays can be done on each supernate to provide an initial characterization of antibody activity; however, such preliminary characterizations may be wasteful of time and effort because many of the positive cultures may fail to yield stable monoclonal antibody-producing cell lines. Whatever detection method is used, the assay must be accurate, reproducible, and rapid, since decisions about which culture wells to save or discard must be made quickly.

17.6   TRANSFER TO ONE-MILLILITER CULTURES (TRANSFER PLATES) AND FREEZING OF HYBRID CELLS

The next step after determining which wells are making antibodies of interest is to transfer the cells into 1-ml cultures in 24-well tissue culture plates. This is the first step in expanding the cell lines for cloning and in generating enough cells for frozen stocks. The transfer is accomplished using BALB/c thymocytes as feeder cells; without thymocyte feeders, most cells will not grow when they are transferred into the 1-ml cultures. BALB/c thymocytes can be used regardless of the H-2 haplotype of the donor spleen cells. (Remember NS-1 is of BALB/c origin.)

MATERIALS AND REAGENTS

Thymocytes (see Section 1.5) from 4–5 week old BALB/c mice (1 thymus/ml of HT medium)
Fetal calf serum (FCS)
Culture medium (see Section 17.2)
HT medium (see Section 17.4)
Dimethyl sulfoxide (DMSO)
24-well tissue culture plates (Costar, #3524; see comment 2, Section 17.3)
Pasteur pipettes and bulb
T flasks
Liquid nitrogen freezer
Freezing vials (Nunc, #N1076-1)

PROCEDURE

1. Place 0.5 ml of HT medium into each well of the transfer plate.

2. Remove thymuses from mouse donors and prepare a cell suspension. Wash the thymocytes at least 3 times and resuspend them at a concentration of 1 thymus/ml of HT medium. Using a Pasteur pipette, add 1–2 drops of this cell suspension to each well of the transfer plate ($1–2 \times 10^7$ thymocytes per well).

3. Resuspend the contents of each antibody-producing master plate well with a Pasteur pipette and transfer the entire suspension into the transfer well containing the thymocytes and HT medium. Resuspend this mixture and then add back 5 drops of this suspension to the original master plate well. This creates duplicate cultures (a master plate and a transfer cell culture), which protects against losing the new cell line.

4. After 2–3 days, feed these cultures an additional 0.5 ml of HT medium (no additional thymocytes are needed).

5. Two days later, feed the cultures again by first removing as much supernate as possible and adding fresh HT medium.

6. When the cells are nearly confluent (about one week), retest the supernate for antibody activity. Because antibody produced in the master plate is carried over into the transfer cultures, it is important to compare titrations of supernate antibody from the master plate and the transfer plate to determine whether the transferred cells are continuing to produce antibody. Residual antibody from the master plate may produce false positive results. (Transferred cells may lose the ability to produce antibody because of a loss of chromosomes, the overgrowth of the culture by nonproducing hybrid cells, or overgrowth by hybrid cells producing antibody of another specificity.)

7. If the culture continues to produce the desired antibody, then clone the cell line immediately. A small fraction of the 1-ml culture is used for this purpose; the procedure is described in the next section. If the antibody-producing wells are not numerous, it is possible to clone directly from the master plate. However, cloning from cultures that continue to produce antibody after transfer reduces the likelihood of working with the less stable cell lines.

8. After removing samples for cloning, expand the remaining cultures in order to have enough cells to freeze and store in liquid nitrogen. Do this by placing the remaining portion of the 1-ml culture into a small T flask containing 5 ml of fresh medium (normal medium may be used at this stage). When this culture becomes dense (approximately $1–2 \times 10^5$ cells/ml), transfer to a larger tissue culture flask and feed 15 ml of medium.

9. Generally for each 10 ml of culture, one vial of cells is frozen. Centrifuge 10 ml of a growing culture containing a total of approximately 2×10^6 cells. Resuspend the cells in 0.5 ml of 90% FCS, 10% DMSO. Transfer the cells to a freezing vial and immediately begin to freeze the cells either by placing the vials into the *gas phase* of a liquid nitrogen freezer or by insulating the vials with styrofoam and placing them in a $-70°C$ freezer; transfer the vials to a liquid nitrogen freezer after 24 hours.

10. To retrieve frozen cells, thaw the cells quickly and wash immediately with 10 ml of medium. After this wash, resuspend the cells in 10 ml of medium in a T flask and place in the incubator. Expand thawed cells slowly. Initially split the cultures 1 : 2 to maintain high cell density (approximately $1–2 \times 10^5$ cells/ml) until they fully recover from being frozen.

17.7 CLONING BY LIMITING DILUTION*

MATERIALS AND REAGENTS

Thymocytes

Culture medium (see Section 17.2)

HT medium (see Section 17.4), for use only when cloning from master plate

Acridine orange-ethidium bromide (AO/EB), for determining cell viability (Section 1.15)

96-well tissue culture plates (Costar, #3596; see comment 2, Section 17.3)

PROCEDURE

The cloning medium consists of 10^7 thymocytes per ml of 15% FCS in RPMI 1640. (If cloning is done directly from the master plate, HT medium is used; see comment 2, Section 17.4.) The thymocytes act as carrier cells in diluting the hybrid cells and also as feeder cells in culture. Again BALB/c thymocytes are used. The objective is to plate 36 wells of a 96-well tissue culture plate with an average of 5 cells/well, 36 wells with an average of 1 cell/well, and the remaining 24 wells with an average of 0.5 cells/well. One of these plating concentrations will yield wells with monoclonal growth. The dilutions are carried out as follows:

1. Remove samples from the 1-ml cultures and determine the concentration of viable cells by staining with AO/EB (Section 1.15). Trypan blue, which is commonly used to determine viability, should be avoided in this instance because the bovine serum albumin in the medium will bind the stain and thereby produce misleading results.

2. Dilute a sample of the culture to be cloned so that 230 live hybrid cells are suspended in 4.6 ml of the thymocyte-containing cloning

---

* Specific antibody-producing hybrid cells can be selected and cloned with the fluorescence-activated cell sorter (FACS; Becton Dickinson FACS Division). Antigen-coated fluorescent microspheres (0.9 μm) are used to stain hybrid cells producing antibody reactive with the antigen. Using the FACS with some electronic modifications (Parks et al. 1979), antigen-binding hybrid cells are sorted and individually deposited into the wells of a 96-well culture plate with thymocytes (10^6 cells/well) as feeder cells. This method has been successfully used to "sorter clone" antibody-producing hybrid cells reactive with mouse immunoglobulin allotypes as early as 16 days after hybridization. When the appropriate antigens are not readily coupled to the microspheres, the FACS can be used to clone cells on the basis of viability.

medium. Plate 36 wells of a 96-well plate with 0.1 ml of this mixture. This will leave 1.0 ml of cell suspension. To this, add an additional 4.0 ml of the thymocyte-containing medium and plate another 36 wells with 0.1 ml. Finally, add 1.4 ml of the thymocyte-containing medium to the remaining cell suspension and plate the last 24 wells.

3. At day 5 and again at day 12, feed the cloning plate by adding 2 drops of medium with a Pasteur pipette. By day 14 the clones should be large enough to test. Depending on culture conditions, cloning efficiencies, and counting and dilution errors, one of the three dilutions plated should yield some wells with no growth (e.g., if an average of 1 cell/well is plated, 37% of the wells should have no growth). Wells appearing to be monoclonal are then tested for antibody activity.

4. Transfer 6 positive clones into separate 1-ml cultures with thymocytes as described above (Section 17.6, except with normal medium). Test the supernates for antibody at the end of a week.

5. Transfer at least 2 of the positive clones into 5-ml flasks and further expand the cultures. Freeze cell stocks as soon as possible (at least 6 vials should be frozen for each clone). It is now possible to grow cultures for antibody production as described in Section 17.8.

COMMENTS

1. Recloning from the original frozen stock may be necessary if no positive clones are recovered.

2. Recloning of established antibody-producing cell lines also becomes necessary when these cells have been continually grown for long periods. Somatic mutation or chromosome loss may cause cells to lose the ability to produce antibody. Keeping a number of vials of clones producing antibodies in liquid nitrogen storage is the best safeguard against such occurrences.

17.8 ANTIBODY PRODUCTION

Antibody production in culture supernates ranges from 10 to 60 μg per ml; therefore, a liter of culture grown in roller bottles or Spinner flasks will yield 10 to 60 mg of antibody. (Growing cells in stationary T flasks is also satisfactory.) To achieve this level of production, the cells are overgrown, that is, grown beyond the time when the culture begins to die. A 1-liter roller bottle seeded with 50 to 100 ml of fully grown cells from a T flask takes four to six days to reach this stage.

Antibody production in mice can be achieved by injecting 2×10^6 healthy hybrid cells into the appropriate H-2 compatible mice. Subcutaneous tumors are nearly always successful and the mice can be continuously bled from the time the tumor first appears, which is anywhere from 10 to 30 days after injection. Analysis by agar or cellulose acetate electrophoresis of serum from these tumor-bearing mice shows a characteristic myeloma protein spike. The concentration of antibody in serum ranges from 1 to 10 mg/ml.

Ascites tumors are sometimes more difficult to induce, but many of the hybrid cell lines will grow this way. "Priming" the mice with 0.5 ml pristane* 10 and 3 days before injecting the hybrid cell lines intraperitoneally may increase the frequency of ascites tumors.

When using mice for antibody production, avoid using a mouse strain that may absorb antibody *in vivo*. This situation may arise when producing antibodies directed against alloantigens. For example, a CWB anti–Ig-5a × NS-1 antibody-producing cell line should not be grown in a (CWB × BALB/c)F$_1$. The BALB/c haplotype will absorb the anti-Ig-5a antibodies. Instead, a (CWB × BAB/14)F$_1$ should be used. BAB/14 is an Ig^b haplotype mouse strain congenic to BALB/c.

17.9 ANTIBODY PURIFICATION: PROTEIN A-SEPHAROSE COLUMN CHROMATOGRAPHY

It is frequently desirable to purify the antibodies synthesized by hybrid cell lines. Several methods of purifying immunoglobulins have been described in Chapters 11 and 12. A recently developed method, which provides rapid purification of immunoglobulins in a single step, utilizes protein A-Sepharose column chromatography. Mouse IgG$_{2a}$, IgG$_{2b}$, IgG$_3$, some IgG$_1$, and some IgM will bind to protein A (Goding 1978). Ey et al. (1978) describe in detail the use of various buffers to elute different classes of mouse immunoglobulin. Elution is done by lowering the pH of the protein A column. The majority of mouse immunoglobulins bind to protein A at pH 8.6 and elute from the column at pH 4.3, or higher; thus harsh acidic elution can be avoided.

---

* Pristane (2,6,10,14-tetramethylpentadecane) is available from Aldrich Chemical.

MATERIALS AND REAGENTS

Protein A-Sepharose CL 4B (Pharmacia Fine Chemicals)

NaN_3. Caution: Sodium azide is extremely toxic.

NaCl, $M_r = 58.4$

NaOH, $M_r = 40.0$

Tris (tris [hydroxymethyl] aminoethane), $M_r = 121.1$

HCl, concentrated

Citric acid monohydrate, $M_r = 210.15$

Trisodium citrate dihydrate, $M_r = 294.12$

Na_2HPO_4, $M_r = 142.0$

NaH_2PO_4, monohydrate, $M_r = 138.0$

Sodium acetate trihydrate, $M_r = 136.1$

Acetate acid, glacial

Glycine-hydrochloride, $M_r = 111.5$

Fraction collector

UV monitor (optional)

Buffers: The molarity of the buffering component may be varied. The important parameter is the pH. Sodium azide may be replaced by any suitable preservative (e.g., pentachlorophenol).

0.05 M Tris, 0.15 M NaCl, 0.02% NaN_3, pH 8.6: For 1 liter of buffer, dissolve 6.06 g of Tris and 8.76 g of NaCl in 800 ml of distilled water. Add 10 M HCl to pH 8.6 and make up the volume to 1 liter with water.

0.05 M phosphate, 0.15 M NaCl, pH 7.0: For 1 liter of buffer, dissolve 4.34 g of Na_2HPO_4, 2.70 g of NaH_2PO_4 monohydrate, and 8.76 g of NaCl in water to 1 liter; buffer pH should be 7.0.

0.05 M citrate, 0.15 M NaCl, pH 5.5: For 1 liter of buffer, dissolve 2.68 g of citric acid monohydrate, 10.96 g of trisodium citrate dihydrate, and 8.76 g of NaCl in water to 1 liter; buffer pH should be 5.5.

0.05 M acetate, 0.15 M NaCl, pH 4.3: For 1 liter of buffer, dissolve 6.8 g of sodium acetate and 8.76 g of NaCl in 800 ml of water. Add acetic acid to pH 4.3 and make up the volume to 1 liter with water.

0.05 M glycine-hydrochloride, 0.15 M NaCl, pH 2.3: For 1 liter of buffer, dissolve 5.6 g of glycine-HCl and 8.76 g of NaCl in 800 ml of water; add 10 M HCl to pH 2.3 and make up the volume to 1 liter with water.

PROCEDURE

Note: Purification is performed at room temperature.

1. Swell 1.5 g protein A-Sepharose CL 4B in Tris-buffered saline, pH 8.6. Pack resin in a suitable column (bed volume is 5–6 ml).

2. Harvest culture supernate and adjust to pH 8.6 by adding dilute NaOH.

3. Apply culture supernate to the protein A column. Wash column with Tris-buffered saline, pH 8.6. (One liter of culture supernate at pH 8.6 containing 10–60 mg of antibody is easily passed through the protein A column.)

4. Carry out step elution with the buffered saline at pH 7.0, 5.5, 4.3, and 2.3 until the hybrid cell antibody is eluted, avoiding low pH buffers whenever possible. A UV monitor is useful in detecting antibody elution from the column.

5. Pool fractions containing antibody and dialyze using an appropriate buffer (e.g., 0.05 M Tris, 0.15 M NaCl, pH 8.1).

6. Regenerate column by washing with the glycine-HCl-buffered saline, pH 2.3, and equilibrating with the Tris-buffered saline, pH 8.6 (including 0.02% NaN_3).

COMMENTS

1. Sometimes two protein peaks will be eluted from a supernate from a monoclonal cell line. By all physical criteria, the protein from both elution peaks may be identical. A possible explanation for this result is that protein A has two binding sites of different affinities for immunoglobulin (Lancet et al. 1978), hence elution conditions for a single protein species may require solutions of different pH.

2. When the antibody produced by a hybrid cell line does not bind to protein A, it is generally easier to purify the antibody from the sera of tumor-bearing mice by standard procedures. The disadvantage of this approach is the presence of normal serum immunoglobulin. Naturally occurring antibodies, for example, antiviral antibodies, may be co-purified with the hybrid cell antibody when affinity chromatography purification methods are precluded by the nature of the antigen, such as with cell surface antigens.

17.10 ANTIBODY CHARACTERIZATION

The monoclonal origins of the antibodies produced by hybrid cell lines must be confirmed by demonstrating the production of homogeneous antibody molecules. When NS-1 is used as the parent myeloma, a monoclonal cell line can produce three species of antibodies, because the cells will synthesize the heavy (H) and light (L) chains of the spleen cell parent as well as the MOPC-21 κ chain (K) of NS-1 origin. In the intracellular process of assembling the immunoglobulin, mixed molecules are made and secreted. These occur as the following four-chain species: H_2L_2, H_2LK, and H_2K_2. Of course, antibody activity is limited to the first two species. In the process of selecting antibody-producing clones, it is possible to select clones that have lost the ability to synthesize the MOPC-21 κ chain. These clones would then produce no mixed molecules, and every immunoglobulin molecule would be an identically active species.

The chain composition of the products of hybrid cell lines can be determined by various gel analyses. A description of these techniques is beyond the scope of this chapter. Two particular systems are recommended and references to these techniques are noted: (1) reducing and nonreducing isoelectric focusing (IEF; Williamson 1978); and (2) two-dimensional analyses using a nonequilibrium pH gradient and size separation (see Chapter 19).

17.11   CELL DISTRIBUTION CENTER

When an investigator generates a hybrid cell line producing an antibody that would have utility and interest to the general scientific community, it is urged that the cell line be made available to other investigators through the Cell Distribution Center at the Salk Institute (P.O. Box 1809, San Diego, CA 92112).

The Center already has available hybrid cell lines producing several anti–I-A^k antibodies (some of which cross-react with I-A antigens of f, r, and s haplotypes), anti-H-$2K^k$, anti-Ig-5a(δ), and anti-Ig-5b(δ); by the time this book is published, it will have even more lines available.

REFERENCES

Ey, P. L., S. J. Prowse, and C. R. Jenkin. 1978. Isolation of pure IgG$_1$, IgG$_{2a}$ and IgG$_{2b}$ immunoglobulins from mouse serum using protein A-Sepharose. *Immunochemistry* 15:429.

Galfre, G., S. C. Howe, C. Milstein, G. W. Butcher, and J. C. Howard. 1977. Antibodies to major histocompatibility antigens produced by hybrid cell lines. *Nature* 266:550.

Galfre, G., C. Milstein, and R. Wright. 1979. Rat × rat hybrid myelomas and a monoclonal anti-Fd portion of mouse IgG. *Nature* **277**:131.

Goding, J. W. 1978. Use of Staphylococcal protein A as an immunological reagent. *J. Immunol. Meth.* **20**:241.

Kearney, J. S., A. Radbruch, B. Liesegang, and K. Rajewsky. A new mouse myeloma cell line which has lost immunoglobulin expression that permits the construction of antibody-secreting hybridomas. *J. Immunol.*, in press.

Köhler, G., and C. Milstein. 1975. Continuous cultures of fused cells secreting antibody of predefined specificity. *Nature* **256**:495.

Lancet, D., D. Isenman, J. Sjödahl, J. Sjöquist, and I. Pecht. 1978. Interactions between staphylococcal protein A and immunoglobulin domains. *Biochem. Biophys. Res. Comm.* **85**:608.

Littlefield, J. W. 1964. Selection of hybrids from mating of fibroblasts *in vitro* and their presumed recombinants. *Science* **145**:709.

Oi, V. T., P. P. Jones, J. W. Goding, L. A. Herzenberg, and L. A. Herzenberg. 1978. Properties of monoclonal antibodies to mouse Ig allotypes, H-2 and Ia antigens. *Cur. Top. in Microbiol. and Immunol.* **81**:115.

Parks, D. R., V. M. Bryan, V. T. Oi, and L. A. Herzenberg. 1979. Antigen-specific identification and cloning of hybridomas with a fluorescence-activated cell sorter. *Proc. Natl. Acad. Sci. (USA)* **76**:1962.

Pontecorvo, G. 1976. Production of indefinitely multiplying mammalian somatic cell hybrids by polyethylene glycol (PEG) treatment. *Somatic Cell Genet.* **1**:397.

Schulman, M., C. D. Wilde, and G. Köhler. 1978. A better cell line for making hybridomas secreting specific antibodies. *Nature* **276**:269.

Williamson, A. R. 1978. Isoelectric focusing of immunoglobulins. In D. M. Weir (Ed.), *Handbook of Experimental Immunology,* third edition, vol. 1. Blackwell Scientific Publications, Oxford.

Solid-Phase Radioimmune Assays

Theta T. Tsu and Leonore A. Herzenberg

18.1   INTRODUCTION

Radioimmune assays (RIAs) combine the exquisite specificity of antigen-antibody reactions with the quantitative accuracy of isotope determinations. They allow sensitive measurement of antibody or antigen concentrations, even in unpurified preparations. Many procedural variations in the RIA have been developed to meet particular clinical or research needs, but the underlying principle of all assays is the same: Bound radioactivity is used as an index of the amount of antigen bound to a given quantity of antibody or of the amount of antibody bound to a given quantity of antigen.

Radiolabel may be bound either directly in the antigen-antibody complex by radiolabeling one of the participants of the reaction (antibody or antigen) or it may be bound indirectly by radiolabeling a reagent, generally a second antibody, which reacts with one of the unlabeled participants to provide an index of the amount of the participant bound in the initial antigen-antibody complex. In each case, the radiolabel bound to the complexes must then be separated from unbound radiolabeled material so that the amount of bound radioactivity can be determined.

In this chapter, we describe several variations of the "solid-phase" RIA in which one of the reactants is immobilized on the plastic inner surface of a 96-well (Microtiter) polyvinylchloride plate to facilitate separation of the antigen-antibody complexes from unbound material. The use of this solid-phase technology has greatly improved the sensitivity, specificity, and practicality of the RIA and has thus substantially expanded the attractiveness of this type of assay for many purposes. The examples we have chosen are intended to demonstrate the versatility of the solid-phase RIA and to serve as prototypes for assays that can be adapted to meet specific needs.

The ultimate precision and sensitivity of the RIA depend on the selection and preparation of suitably specific antibody reagents and the careful determination of optimal reagent concentrations. While guidelines for the preparation and use of reagents are presented in this chapter, it is necessary to determine empirically the exact experimental conditions for each antibody-antigen system. Generally accurate measurements for antigen or antibody in the nanogram range can be obtained with careful technique. Similar results with perhaps slightly less sensitivity and precision may be obtained in assaying the reactions of cell surface determinants and their specific antibodies when employing cell-binding RIA methods (analogous to solid-phase RIAs).

The cell-binding assays require centrifugation to separate the complexes of cells and bound reagents from unbound material. Aside from this procedural modification, however, cell-binding RIAs and solid-phase RIAs follow essentially the same general protocol. In the introductory text that follows, we present a general description of the procedure to provide an overview of the assay. In subsequent sections, we describe in detail specific protocols for preparing reagents and for using several variations of these methods.

1. Coating the Plate

Proteins and other macromolecules in solution tend to stick nonspecifically to plastic. The adsorption is essentially irreversible in buffered salt solutions such as phosphate-buffered saline (PBS), pH 7.4. Thus, incubation of an antigen or antibody solution in Microtiter wells results in deposition of a coat which persists throughout repeated washing.

The amount of antigen or antibody deposited depends on its concentration in solution, its inherent "stickiness," and the amount of contaminating material in solution capable of competing for sites on the plastic. Purified coating reagents yield more efficient coating. Titration curves based on the binding of the radiolabeled reagent to be used in the assay should be obtained to determine the most efficient coat concentration, taking into consideration the potential problem of increases in assay backgrounds due to nonspecific binding of radiolabeled reagents, which may occur at high coat concentrations.

2. Blocking the Plate

After the coat has been deposited, the plate must be "blocked" to prevent nonspecific adsorption of subsequently added reagents. Several washings of the coated wells with a concentrated protein solution, for example, 1% bovine serum albumin in PBS (RIA buffer) are quite satisfactory for this purpose. No incubation time is required for this step other than that involved in the washing process.

3. Washing the Plate

Plates are washed by filling the wells and dumping or "flicking" the contents of the wells into a sink or other suitable receptacle. The last drops of wash fluid are removed by throwing the plate, face down, onto several layers of absorbent material on a table.

4. Binding the Radiolabeled Reagent

Here, assays adapted for different purposes vary considerably (see Table 18.1):

a. In direct binding (one-step) assays, labeled reagent is simply added to the coated well and allowed to incubate.

b. In indirect (two-step) assays, unlabeled "first-step" antibody (or antigen) is incubated in the well for a period of time, and the well is then washed with RIA buffer to remove all unbound material. Radiolabeled reagent specific for the first-step reagent is then added and incubated.

c. In blocking assays, a solution containing material potentially similar to the coating antigen (or antibody) is mixed with the radiolabeled reagent and the mixture is added to the well and incubated. Alternatively, the blocking agent and then the radiolabeled reagents are added sequentially to the well prior to incubation.

In each procedure, the final incubation allows binding of radiolabeled reagent either to the coat antigen or to the first-step reagent bound to the

TABLE 18.1
Adaption of solid-phase radioimmune assays for different purposes

Well coat	First step	Second step	Use	Refer to
		One-Step Assay		
Ag	^{125}I-Ab	—	Measure reactivity of antibody	Section 18.3
Ab	^{125}I-Ag	—	or antigen	
Ag	Ag + ^{125}I-Ab	—	Measure or compare Ag-blocking assay	Section 18.5
Ab	Ag + ^{125}I-Ag	—	Measure or compare Ag-blocking assay	Section 18.5
		Two-Step Assay		
Ag	Ab	^{125}I-anti-Ig	Measure reactivity of Ab or Ag; determine isotype or allotype of Ab	Section 18.4
Ab	Ag	^{125}I-Ab (to Ag; must not react with Ab)	Measure reactivity of Ab or Ag	
Ag	Ab + Ag	^{125}I-anti-Ig (must not react with Ag)	Measure or compare Ag-blocking assay	

coat antigen. Excess radiolabeled reagent is removed from the wells after incubation and the wells are washed with RIA buffer to remove any additional unbound label.

5. Counting the Radioactivity Bound to the Wells

In general, ^{125}I-labeled reagents are used for these assays. The wells need only be severed from each other and dropped into carrier tubes, which can be counted in a gamma scintillation counter.

Severing the wells of the soft plastic plates recommended for use here can be accomplished simply by cutting them apart with a scissors or knife; however, if large numbers of wells are to be processed, wells can be severed by a more orderly and less time-consuming procedure. Adhesive plastic sheets (designed originally as nonpermeable covers for the Microtiter plates) can be firmly adhered to the *bottom* of the plates such that each well is anchored at its base. The top of the plate can then be cut away with a hot wire, leaving the anchored wells free to be plucked from their adhesive support and placed in counting tubes. A hot wire cutter has been especially designed for this purpose (see Materials and Reagents, Section 18.3).

6. Converting Counts to Quantitative Data Comparable from Experiment to Experiment

Since ^{125}I decays with a half-life of 60 days, expressing data as counts per minute (cpm) is often inadequate for a series of experiments conducted over a long period of time. Similarly, because assay conditions may vary slightly from day to day, raw count values may be misleading. We have found it helpful to include a standard curve with each assay and to express data in terms of standard equivalents (mg or μl) per milliliter of test serum. Use of standard curves also allows correction for nonlinearity of binding and thus gives a more accurate representation of the amount of antibody (or antigen) in the test serum.

18.2 PREPARATION OF RADIOLABELED REAGENTS FOR RIA

Editors' Note: Safety precautions necessary for work with sodium ^{125}iodide and iodinated material are described in Section 14.2.

Any of the standard iodination procedures are satisfactory for preparing ^{125}I-RIA reagents as long as most of the labeled protein in the preparation proves to be active in the specific binding reaction. We use a solid-phase radiolabeling method in which the antibody is iodinated while bound to antigen insolubilized by covalent binding to Sepharose beads, as described by Miles and Hales (1968). This method allows minimal losses in the labeling of small amounts of antibody because the antibody binding sites are protected during the labeling, and absorptions and elutions can be carried out in the presence of protein (e.g., BSA) to guard against nonspecific losses on glassware during the procedure. In addition, the method is reliable, reproducible, and economical since it does not require a separate antibody purification step prior to labeling.

Reagents prepared in this fashion usually contain more than 60% ^{125}I-labeled specifically bindable antibody; however, occasionally the procedure yields substantially less bindable antibody. In these instances, the labeled antibody is readsorbed on the antigen-Sepharose and re-eluted to bring the reagent up to standard for use in the RIA.

Soluble iodination is also used in our laboratory, mainly when antigen-

Sepharose conjugates are unavailable (e.g., for labeling antibody reactive with cell surface determinants or when determination of the specific activity of the labeled protein is required).

The procedure described below is for labeling antibodies to immunoglobulins. Appropriate modifications are required if other kinds of antibodies or if antigens are to be labeled.

MATERIALS AND REAGENTS

Antiserum to be labeled: Antiallotype and other antisera are made as described by Herzenberg and Herzenberg (1978a).

Antigen conjugated to Sepharose 4B: Couple purified antigen (myeloma protein) to Sepharose using CNBr-activated Sepharose 4B (Pharmacia Fine Chemicals) and the method described in a booklet available from Pharmacia—*Affinity Chromatography: Principles and Methods*. The protein-to-Sepharose ratio is 5 mg/ml gel. Store conjugate in PBS with 0.02% NaN_3 at 4°C.

Phosphate-buffered saline (PBS; see Appendix A.8)

Airfuge, air-driven ultracentrifuge (Beckman Instruments)

Sero-Fuge (Clay Adams, #0511)

PD-10 column, Sephadex G-25M (Pharmacia Fine Chemicals)

Pipetman, 20 μl and 200 μl (Rainin Instrument Co.)

Tube, 10 × 75 mm

Pasteur pipette, sealed, long tip (used as a stirring rod)

Gamma counter

Buffers and solutions

0.5 M phosphate buffer, pH 7.5: Dissolve 1.12 g KH_2PO_4 and 5.96 g Na_2HPO_4 anhydrous in 100 ml distilled water. For 0.05 M phosphate buffer, dilute 0.5 M buffer 1 : 10 with distilled water.

0.2 M glycine-HCl buffer, pH 2.3: Add 1.5 g glycine to approximately 90 ml distilled water, and adjust to pH 2.3 with concentrated HCl; add distilled water to bring volume up to 100 ml.

Bovine serum albumin (BSA): 1% (w/v) in PBS, containing 0.02% (w/v) NaN_3. Caution: Sodium azide is extremely toxic.

Trichloroacetic acid (TCA): 15% (w/v)

Chloramine "T": 10 mg/5 ml of 0.05 M phosphate buffer, pH 7.5

Sodium metabisulfite: 10 mg/5 ml of 0.05 M phosphate buffer, pH 7.5

Sodium ^{125}I in 0.1 M NaOH, carrier-free: 10 mCi/0.1 ml

PROCEDURE

1. Deaggregate antiserum in Airfuge (22 psi for 10 min).
2. Place 20 μl immunoadsorbent in a 10 × 75-mm tube. Wash once

(tube volume) with 0.2 M glycine-HCl, pH 2.3, by centrifugation in Sero-Fuge for 1 min.

3. Wash immunoadsorbent 2 times with PBS to neutralize (pH should be approximately 7.2). Pellet immunoadsorbent by centrifugation.

4. Add 75 μl of antiserum to the pelleted immunoadsorbent. Incubate at room temperature for 20 minutes (mix twice over the 20-minute period).

5. Wash immunoadsorbent 3 times with PBS and pellet by centrifugation.

6. Add 50 μl of 0.5 M phosphate buffer, pH 7.5, followed by 1 mCi ^{125}I (use within 2 weeks of arrival). Then add 10 μl chloramine "T". Mix for 30 seconds at room temperature with a sealed, long-tip Pasteur pipette.

7. Add 10 μl sodium metabisulfite solution. Mix for 30 seconds.

8. Add 1.4 ml 0.2 M glycine-HCl, pH 2.3, and pipet mixture onto a PD-10 column (equilibrated with 25 ml of 1% BSA in PBS and 0.02% sodium azide). Discard effluent.

9. Rinse tube with 1.0 ml of 0.2 M glycine-HCl, pH 2.3, and wash onto PD-10 column. Discard effluent (void volume is approximately 2.5 ml).

10. Add 3.0 ml of PBS onto the PD-10 column. Collect the effluent (which contains the radiolabeled antibody).

11. Determine the percentage of radiolabel precipitable by TCA:

    a. Place a 2-μl sample of the radiolabeled antibody into 150 μl 1% BSA in PBS. Count sample in gamma counter (Count A).

    b. Add 150 μl 15% TCA into counted sample (a) to precipitate protein. Centrifuge sample (290 $\times$ g, 10 min) and remove 75 μl of the supernate. Count sample in gamma counter (Count B).

$$\% \text{ TCA ppt} = 100\% - \frac{(4 \times B \times 100\%)}{A}$$

12. Store radiolabeled antibody at 4°C.

COMMENTS

1. When recovered sample is reapplied to a second Sepharose immunoadsorbent and eluted, 30–50% is usually recovered.

2. ^{125}I-labeling in solution: Labeling with ^{125}I in solution is identical to solid-phase ^{125}I-labeling except that steps 2–5 (immunoadsorbent

binding) are skipped. Also, PBS can be substituted for the 0.2 M glycine-HCl, pH 2.3, eluting buffer in steps 8 and 9. This method can be used when there are sufficient quantities of purified proteins. We routinely use this method to label: (a) purified mouse myeloma protein; use approximately 7.5 μl at 20 mg/ml = 150 μg; (b) staphylococcal protein A; use 10 μl at 1 mg/ml = 10 μg.

18.3 ONE-STEP SOLID-PHASE RIA: SPECIFICITY TESTING OF ^{125}I-LABELED ANTIALLOTYPE REAGENTS

After labeling an antiallotype sera, we test the specificity of the labeled antiallotype by coating 96-well Microtiter plates with myeloma proteins of known class and allotype (e.g., Ig-1a, Ig-1b, Ig-4a, Ig-4b)* and measuring the binding of the ^{125}I-labeled antiallotype. When properly prepared, the reagent should bind only to the appropriate myeloma protein.

If the reagent appears to be nonspecific (i.e., binds to the wrong myeloma protein), the coat concentration of the myeloma protein may be at fault. Purified myeloma proteins are frequently contaminated with small amounts of other Ig; thus, too high a coating concentration may result in coating the wells with a sufficient amount of a contaminating Ig class to allow detection of antibody bound to the contaminant. For example, wells coated with a 1 mg per milliliter solution of Ig-1a myeloma protein contaminated with 1% Ig-1b (e.g., from growth of the tumor in BALB/c Ig^b mice) will bind significant levels of ^{125}I-anti-Ig-1b because of the contaminant. (This antibody is known not to bind to Ig-1a because of the mouse strain combination used in the immunization.) Reduction of the coating concentration to 0.01 mg per ml in this case prevents detection of binding to the contaminant but does not interfere with detection of binding to the Ig-1a myeloma protein by reagents specific for it (e.g., anti-Ig-1a).

MATERIALS AND REAGENTS

Myeloma proteins: Ascites and sera from myeloma-bearing mice are purified by ammonium sulfate precipitation (Section 12.2) and column chromatography (e.g., DEAE Sephadex CH-6B or protein

---

* Nomenclature of mouse immunoglobulin isotypes and allotypes is presented in Herzenberg and Herzenberg (1978a).

A-Sepharose CL-4B; Pharmacia Fine Chemicals; see Sections 12.3 and 17.9).

^{125}I-labeled antiallotype sera

Phosphate-buffered saline (PBS), pH 7.4 (Appendix A.8)

Microtiter plates, "U" bottom, disposable, flexible, nonsterile (Cooke Laboratory Products, 96-2311 plates, #220-24)

Parafilm

Pipetman, 20 μl and 200 μl (Rainin Instrument Co.)

CHUX disposable diapers, used as absorbent paper for drying plates

Pasteur pipettes or apparatus for vacuum aspiration

Hot wire cutter (D. Lee, Inc.)

Gamma counter

RIA buffer, 1% bovine serum albumin (BSA) in PBS, 0.02% NaN$_3$: For 20 liters, add 200 g BSA (Fr V) to 20 liters PBS. Stir slowly until BSA completely dissolves. Filter solution by positive pressure through a 0.45-μm Millipore filter. Collect into 500-ml bottles (500 ml/bottle), adjust to pH 7.4, and add 1.0 ml of 10% NaN$_3$ to each bottle. Store at 4°C. Caution: Sodium azide is extremely toxic.

PROCEDURE

1. Dilute myeloma proteins (e.g., Ig-1a, Ig-1b, Ig-4a, Ig-4b) in PBS to subsaturating coating concentrations (0.1 mg/ml–0.01 mg/ml).

2. Add 50 μl of protein solution to an appropriate number of wells. All tests should be done in duplicate. Put RIA buffer in 2–4 wells for negative controls.

3. Cover the plate with Parafilm and incubate for 1 hour at room temperature.

4. Dump fluid from the wells and wash wells 3 times with RIA buffer.

5. After dumping the third wash, dry the plate by throwing it face down onto absorbent paper.

6. Add 20 μl of ^{125}I-labeled antiallotype reagent.

7. Cover plate with Parafilm and incubate 1 hour at room temperature.

8. Remove radioactive supernate from the plate by vacuum aspiration (or with a Pasteur pipette) and discard the supernate appropriately. Wash plate 3 times with RIA buffer and dry as above.

9. Cut wells apart with hot wire cutter or scissors and count in gamma counter (as described in the introduction to this chapter).

18.4 TWO-STEP SOLID-PHASE RIA: ESTIMATION OF ISOTYPE AND ALLOTYPE REPRESENTATION IN AN ANTIBODY RESPONSE, E.G., RESPONSE TO THE DINITROPHENYL HAPTEN (DNP) ON A CARRIER PROTEIN

Two-step solid-phase RIAs are easily adaptable to the measurement of antibody responses to soluble antigens and cell surface determinants. Since these assays are very sensitive, very small amounts of sera from responding animals (or of supernate from hybridoma cultures; see Chapter 17) are required for each test; however, because of this sensitivity, care must be exercised to assure that samples are adequately diluted (in RIA buffer) to place them within the accurate range of the assay (i.e., well below saturation). Usually, this range falls within the reasonably linear portion of the standard curve (titration of purified antibody or standard antiserum) that is run along with each assay to provide a reference for expressing antibody levels in the test sera.

For these two-step solid-phase assays, antigen is coated on (or placed in) the wells of 96-well Microtiter plates. Coating concentrations below 100 μg/ml are usually used to decrease assay backgrounds. After the appropriate washing of coated wells, dilutions of test or standard first-step antisera are incubated in the wells. After appropriate washing, ^{125}I-labeled anti-Ig (second-step) reagents are incubated in the wells to provide an index of the amount of first-step antibody bound. Choice of the second-step reagent(s) determines which isotype(s) or allotype(s) represented in the response are measured.

We have used this type of RIA extensively to measure the adoptive secondary response of allotype heterozygotes to DNP conjugated to keyhole limpet hemocyanin (DNP-KLH; Tokuhisa, Black, Tsu, Ledbetter, Hayakawa, Gadus, and Herzenberg, unpublished observations). In this kind of study, sera are taken from mice 7–21 days after the adoptive transfer. The sera are tested on plates coated with DNP-BSA to avoid measurement of anti-KLH antibody. Four tandem assays are performed for each serum to allow individual measurements of Ig-1a, Ig-1b, Ig-4a, and Ig-4b anti-DNP antibody in the serum. Each serum is tested in duplicate, generally at each of two dilutions, for initial screening. Those test sera falling outside the valid range of the assay are then diluted appropriately and retested to obtain accurate measurements. Responses are expressed as a percentage of the antibody present in a standard serum prepared by pooling sera from a large number of responding (control) recipients in an adoptive transfer similar to those transfers from which the test recipients are drawn. (Other standards can be used, but we have found it is wise to match test and standard sera as closely as possible.)

A wide variety of specific second-step reagents can be used in these assays, including antiallotype, anti-idiotype, anti-isotype, and anti–light chain. The amount of labeled reagent required must be determined for each system but will usually be approximately 20 000 cpm in a freshly labeled preparation (using the labeling techniques described in Section 18.2). Once established, the same concentration of labeled reagent should be maintained throughout its use, despite decay of radioactivity; this is helpful for comparing results obtained in different assays.

Polyvalent anti-Ig reagents composed of mixtures of specific reagents can also prove useful for RIA; however, these reagents (especially polyvalent anti-Ig in which the proportion of antibodies specific for different isotypes or allotypes is unknown) must be used with caution. One of the component antibodies in such a reagent may be limiting and thus fail to completely reveal a significant proportion of first-step antibody binding even though the overall second-step antibody concentration appears adequate. The presence of antibody reactive with IgM in these polyvalent anti-Ig second-step reagents may give disproportionately high values because IgM antibody is pentameric and thus potentially binds five times as much radiolabel per mole of antibody.

One last caution: Solid-phase RIAs, like all antibody assays, cannot detect antibody whose avidity is below a certain level. Ignorance of the lower limit of avidities detectable in an assay (e.g., measurement of pri-

TABLE 18.2
Low-avidity anti-DNP antibody is revealed better by binding on plates coated with highly conjugated DNP-BSA

Source of α-DNP antibodies	Expected average avidity	α-DNP binding* (RIA plate coat)	
		DNP_{12}-BSA	DNP_{42}-BSA
In situ primary	low	2	16
Adoptive primary			
KLH 1° spleen	low	3	19
KLH 1° nylon T	low	0	6
Adoptive secondary†			
2-week DNP 1° B (+ KLH 1° T)	low	13	34
8-week DNP 1° B (+ KLH 1° T)	high	150	150
DNP-KLH 1° spleen (assay standard)	high	100	108
In situ hyperimmune	high	360	350

* Binding expressed as units of α-DNP activity per ml of sample serum relative to the binding of the assay standard on DNP_{12}-BSA. Standard binding is arbitrarily set at 100 units/ml; thus a serum with 1 unit/ml has 1% of the α-DNP binding activity present in the standard.
† Sera obtained 7 days after adoptive transfer and 2° immunization. Two week DNP 1° B cells were from mice primed 2 weeks before transfer; 8 week DNP 1° B cells were from mice primed 8 weeks before transfer. KLH 1° T cells and DNP-KLH 1° spleen cells were from mice primed 6 or more weeks before transfer.

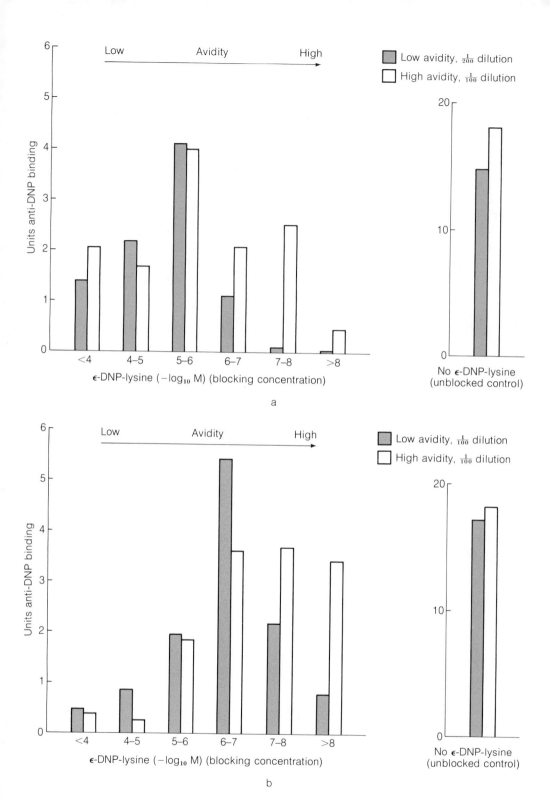

mary (low-avidity) antibody responses) can lead to falsely negative results.

In the anti-DNP assay performed as described here with DNP_{12}-BSA as coat antigen, we have found that primary responses to DNP-KLH on alum, with or without adjuvants, are only poorly detected. However, it is possible to extend the range of avidities detected by using DNP-BSA conjugates with higher hapten substitution ratios. Thus, coating with DNP_{19}-BSA or DNP_{42}-BSA allows detection of primary and similar low-avidity secondary responses, whereas coating with DNP_5-BSA and DNP_{12}-BSA allows detection of only the relatively high avidity components in a secondary response (see Table 18.2). Backgrounds are not substantially increased with the more highly conjugated antigens.

The differences in the avidity of the antibody detected were established using a hapten-inhibition RIA. In this assay, ε-DNP-lysine in $\log_{10}$ dilution steps was preincubated for one hour with a constant dilution of antibody in a separate plate. A constant volume ($20\mu l$) of each of the incubated mixtures was then transferred to antigen-coated wells, and the assay was continued in the usual manner. Antibody dilutions were established to give a standard number of second-step (anti-Ig) counts bound for all samples in the absence of hapten inhibitor. Since the amount of second-step binding reflects the amount (μg) of first step bound, standardizing samples in this way allows comparison of avidities of different antibody samples for most sera without determination of the actual number of micrograms per milliliter of antibody in the serum.

This assay gives typical hapten inhibition curves (see Figure 18.1); however, the counts bound must be converted into units of antibody (see above) before plotting the curves, to correct for the nonlinearity of the original antibody titration.

As a routine screening procedure for high- and low-avidity antibody in responses, we have found that subtraction of units of antibody bound to DNP_{12}-BSA from units bound to DNP_{42}-BSA gives a reliable estimate of the low-avidity component in the sample.

The procedures described above for measuring low- and high-avidity

FIGURE 18.1

Avidity distributions of low- and high-avidity anti-DNP serum pools measured on RIA plate coats of (a) DNP_{42}-BSA and (b) DNP_{12}-BSA. Bars in the figure represent units* of anti-DNP antibody not blocked by the lower ϵ-DNP-lysine concentration but blocked by the higher. The low-avidity pool contained 17 units anti-DNP activity measured on DNP_{12}-BSA and 30 units measured on DNP_{42}-BSA; the high avidity-pool contained 18 units anti-DNP activity on either coat. Antibody dilutions used were adjusted to equalize binding between low- and high-avidity pools for each plate coat.

* Binding is expressed as units of α-DNP activity per ml of sample serum relative to the binding of the assay standard on DNP_{12}-BSA. Standard binding is arbitrarily set at 100 units/ml; thus a serum with 1 unit/ml has 1% of the α-DNP binding activity present in the standard.

antibody were developed by Takeshi Tokuhisa, Kyoko Hayakawa, Tim Gadus, Jeff Ledbetter, Sam Black, and the authors.

Figure 18.2 depicts a sample work sheet used to screen supernates from hybridoma cell lines for antibody against antigens on cell surfaces (see Section 18.6) or antigen coated on Microtiter plates.

MATERIALS AND REAGENTS

As described in Section 18.3 (except for the deletion of myeloma proteins), with the following additions:

DNP-BSA, made as described by Iverson (1978): Adjust stock concentration to 10 mg/ml in PBS as determined by Bio-Rad protein assay (Bio-Rad Laboratories, #500-0001). Conjugation ratios are determined by the spectrophotometric method described by Iverson (1978). Aliquot DNP-BSA into small plastic tubes and store at $-20°C$. Dilute solution 1 : 100 in PBS to 0.1 mg/ml prior to use.

Normal mouse serum (NMS)

Anti-DNP serum for preparing standard curve (e.g., serum from an anti-DNP adoptive secondary response as described by Okumura et al. 1976)

PROCEDURE

1. Dilute DNP-BSA to 0.1 mg/ml in PBS and add 50 μl to an appropriate number of wells (all tests should be run in duplicate).

2. Cover plate with Parafilm and incubate for 1 hour at room temperature.

3. Dump plate and wash 3 times with RIA buffer. Dry plate after last wash by throwing plate face down onto absorbent paper.

4. Add 20 μl of appropriately diluted test or standard control serum to each well. Each assay should include a standard curve in dilutions (1 : 1000 to 1 : 32 000, depending on the antiserum) of an adoptive secondary or other anti-DNP serum pool. Test sera should be diluted at least 50-fold (1 : 50) to avoid background problems. Wells with NMS (1 : 50) and RIA buffer should be included in the assay as negative controls.

5. Cover plates with Parafilm and incubate 1 hour at room temperature.

6. Dump plates and wash 3 times with RIA buffer. Dry after the last wash by throwing plate face down onto absorbent paper.

7. Add 20 μl of ^{125}I-labeled second-step reagent (10 000 to 20 000 cpm/well). (Note: Place a 20 μl sample of the ^{125}I-labeled reagent

Expt. # _____   Hybr.-plate no. _____   Date _____

Cell type _____   Strain _____   Cells/well _____

Coat antigen _____   Super. vol/well _____   Super. date _____

Labeled reagent _____ ID # _____ cpm/vol. added _____

	1	2	3	4	5	6	7	8	9	10	11	12
A												
B												
C												
D												
E												
F												
G												
H												

A
B
C
D
E
F
G
H

Expt. # _____   Hybr.-plate no. _____   Date _____

Cell type _____   Strain _____   Cells/well _____

Coat antigen _____   Super. vol/well _____   Super. date _____

Labeled reagent _____ ID # _____ cpm/vol. added _____

FIGURE 18.2
Sample work sheet used to screen supernatants from hybridoma cell lines for antibody
activity.

in a counting tube at this time. Count this tube to determine the total cpm/well actually added in the assay.)

8. Cover plates with Parafilm and incubate 1 hour at room temperature.

9. Aspirate the radioactive supernate and discard appropriately. Wash plates 3 times and dry after last wash.

10. Cut wells apart and count in gamma counter (as described in Introduction).

11. Plot standard curve on linear scale (counts vs μl of standard/well; see Figure 18.3). Generally, the curve will have an initial "linear" portion before flattening towards saturation. Whenever possible, read diluted test sera values from this linear portion since it gives the most accurate readings. (It is often wise to repeat tests on sera that do not test within the "linear" range of the assay, using a more diluted sample of each test serum, if highly accurate readings are desired.) Values read from the curve will indicate the microliter equivalent of the standard in the diluted test sample. Correct for dilution to obtain μl of standard equivalent/μl undiluted test serum. Results can also be expressed as a percentage of the standard.

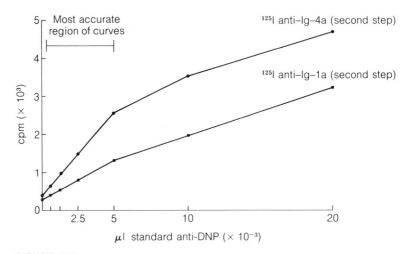

FIGURE 18.3
Anti-DNP standard curves with different antiallotype second-step reagents. First step: 20 μl standard anti-DNP. Second step: 20 μl ^{125}I-antiallotype. Plate coat: 50 μl DNP$_{12}$-BSA at 0.1 mg/ml.

18.5 RADIOIMMUNE BLOCKING ASSAY: MEASUREMENT OF IMMUNOGLOBULIN LEVELS

The quantitation of immunoglobulin (Ig) levels in this assay is based on competition between bound and soluble Ig for radiolabeled antibody. The wells of a Microtiter plate are first coated with saturating amounts of antigen (e.g., Ig of a given class or allotype such as an Ig-1a myeloma protein). After excess coating antigen is removed by washing, a second volume of antigen is added to the wells. Some of the wells receive graded concentrations of the known standard, making it possible to construct a standard curve for reference; others receive the unknown test samples. Negative control wells receive no antigen (or receive antigen that does not cross-react with the coat antigen). All wells then receive ^{125}I-labeled antibody (e.g., anti–Ig-1a) at a fixed, limiting concentration. After incubation, plates are washed and the wells counted in a gamma scintillation counter.

Wells with no antigen added as competitor bind the maximum bindable fraction of the counts (antibody) added. Wells containing competitor antigen bind fewer counts because the soluble antigen binds some of the added counts so that those counts are not available for binding to the antigen on the well. (Complexes of soluble antigen and radiolabeled antibody apparently do not adhere to the precoated well.) A standard curve is drawn from the titration of the known standard. Amounts of antigen in the test samples are then calculated from this standard curve. Plotting the log of the amount of myeloma protein (or normal serum standard) against the number of counts bound generally yields a straight line, often over a thousandfold concentration range (depending on the labeled reagent used). The linearity of this curve makes it easy to interpolate to determine the quantity of the antigen in the test serum and to express this quantity in terms of milligrams per milliliter or a percentage of the normal serum standard.

MATERIALS AND REAGENTS

As described in Section 18.3, with the following additions:

Test serum
Negative control serum containing the wrong allotype

PROCEDURE

1. Dilute myeloma protein to 20 μg/ml in phosphate-buffered saline (PBS). Add 50 μl to an appropriate number of wells. Run all tests in duplicate.

2. Cover plates with Parafilm. Incubate for 1 hour at room temperature.

3. Dump the plate and wash twice with RIA buffer.

4. Refill the plate with RIA buffer. Leave this third wash on the plate for 1 hour at room temperature to allow any loosely bound protein to escape. Dump plate and dry.

5. Add 20 μl of standard myeloma protein solution (or normal mouse serum known to contain immunoglobulin of the appropriate allotype) to the appropriate number of wells. To obtain a standard curve, use serial dilutions of the original myeloma protein coat (starting at 20 μg/ml and decreasing to 0.02 μg/ml) or the normal mouse serum (starting at 1 : 10).

6. Add 20 μl of test serum or negative control serum to the other wells. Test serum dilutions of between 1 : 100 and 1 : 500 usually fall in the range of the standard curve. The negative control serum is tested at the same dilutions.

7. After adding all of the sera in steps 5 and 6, add 20 μl of ^{125}I-labeled antibody reactive with the myeloma protein coated to the plate (40 000 cpm/well). Incubate for 1 hour at room temperature.

8. Aspirate radioactive supernate and discard appropriately. Wash plates 3 times and dry.

9. Cut wells apart and count in gamma counter (as described in Section 18.1).

10. Plot standard curve on semilog paper (counts vs log of blocking protein concentration; see Figure 18.4). Read amounts in test serum dilutions from standard curve. Correct for dilution to obtain mg/ml in undiluted test serum.

18.6 CELL BINDING ASSAY: CELL SURFACE ANTIGENS ON LYMPHOCYTES

Antibodies to cell surface antigens can be detected in a two-step assay in Microtiter plates by binding antibody to target cells and then detecting bound antibody with ^{125}I-labeled second-step reagents (e.g., antiallotype or staphylococcus protein A). This assay can also be used to determine the presence or absence of a cell surface determinant in a cell population or to determine the *average* amount of a surface antigen expressed on cells in a population. Because the procedure deals with a total population, it does not allow determination of the distribution of cells carrying different

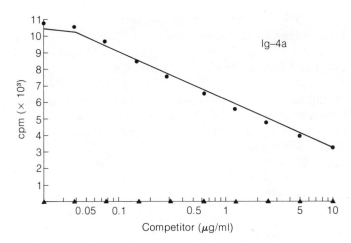

FIGURE 18.4
Standard curve for the RIA blocking assay. When counts per minute (cpm) are plotted against the logarithm of the concentration of antigen added to the wells to compete with the plate coat, a straight line is obtained. In this assay, MOPC-21 was used as the plate coat and the competitor.

amounts of the surface antigen within the population. Thus, with this assay, a population of many cells each carrying a small amount of antigen cannot be distinguished from a population of a few cells carrying a large amount of antigen among many antigen-negative cells. Data on the distribution of cells carrying different amounts of surface antigen within a population require the use of methods in which cells are examined individually, for example, analysis with the fluorescence-activated cell sorter (FACS) as discussed by Herzenberg and Herzenberg (1978b).

MATERIALS AND REAGENTS

Target cells (e.g., spleen; see Chapter 1 for general procedures for obtaining mouse cell suspensions)

Positive control antiserum, known to bind to target cells and detectable by the second-step reagent

[125]I-labeled second-step reagent (e.g., anti-Ig or staphylococcus protein A; Section 18.2)

Phosphate-buffered saline (PBS; Appendix A.8)

RIA buffer, 5% FCS in PBS, 0.02% NaN_3: Prepare as described in Section 18.3, except add 5% FCS instead of BSA.

Microtiter plates, "U" bottom (Cooke Laboratory Products, 96-2311 plates, #220-24)

Microtest II plate lids (Falcon, #3041 or similar)
Microtiter mixer (Cooke Laboratory Products)
Plate holder, rubber (Cooke Laboratory Products, #220-26)
Pipetman, 20 μl and 200 μl (Rainin Instrument Co.)
Nitex monofilament screen cloth, 42 in. × 5 yd (TETKO, #HD-3-85)
Glass wool column: Fill a 3-ml disposal syringe barrel with approxi-
    mately 0.75 ml glass wool for each spleen to be filtered. Incubate
    the column with RIA buffer for 15 minutes prior to use.
Heat lamp to dry Microtiter plates
Hot wire cutter (D. Lee)
Glass slides, 1 × 3 in., frosted end
Gamma scintillation counter

PROCEDURE

1. Remove target cell organs (e.g., spleen) from mice and make a
   single-cell suspension in RIA buffer by gently squeezing organs
   between frosted ends of 1 × 3-in. glass slides and passing cells
   through nylon monofilament cloth.

2. Centrifuge at 290 × g for 10 minutes (1000 rpm in an IEC centrifuge), wash cells with RIA buffer, and resuspend cells in 1.0 ml
   RIA buffer per spleen.

3. Remove dead cells by filtration through glass wool (Section 1.21).
   Apply the cell suspension to the column (avoiding a pressure
   head) and immediately follow with 10 ml of RIA buffer at room
   temperature. Collect all the effluent.

4. Centrifuge and resuspend as in step 2 (cell concentration will be
   approximately 1 × 10⁸ cells/ml). Count cells and adjust to 2 × 10⁷
   cells/ml.

5. Add 20 μl of the cell suspension to Microtiter wells (20 μl of 2 ×
   10⁷ cells/ml = 4 × 10⁵ cells/well). Tape rubber plate holders to the
   Microtiter plates to provide support.

6. Add 20 μl of the test solution (containing antibody appropriately
   diluted in RIA buffer) to the cell suspension in the wells. Mix
   plates thoroughly on a Cooke Microtiter mixer, cover the plates
   with lids, and incubate the plates for 30 minutes at 4°C. Mix the
   plates again and incubate for an additional 30 minutes.

7. After the second incubation, add 100 μl of RIA buffer to each
   well. Centrifuge plates at 290 × g for 3 minutes (1000 rpm in an
   IEC centrifuge with Cooke centrifuge carriers).

8. Aspirate supernate with a blunt-end, 23-gauge needle attached

to a vacuum. Add 200 μl of RIA buffer to each well. (Directing the buffer stream at the pellet facilitates resuspension.) Mix plates and check visually to see that the cells are thoroughly resuspended. Centrifuge plates at 290 × g for 3 minutes.

9. Aspirate the supernate. Add 50 μl of ^{125}I-labeled (10 000–20 000 cpm) second-step reagent. (Note: Place a 50-μl sample of the ^{125}I-labeled reagent in a counting tube at this time. This tube will be counted to determine the total cpm/well actually added in the assay.) Mix plates thoroughly. Incubate the plates for 30 minutes at 4°C, mix again, and incubate for an additional 30 minutes at 4°C.

10. Repeat steps 7 and 8, with an extra 200-μl cycle, to wash away the unbound radiolabeled reagent. Collect the first wash, containing the bulk of the radioactivity, into a special container for appropriate disposal.

11. After the last wash, aspirate the supernate and dry the plates for about 5 minutes under a heat lamp.

12. Cut the wells apart, place wells in counting tubes, and count in a gamma scintillation counter.

COMMENTS

1. We routinely include 6 negative controls composed of RIA buffer plus target cells and 6 positive controls composed of an antibody known to bind to the target cells plus the target cells themselves. This positive control antibody also must be known to be detectable by the second-step (radiolabeled) reagent.

2. The second-step reagent must not, by itself, bind appreciably to the target cells. Otherwise, background values will be too high to assess binding of the first-step reagent. Thus, anti-IgM and anti–Ig light chain reagents cannot be used when spleen cells are used as targets because of the large amount of surface IgM and IgD on splenic B cells. Fortunately, very little surface IgG is present on these cells; therefore, it is possible to use specific anti-IgG second-step reagents without generating appreciable backgrounds.

3. Occasionally, cells appear (by eye) to disappear during the assay. Despite this occurrence we recommend that the assay be carried out to completion as the assay can still give interpretable values.

4. To make the cell pellet more visible, "carrier" erythrocytes can be added. Controls should then also include wells with the carrier cells alone.

5. Preliminary data suggest that antibodies to H-2, Ia, and other lymphocyte cell surface antigens are detectable in plate binding as well as cell binding assays. Plates are coated with isolated cell surface membranes prepared and suspended in detergent-free aqueous buffers containing Mg^{2+}. Assays for antibody are then conducted as described in previous sections. Optimal protocols are currently under development (S. Qasim Mehdi, Department of Radiology; Frank Howard, Department of Chemistry; and Jeffrey Ledbetter, Department of Genetics; all at Stanford University).

18.7 AUTOMATED PIPETTING DEVICE

Assaying large numbers of samples (many plates per day) can be considerably facilitated by the use of automated pipetting devices; however, such devices must meet the standards of accuracy desired in the assay. In a rough survey of equipment available on the market in 1977, we were unable to find equipment that satisfied our needs. We therefore constructed the following device.

We ordered a special programmable pipetting apparatus* that had gauged peristaltic pump heads capable of handling up to 12 individual pipetting lines in parallel. We connected each of these lines to a plastic fitting milled to hold the standard plastic tips used on a Pipetman. The 12 fittings were then mounted in a "wand" so that they could be moved from plate to plate as one unit. The fittings were rigidly aligned in the wand such that the tips were centered over the 12 wells in one row of a Microtiter plate. Thus 12 samples (one row) could be simultaneously withdrawn or added to a plate (see Figure 18.5).

For operation, a set of plastic tips are affixed to the fittings in the wand, the lines are seated in the peristaltic pumps, and the free ends are placed in a reservoir containing RIA diluent. The lines are then filled with RIA buffer and the bubbles removed if necessary. The apparatus is then ready for use. The diluent is maintained in the line and driven through before each new sample is pipetted to prevent carry-over between samples (i.e., tips are washed from within). The entire set-up procedure takes about five minutes.

To control the volume of fluid pipetted and the sequence of pickups,

---

* 12-Channel Programmable Micro-Pipetting Pickup and Delivery System, Innovative Medical Systems, Harleysville, PA.

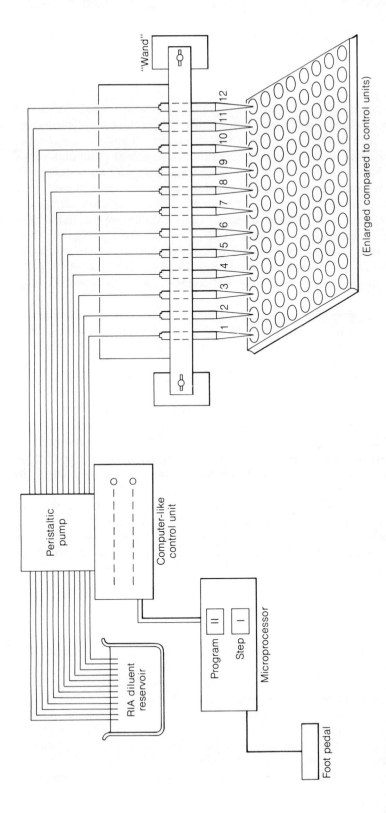

FIGURE 18.5
Schematic diagram of automated pipetting device.

deliveries, and washes as samples are transferred from "supply" wells on one plate to "test" wells on another, the programmable pipetting apparatus (which in itself can control volume) is placed under the control of a microprocessor unit that can be programmed to repeat a complex series of steps, with each successive step being triggered by a foot pedal signal. We have written programs for the standard assay protocols in use in the laboratory. One such program, for example, allows duplicate samples to be pipetted from rows of supply wells with intervening washes in between rows; the program dictates: Take in 30 μl air (to separate sample from diluent in line), pick up 20 μl from supply wells, deliver 20 μl to test wells, pick up 20 μl from supply wells, deliver 20 μl to (duplicate) test wells, deliver 200 μl diluent to waste collection vessel (to wash), restart sequence.

Over a long period of use, we have found the accuracy of work with this apparatus equal to or greater than the accuracy of pipetting samples with a Pipetman if we change Pipetman tips between samples. If we merely rinse the Pipetman tips between samples, the accuracy of the "automatic" apparatus is greater because of occasional carry-over between samples transferred with a Pipetman.

We are currently building a fully automated system based on the above principles, where supply and test plates are shuttled into position under the wand and the wand raised and lowered into the wells as required. In this version of the system, the programmable pipetting control system has been eliminated and the microprocessor is used to directly control the peristaltic pumps (i.e., the volumes delivered).

Personnel involved in designing the manual and automated systems include: William Harlow, Tom Nozaki, Jr., Wayne Moore, David Parks, and Leonore Herzenberg, with assistance from facilities in our laboratory operated under the direction of Richard Sweet and Leonard Herzenberg.

REFERENCES

Herzenberg, L. A., and L. A. Herzenberg. 1978a. Mouse immunoglobulin allotypes: Description and specific methodology. In D. M. Weir (Ed.), *Handbook of Experimental Immunology,* third edition. Blackwell Scientific Publications, Oxford.

Herzenberg, L. A., and L. A. Herzenberg. 1978b. Analysis and separation using the fluorescence-activated cell sorter (FACS). In D. M. Weir (Ed.), *Handbook of Experimental Immunology,* third edition. Blackwell Scientific Publications, Oxford.

Iverson, G. M. 1978. Assay methods for antigen-mediated cell cooperation. In D. M. Weir (Ed.), *Handbook of Experimental Immunology,* third edition. Blackwell Scientific Publications, Oxford.

Miles, L. E. M., and C. N. Hales. 1968. Labelled antibodies and immunological assay systems. *Nature* **219:**186.

Okumura, K., L. A. Herzenberg, D. B. Murphy, H. O. McDevitt, and L. A. Herzenberg. 1976. Selective expression of *H-2* (*I*-region) loci controlling determinants on helper and suppressor T lymphocytes. *J. Exp. Med.* **144:**685.

19

Analysis of Radiolabeled Lymphocyte Proteins by One- and Two-Dimensional Polyacrylamide Gel Electrophoresis

Patricia P. Jones

19.1 INTRODUCTION

The cell surface proteins of lymphocytes play important roles in the generation of immune responses, serving as specific receptors for antigens, other molecules, and possibly other cells. Surface antigens are also valuable as distinctive markers of lymphocyte subpopulations. Biochemical characterization of lymphocyte antigens is often desirable to provide information about the genetics, structure, and functions of these molecules. Although the direct purification of membrane proteins is difficult to achieve because of their low concentration in the cell, labeling the antigens with radioactive isotopes has made such studies possible. Specific antisera against the antigens can be used to isolate the radiolabeled proteins from detergent extracts of the cells and the proteins can then be characterized by a variety of electrophoretic procedures. This approach was first used in the early 1970s to examine lymphocyte surface immunoglobulin (Baur et al. 1971). Since then the technology has become much more advanced, and many different lymphocyte membrane antigens have been examined in this way.

This chapter describes a number of procedures that have proven successful for the analysis of a variety of lymphoid cell products (Jones 1977;

Oi et al. 1978). The methods included for radiolabeling, extracting, and immunoprecipitating cell proteins are fairly standard. Two different methods are outlined for radiolabeling cells: lactoperoxidase-catalyzed labeling of cell surface proteins with ^{125}I and biosynthetic labeling of cell proteins with radioactive amino acids. After being labeled, the cells are extracted with the detergent Nonidet P40, a non-ionic detergent that effectively solubilizes membrane proteins without destroying their antigenicity. Antisera are added to the extracts to bind the desired antigen. The antigen-antibody complexes are then removed from solution by a protein A-bearing *Staphylococcus aureus* bacteria adsorbent.

Two procedures for characterizing the immunoprecipitated antigens are described. The first is two-dimensional polyacrylamide gel electrophoresis (2-D PAGE), a method developed initially by O'Farrell (1975). In this system proteins are first separated in narrow cylindrical gels according to their charge; these gels are then placed on top of a sodium dodecyl sulfate (SDS) slab gel for the second dimension separation according to size. This procedure resolves each protein as a single spot, visualized by protein stains or by autoradiography. The equipment and methodology of 2-D PAGE initially may seem very complex. However, the great power of this technique (i.e., the ability to separate heterogeneous mixtures of protein into their component species) makes it well worth the initial expense and effort. Once the system is established it works consistently and the gel patterns produced are so reproducible that they actually represent "molecular fingerprints" of the proteins in the sample.

The second technique presented for analyzing radiolabeled proteins is one-dimensional SDS polyacrylamide gel electrophoresis (SDS-PAGE) in slab gels. This method is virtually identical to the second step of the 2-D PAGE system; it provides less information than the two-dimensional system but is faster and enables more samples to be processed at one time.

The procedures described below work well for the radiolabeling, isolation, and characterization of a variety of cell surface proteins by polyacrylamide gel electrophoresis in denaturing conditions. However, because analysis of other proteins may require different approaches, the reader is encouraged to adapt the described procedures to suit his or her own needs.

19.2 RADIOLABELING AND EXTRACTION OF CELL PROTEINS

The two methods described below for labeling cell surface proteins differ in that lactoperoxidase-catalyzed radioiodination of intact cells labels only those proteins that are on the cell surface, while incorporation of radioactive amino acids labels both cytoplasmic and cell surface proteins. The choice of labeling procedure depends on both the purpose of the experiment and the nature of the membrane protein.

There are several advantages to labeling cellular proteins with amino acids. First, since all biosynthetic forms of a protein become labeled, the 2-D PAGE pattern generated by this protein would be more complex than if only cell surface protein had been labeled with [125]I. The more complex the gel pattern, the more characteristic it is of a given protein. Thus, if one wants to determine whether two proteins are identical or different using 2-D PAGE, biosynthetic labeling is recommended. Second, biosynthetic labeling can also reveal whether a protein exists in multiple molecular forms, as is usually true for membrane proteins that are glycosylated on the way to the cell surface. A further advantage of biosynthetic labeling is that most proteins can be labeled by such a procedure, while not all membrane proteins label with [125]I. For example, some Ia antigens of mouse, guinea pig, and human lymphocytes do not label with ^{125}I, perhaps because they have no exposed tyrosine residues (Schwartz et al. 1976; Jones 1977).

However, there also are advantages to cell surface radioiodination. For some purposes, one wants to examine only those molecules that are on the cell surface, not those inside the cell. Also, membrane proteins that turn over slowly may not label well biosynthetically, whereas enough molecules might be present on the cell surface to be detected by radioiodination. IgD molecules on B cell membranes are difficult to detect following incorporation of radioactive amino acids, perhaps for this reason. In contrast, labeling IgD with ^{125}I works well. If one does not know about the labeling behavior of a particular antigen, it is probably advisable to try both approaches.

A. Biosynthetic Incorporation of Radioactive Amino Acids

The choice of which radioactive amino acid to use depends on several factors. The most important is the method that will be used to analyze the separated proteins. If autoradiography will be used, as is recommended in this chapter, then ^{35}S-methionine is the isotope of choice.* The energy of β particles emitted from ^{35}S is much higher than those of ^{3}H, so they are more efficient for autoradiography. While the energy of ^{14}C emission is comparable with that of ^{35}S, the low specific activity and high cost of

---

* ^{35}S-cysteine is now available at reasonably high specific activity and may be used in place of (or simultaneously with) ^{35}S-methionine. Medium lacking cysteine must be used when one is labeling with ^{35}S-cysteine.

^{14}C-amino acids make their use impractical. It is possible to increase the efficiency of detecting ^{3}H and ^{14}C by using fluorography (see Section 19.7); however, this method is much more tedious than autoradiography. ^{35}S-methionine can be obtained at very high specific activities (approximately 1000 Ci/mmol) so it is relatively inexpensive to label proteins to high specific activities. A note of reassurance: It is worth mentioning that despite the relatively infrequent occurrence of methionine in proteins, we have not detected any proteins that label abnormally high or low with ^{35}S-methionine compared to their labeling with a mixture of ^{3}H-amino acids (P. Jones, unpublished observations).

Normal lymphocytes are usually labeled for 4–5 hours; incorporation of radioactive amino acids into protein is linear during this period. The amount of ^{35}S radioactivity incorporated into protein generally ranges from 50 000–100 000 cpm per 10^5 cells. If shorter labeling times are desired, it may be necessary to increase the amount of ^{35}S-methionine. If this is done, the ^{35}S-methionine to be used should probably be freeze-dried prior to addition to cultures, to avoid excessive dilution of the labeling medium. Tumor cells and other rapidly growing cells may need less time to attain the same level of labeling since their overall rate of protein synthesis is generally higher than that in the resting lymphocytes.

MATERIALS AND REAGENTS

Fetal calf serum (FCS)

Tissue culture medium, lacking methionine: RPMI 1640, Eagle's minimum essential medium, or Dulbecco's minimum essential medium (special order from Grand Island Biological or other tissue culture supply company)

Phosphate-buffered saline (PBS; Appendix A.8) or balanced salt solution (BSS; Appendix A.3)

Stock solutions for Tris-buffered ammonium chloride (Section 1.17) or hemolytic Gey's solution (Section 1.18)

Materials and reagents to determine cell viability (see appropriate sections in Chapter 1)

^{35}S-methionine, 500–1000 Ci/mmol (New England Nuclear or Amersham)

Centrifuge tubes, 15 ml

Disposable plastic tubes, 17×100 mm and 12×75 mm (Falcon or similar)

5% CO_2-in-air gas mixture

37°C humidified CO_2 incubator

Refrigerated centrifuge

Washing buffer: PBS or BSS containing 2 mg/ml nonradioactive methionine and 0.02% sodium azide. Caution: Sodium azide is extremely toxic.

PROCEDURE

All steps should be done under sterile conditions.

1. Prepare cells from desired lymphoid tissue as described in Chapter 1 in PBS or BSS containing 5% FCS.
2. Lyse red blood cells with Tris-buffered ammonium chloride (Section 1.17) or hemolytic Gey's solution (Section 1.18).
3. Determine viable cell count (see appropriate section in Chapter 1).
4. Transfer 5×10^7 viable cells to a 17×100-mm plastic tube, and centrifuge.
5. Remove supernate and resuspend in 2 ml of labeling medium (tissue culture medium lacking methionine, containing 5% FCS)
6. Add 0.5 mCi ^{35}S-methionine (usually 100–200 μl).
7. Gas tube with 5% CO_2 in air mixture for at least 10 seconds to prevent medium from becoming too basic.
8. Place tube in CO_2 incubator.
9. Incubate 4–5 hours, flicking the tube at least once each hour to resuspend the cells.
10. Add 3 ml cold washing buffer and centrifuge in refrigerated centrifuge.
11. Wash two additional times with 5 ml cold washing buffer. The last wash should be in a 12×75-mm plastic tube.

COMMENTS

1. If more than 5×10^7 cells are to be labeled, set up additional tubes of 5×10^7 cells in 2 ml of labeling medium. Do not increase the volume per tube; the cells settle out and large volumes prevent good pH regulation.
2. Once the incorporation has been stopped, the cold azide-containing washing buffer prevents the radioactivity from being degraded or "chased" from one form to another.

B. Radioiodination of Cells

In this procedure the formation of the active iodine molecule, which is capable of iodinating proteins, from ^{125}I-iodide is catalyzed by the enzyme lactoperoxidase in the presence of hydrogen peroxide. This reaction occurs on the outside of living cells, so no cytoplasmic proteins are normally labeled. However, if dead cells are present internal proteins will be iodinated. Therefore, it is important that the cell preparations contain a high percentage (>95%) of viable cells. Also, care must be taken to remove all traces of serum proteins which, if present, also would be iodinated. The procedure outlined below was developed by Dr. Samuel Black at Stanford and is similar to those described previously by others (Cone and Marchalonis 1974; Kessler 1975). It generally produces 20 000–60 000 cpm of ^{125}I radioactivity in the protein from 10^5 cells.

MATERIALS AND REAGENTS

Fetal calf serum (FCS)

Materials and reagents to determine cell viability (see appropriate section in Chapter 1)

Phosphate-buffered saline (PBS; Appendix A.8) or balanced salt solution (BSS; Appendix A.3)

Stock solutions for Tris-buffered ammonium chloride (Section 1.17) or hemolytic Gey's solution (Section 1.18)

^{125}I-sodium iodide, carrier-free (Amersham)

Hydrogen peroxide (H_2O_2): 30% solution (obtainable from drug stores or chemical supply companies)

Centrifuge tubes, 15 ml, plastic, conical

Pipetman, 200-μl and 20-μl capacity (Rainin Instrument)

Fume hood for handling ^{125}I solution

Beaker containing water at 30°C

Disposable plastic tube (Falcon 12 × 75 mm or similar)

Phosphate buffer, 0.5 M, pH 7.0: Dissolve 6.9 g $NaH_2PO_4 \cdot H_2O$ in 50 ml distilled water. Adjust to pH 7.0 with 1 M NaOH. Bring volume to 100 ml with distilled water.

Lactoperoxidase solution: 2 mg/ml lactoperoxidase (Calbiochem) in PBS

Washing buffer: Phosphate-buffered saline (PBS; Appendix A.8) or balanced salt solution (BSS; Appendix A.3) containing 0.02% sodium azide and 2 mM (0.32 mg/ml) potassium iodide. Caution: Sodium azide is extremely toxic.

PROCEDURE

Note: Refer to Section 14.2 for safety procedures recommended while handling ^{125}I.

1. Prepare cells from desired lymphoid tissue as described in Chapter 1 (sterile conditions are not necessary).

2. Lyse red blood cells with Tris-buffered ammonium chloride (Section 1.17) or hemolytic Gey's solution (Section 1.18). Be sure to wash cells several times with PBS or BSS without fetal calf serum to eliminate red blood cell membranes and serum proteins.

3. Determine viable cell count (see appropriate section in Chapter 1). If viability is less than 95%, remove the dead cells by filtration through a glass wool column (Section 1.21).

4. Place 5×10^7 cells in 150 μl of PBS into a 15-ml plastic conical centrifuge tube; put the tube into the 30°C water bath.

5. Add 50 μl of lactoperoxidase solution and 10 μl of 0.5 M phosphate buffer, pH 7.0.

6. In the fume hood, transfer 1 mCi of ^{125}I to the cell suspension.

7. Dilute the H_2O_2 to 0.03% in PBS (1:1000), mix, and transfer 20 μl to the cell suspension.

8. Mix vigorously, and incubate 4 minutes at 30°C.

9. Add an additional 20 μl of 0.03% H_2O_2 to tube, mix vigorously, and incubate 10 minutes at room temperature.

10. Dilute with 5 ml cold washing buffer, and centrifuge. (Discard wash fluids appropriately.) All subsequent steps should be done in the cold.

11. Wash cells once with washing buffer.

12. Resuspend cells in 1 ml of washing buffer, underlay with 2 ml FCS, and centrifuge.

13. Wash two additional times with washing buffer; the final wash should be in a 12×75-mm plastic tube.

COMMENT

^{125}I emits high-energy gamma rays, so care must be taken during its use (see Section 14.2). The main dangers in using amounts of the order of several millicuries are inhalation of radioactive vapors and absorption through the skin. Therefore, rubber gloves should be worn, and transfers of ^{125}I from the primary stock bottle should be done in a fume hood. Moreover, it is advisable to carry out manipulations on disposable absorbent paper and behind lead shielding (lead sheeting $\frac{1}{16}$ inch thick is sufficient to protect against this level of irradiation). All radioactive waste such as tubes and supernatant fluid should be disposed of appropriately.

C. Extraction of Radiolabeled Cell Proteins

The procedure described below is used to extract proteins from cells labeled with either amino acids or [125]I. The concentration of Nonidet P40 (NP40) detergent recommended, 0.5%, is the standard concentration for extraction of a number of lymphocyte antigens, including cell surface immunoglobulin, H-2, and Ia antigens. However, extraction of other antigens may require different concentrations of NP40; for example, extraction of immunoglobulin-like molecules from T cells has been reported to occur at 0.1% but not at 0.5% (Cone and Marchalonis 1974). Also, the efficiency of extraction is highly dependent on the ratio of detergent to protein. The conditions described below work well for normal lymphocytes, which are relatively small cells. If the cells being used are large, as are cells from lymphoid tumors and tissue culture lines, the amount of NP40 extraction buffer used for extraction should be increased proportionately.

MATERIALS AND REAGENTS

Vortex mixer
Plastic centrifuge tubes, 12 × 75 mm (Falcon)
Plastic microfuge tubes
Drawn-out Pasteur pipettes
High speed centrifuge (20 000 rpm)
Liquid nitrogen or −70°C freezer
Extraction buffer: 10 mM Tris-Cl, pH 7.2, 0.15 M NaCl, 0.02% NaN$_3$ (toxic), 0.5% (w/v) Nonidet P40 (NP40; Particle Data Laboratories)
> Note: NP40 is a liquid and must be weighed. To make up 100 ml of buffer, mix 0.5 g NP40, 0.12 g Tris base (Sigma Chemical), 0.87 g NaCl, 0.02 g NaN$_3$, 80 ml deionized water. Adjust to pH 7.2 with concentrated HCl. Adjust volume to 100 ml with deionized water. Can be stored indefinitely in the refrigerator.

PROCEDURE

All steps must be done in the cold.

1. Prior to extraction, centrifuge the washed radiolabeled cells in 12 × 75-mm Falcon plastic tubes and remove the supernate completely.
2. Add 0.5 ml of extraction buffer.
3. Vortex and let mixture sit 15 minutes on ice.
4. Transfer to plastic microfuge tubes.

5. Centrifuge at high speed (speed is not critical; approximately 27 000 × g in SS-34 rotor in a Sorvall centrifuge for 20 minutes).

6. Carefully collect supernates with drawn-out Pasteur pipette, and place in clean microfuge tubes. Discard pellets, which include nuclei.

7. Take samples for determination of radioactivity in cell proteins (see below).

8. Store extracts in liquid nitrogen (if not available use a −70°C freezer). Avoid repeated freezing and thawing.

D. Determination of Acid-Insoluble Radioactivity

This procedure is designed to determine how much ^{35}S or ^{125}I radioactivity has been incorporated into protein.

MATERIALS AND REAGENTS

Micropipettes, 1 μl
Glass test tubes, 12 × 75 mm
Saline-FCS: 0.15 M NaCl containing 0.5% FCS
10% trichloroacetic acid (TCA) containing 2 mg/ml methionine and/or 0.3 mg/ml potassium iodide
Filters, 0.45 μm, 25 mm diameter (Millipore, HAWP02500)
Filter holder and vacuum flask for filtration
5% TCA in squeeze bottle
For ^{35}S-methionine:
    Scintillation vials
    Scintillation fluid
    Scintillation counter
For ^{125}I:
    Tubes for gamma counter
    Gamma counter

PROCEDURE

1. Pipet 1-μl samples of radioactive preparations into glass test tubes containing 0.5 ml of saline with 0.5% FCS as carrier protein (this should be done in duplicate).

2. Mix, and add 0.5 ml of 10% TCA containing methionine and/or potassium iodide as cold competitors for any free ^{35}S-methionine or ^{125}I that might be present.

3. Mix and let stand at least 30 minutes at room temperature or overnight in the refrigerator. The solution should appear faintly cloudy.

4. Collect the precipitate on a Millipore filter, rinsing out the glass tube and washing the filter with several squirts of 5% TCA, totaling 10–12 ml.

5. Allow the filter to dry at room temperature or briefly under a heat lamp or in an oven.

6. For ^{35}S-labeled samples, place the filter in a scintillation vial, add enough scintillation fluid to cover the filter, and count in a scintillation counter. Counter settings for ^{14}C are appropriate for ^{35}S.

7. For ^{125}I-labeled samples, place the filter in a tube and count in a gamma counter.

19.3 IMMUNOPRECIPITATION OF CELL PROTEINS

The availability of highly specific antisera greatly facilitates the isolation of radiolabeled proteins from detergent extracts. In general, precipitation of sufficient protein for analytical studies requires only small amounts of specific antiserum followed by an agent that will bind the antigen-antibody complexes and allow their recovery. Two types of reagents are commonly used for this purpose. The first is an anti-immunoglobulin antiserum that will react with the antibodies bound to the antigens of interest, resulting in an insoluble immunoprecipitate. This approach is satisfactory, but it has several disadvantages. The large amounts of immunoglobulin protein present in the sample cause distortion of the gel in the regions where the immunoglobulin chains migrate. Also, the procedure is relatively slow, since enough time must be provided for precipitation to occur. Finally, this "indirect" immunoprecipitation procedure requires fairly large amounts of second-step anti-immunoglobulin antiserum for complete precipitation of the antigen-antibody complexes.

Because of these problems, a different approach for recovering antigen-antibody complexes has become popular since the mid-1970s. This procedure takes advantage of the presence on the surface of some *Staphylococcus aureus* (e.g., *S. aureus* Cowan I strain) bacteria of a protein called protein A, which binds to IgG molecules via their Fc region. Formalin-fixed, heat-killed *S. aureus* bacteria function very effectively as an insoluble adsorbent for bringing down antigen-antibody complexes, avoiding some of the disadvantages of indirect antibody immunoprecipitation (Kessler 1975; Cullen and Schwartz 1976). The amount of immunoglobulin in the final samples is limited to what was present in the first-step antiserum, so there is little or no distortion of the gel. The reaction of *S. aureus* with IgG is very fast, and the bacteria carrying the antigen-antibody complexes can be pelleted easily by centrifugation. Finally, *S. aureus* can be grown in large quantities fairly easily (Kessler 1975), or purchased commercially in a form ready to be used for immunoprecipitation (e.g., Pansorbin from Calbiochem; IgGsorb from Enzyme Center). Because of these advantages, only the *S. aureus* method for immunoprecipitation of radiolabeled cell proteins will be described below. After the antigen-antibody-*S. aureus* complexes are washed, they are dissociated by the addition of denaturing electrophoresis sample buffers.

The amounts of extract, antiserum, and *S. aureus* adsorbent (SaC) required for isolation of adequate amounts of a protein for analysis can be quite variable. These parameters are highly dependent on the level of radioactivity in the protein of interest and the strength of the antiserum. Theoretically, each antiserum should be titrated to determine the amount required for optimal precipitation; the amount of SaC should also be varied. This is difficult and expensive to do, however, when many different antisera are being tested. Fortunately, for many purposes it is not absolutely essential that 100% of the antigen be precipitated, so following some general guidelines can save time and precious reagents. Some examples are given below.

	Antigen		
	H-2, Ia	Membrane immunoglobulin*	
Volume of extract	100 μl	100 μl	100 μl
Type of antiserum	Alloantiserum	Alloantiserum	Heterologous
Volume of antiserum	10–50 μl	2–30 μl	2 μl
Volume of SaC (10% suspension)	200 μl	200 μl	200 μl
Volume of sample buffer	50 μl	50 μl	50 μl

Because the binding of antigen-antibody complexes to SaC is stronger than the binding of free IgG molecules (Kessler 1975), the amount of SaC required depends more on the amount of antigen-antibody complexes present than on the total amount of serum immunoglobulin. The volume of electrophoresis sample buffer needed for dissociation of the antigen-antibody-SaC complexes depends on the amount of SaC used.

* Recommendations for precipitation of membrane immunoglobulin were made by Dr. J. Goding, Stanford University School of Medicine.

MATERIALS AND REAGENTS

Staphylococcus aureus adsorbent (SaC): 10% (w/v) suspension of heat-killed, formalin-fixed bacteria (see introduction to this section)

Antisera and normal control sera

Plastic tubes, disposable, 12×75 mm

Glass tubes, 6×50 mm

Isoelectric focusing (IEF) or sodium dodecyl sulfate (SDS) sample buffer (see Section 19.4)

Drawn-out Pasteur pipettes

Plastic microfuge tubes

Sonicator, with microprobe

SaC buffer: Phosphate-buffered saline (PBS; Appendix A.8) containing 0.5% NP40, 2 mM methionine (0.3 mg/ml) and/or 5 mM potassium iodide (0.8 mg/ml), and 0.02% sodium azide.

Ovalbumin: Prepare a 1 mg/ml ovalbumin solution in SaC buffer.

PROCEDURE

All steps should be done *on ice,* unless otherwise specified.

1. Thaw just enough SaC 10% suspension for use (e.g., 200 μl per sample for H-2 immunoprecipitates).

2. If clumped, sonicate the SaC with a microprobe for two bursts of 5 seconds each.

3. Wash SaC twice in 10 ml of SaC buffer, centrifuging for 10 minutes at the minimum speed required to pellet the bacteria (700–1000 $\times$ g).

4. Resuspend SaC to initial volume in SaC buffer containing 1 mg/ml ovalbumin to prevent nonspecific protein binding.

5. To 12×75-mm plastic tubes, add appropriate amounts of extract and antisera; vortex and allow to stand 30 minutes.

6. Add appropriate amounts of washed 10% suspension of SaC in SaC buffer containing 1 mg/ml ovalbumin, vortex, and allow to stand about 15 minutes with occasional mixing.

7. Dilute with 2.5 ml SaC buffer (without ovalbumin) and centrifuge at 700 $\times$ g for 10 minutes.

8. Pour off each supernate into appropriate container for radioactive waste, resuspend pellet in 3 ml SaC buffer by pipetting, transfer to a new plastic tube (tube transfers help to reduce background), and centrifuge.

9. Repeat step 8.

10. Pour off supernate, resuspend in 0.3 ml SaC buffer, and transfer to 6 × 50-mm glass tubes.

11. Centrifuge, and carefully remove all the supernate from the pellet with a drawn-out pipette.

12. Samples to be run on 2-D gels should be processed from here on at room temperature (to prevent the urea in the sample buffer from crystallizing); samples to be run on SDS slab gels can continue to be processed at 4°C.

13. To the pellet add an appropriate amount (e.g., 50 μl) of either IEF or SDS sample buffer, vortex to resuspend the pellet, and centrifuge at 700 × g for 5 minutes.

14. Remove the supernate with a drawn-out pipette and transfer to plastic microfuge tube.

15. Take duplicate 1-μl samples for determination of amount of radioactivity in the supernate (Section 19.2D).

16. Store the samples at −70°C or in liquid nitrogen.

COMMENTS: BACKGROUND RADIOACTIVITY

When used with spleen cell extracts, the procedure described above generally gives low backgrounds; 0.5–1.0% of the total acid-insoluble radioactivity in the extract binds to the SaC in the absence of specific antibodies. A considerable portion of this radioactivity is present in immunoglobulin chains and in actin, which bind to the SaC. This level of background radioactivity usually does not interfere with detection of the specifically precipitated antigens because the proteins are separated in two dimensions. In fact, it is sometimes advantageous to have these background spots present because they provide electrophoretic mobility markers that allow different gels to be compared accurately. However, reduction of background below the 0.5–1.0% level may sometimes be desired. Three approaches for lowering background are outlined below.

1. *Isolation of glycoproteins by lentil lectin affinity chromatography:* Most membrane antigens are glycoproteins; thus, an enriched glycoprotein fraction can be obtained by passing the extract through a lentil lectin affinity column (Hayman and Crumpton 1972). The glycoproteins which are bound by the lectin can be eluted with free sugar, providing a highly enriched fraction for immunoprecipitation. However, the recoveries of cell surface proteins are never complete and it is not known whether the losses are qualitative or just quantitative. For example, nonglycosylated

cytoplasmic precursors probably do not bind to the affinity column.

2. *Preclearing the extracts with SaC prior to the addition of antisera:* Incubation of the extracts with SaC can be done either in bulk on a large quantity of extract or on a tube by tube basis. In general, 20 μl of packed, prewashed SaC is sufficient to absorb 100 μl of extract. It is recommended that the extract be added to packed SaC to prevent dilution of the extract with SaC buffer. After vortexing, the tubes are allowed to sit for 15 minutes at 4°C and then centrifuged for 10 minutes at $700 \times g$. The supernatant extracts are then transferred to fresh tubes for the immunoprecipitation. The main disadvantage of this preclearing step is that it uses up considerable amounts of the SaC.

3. *Washing nonspecifically bound protein from the SaC:* Some of the proteins that bind nonspecifically to the SaC can be removed by washing the SaC with special buffers after the antigen-antibody complexes have been allowed to bind. The addition of 0.1% SDS to the SaC buffer has been used successfully for this purpose. Alternatively, high pH-high salt buffers also have been reported to reduce backgrounds. One such buffer, suggested by Dr. J. Goding of Stanford is 0.5% NP40, 0.4 M NaCl, and 0.1 M Tris-HCl, pH 8.0. It is important, however, that controls be done to test whether either of these special washing buffers affects the immunoprecipitation of the desired antigens, either qualitatively or quantitatively.

19.4 PREPARATION OF SAMPLES

It is important that samples for electrophoresis be prepared properly to guarantee both the complete solubilization and denaturation of the proteins and the appropriate chemical makeup of the samples. Therefore, proteins to be run on the first dimension of 2-D PAGE should be prepared in the isoelectric focusing (IEF) sample buffer which, as described by O'Farrell (1975), contains urea, NP40, 2-mercaptoethanol, and Ampholines for establishing the pH gradient. Samples to be run on SDS slab gels should be prepared in SDS sample buffer (O'Farrell 1975), which contains sodium dodecyl sulfate (SDS), Tris buffer, glycerol (for increased density), and 2-mercaptoethanol. Both sample buffers can be prepared without 2-mercaptoethanol if proteins are to be run without reducing disulfide bonds.

Proteins immunoprecipitated as described in Section 19.3 are eluted from the *S. aureus* adsorbent (SaC) with the appropriate sample buffer and are ready for electrophoresis. If all of the proteins in the cell are to be analyzed, intact cells can be centrifuged and the pellet simply dissolved in sample buffer and electophoresed without any further treatment. However, in some cases, such as when proteins are in dilute solution, it is necessary to add extra denaturant or detergent to insure that the proteins are effectively solubilized. Also, samples prepared in IEF sample buffer can be run on SDS gels and vice versa if the appropriate additions are made to the samples. Procedures for preparing samples are presented below, along with some guidelines concerning sample size.

A. Samples for Two-Dimensional PAGE

MATERIALS AND REAGENTS

Individual suppliers are named *only* if their product is essential for the quality of the gels (supplier followed by an asterisk*) or if the item is not generally available.

Urea, ultrapure (Schwartz/Mann*)
Ampholines, pH 5–7 and pH 3.5–10 (LKB Instruments*)
Nonidet P40 (NP40; Particle Data Laboratories)
2-mercaptoethanol (2-ME)

IEF sample buffer, 50 ml:

	Amount	Final concentration
Urea	28.5 g	9.5 M
NP40	1.0 g	2.0% (w/v)
pH 5–7 Ampholine	2.0 ml	1.6 %
pH 3.5–10 Ampholine	0.5 ml	0.4 %
2-ME	2.5 ml	5.0%

Add deionized water to 50 ml. Store solution in 0.2–0.5 ml aliquots at −70°C.

PROCEDURE

1. *Sample size:* In 130-mm gel tubes, 25–30-μl sample volumes can be accommodated over a 12.5-cm gel. For larger samples, shorter gels can be poured; alternatively, longer gel tubes can be used. Samples of 200 μl have been run successfully. For samples con-

sisting of radiolabeled cells or cell extracts that contain many proteins, at least $3–5 \times 10^5$ cpm of ^{35}S radioactivity or $1–3 \times 10^5$ cpm of ^{125}I radioactivity should be run. Samples consisting of proteins specifically isolated by immunoprecipitation or other means require far less radioactivity. The amount varies from protein to protein, depending on how many molecular species are present. For spleen cell H-2, Ia, and immunoglobulin molecules the amount of ^{35}S or ^{125}I radioactivity in proteins precipitated from $3–5 \times 10^6$ cells is generally sufficient. Thus, if 100 μl of extract prepared from 10^7 cells is used for a single precipitation, as described in Section 19.3, enough sample is obtained for two 2-D gels. If proteins are to be detected by Coomassie blue staining instead of by autoradiography, much more protein needs to be included in the sample. A Coomassie blue-stained protein will be detectable down to 0.1 μg or less; however, it is advisable that each protein in the sample be present in amounts of 1 μg or more. It should be remembered that if the amount of a single protein exceeds about 10 μg, significant distortion of the gel pattern will occur in the vicinity of that protein.

2. *Sample preparation:* The requirements for levels of radioactivity or protein considered above place restrictions on how the samples can be prepared. The IEF sample buffer should not be diluted by more than 10% without adding crystalline urea to maintain the high urea concentration.

   a. *Concentrated samples:* Samples that are highly concentrated (i.e., cell pellets or concentrated aqueous samples) can be readied for electrophoresis by the addition of IEF sample buffer at a ratio of approximately 1:10. For example, 5×10^6 packed lymphocytes (with *all* of the supernate removed) or 5 μl of protein plus 45 μl of IEF sample buffer will provide enough sample for two gels.

   b. *Dilute samples:* Because it is necessary to use more of a dilute sample, precautions must be taken to prevent excessive lowering of the urea concentration in the sample. Use the following proportions:

Aqueous sample	10 μl
Crystalline urea	10 mg
IEF sample buffer	10 μl
Final volume	~30 μl

   c. *Samples in SDS sample buffer:* Samples already in SDS sample buffer can be adapted for IEF or NEPHGE using the following proportions:

SDS sample	10 μl
NP40 (undiluted)	5 μl
IEF sample buffer	10 μl

The large amount of NP40 is added so that the SDS bound to the protein will be exchanged by NP40, a non-ionic detergent. Ames and Nikaido (1976) reported that the ratio of NP40 to SDS must be at least 8 : 1 to prevent streaking of the proteins in the first dimension. The proportions given above will result in a final NP40 : SDS ratio of about 16 : 1.

3. *Sample storage:* Samples in IEF sample buffer should be stored in tightly sealed tubes (to prevent evaporation) at $-70°$C or in liquid nitrogen. *Never* heat the samples since such treatment causes modifications of the proteins (Steinberg et al., 1977). The samples can be thawed at room temperature or by holding at 37°C *just until* samples are thawed. Do not freeze and thaw repeatedly.

B. Samples for One-Dimensional SDS Slab Gels

MATERIALS AND REAGENTS

Individual suppliers are named *only* if their product is essential for the quality of the gels (supplier followed by an asterisk*) or if the item is not generally available.

Tris base (TRIZMA, Sigma Chemical)
Glycerol. Note: Glycerol is a liquid and must be weighed.
Sodium dodecyl sulfate (SDS; sodium lauryl sulfate,† BDH*)
HCl, concentrated
2-mercaptoethanol (2-ME)
Glass tubes, 10 × 75 mm
Boiling water bath

Solutions:
    10% SDS: 10 g SDS and deionized water to 100 ml.

---

† BDH refers to sodium dodecyl sulfate as sodium lauryl sulfate in their catalogue.

1× SDS sample buffer, 1000 ml:

	Amount	Final concentration
Tris base	7.57 g	0.0625 M
Glycerol	100.0 g	10.0 % (w/v)
2-ME	50.0 ml	5.0 %
SDS	23.0 g	2.3 %

Add to 750 ml deionized water. Adjust to pH 6.8 with concentrated HCl. Add deionized water to 1000 ml and store in refrigerator.

2× SDS sample buffer, 100 ml:

	Amount	Final concentration
Tris base	1.51 g	0.125 M
Glycerol	20.0 g	20.0 % (w/v)
2-ME	10.0 ml	10.0 %
SDS	4.6 g	4.6 %

Add to 75 ml deionized water. Adjust to pH 6.8 with concentrated HCl. Add deionized water to 100 ml and store in refrigerator.

PROCEDURE

1. *Sample size:* The maximum sample volume possible is determined by the size of the sample well that is formed in the stacking gel. With the procedures described in Section 19.6, samples of 25–30 μl are recommended, and volumes should not exceed 40 μl. In general, samples for SDS slab gels require only 25–50% of the radioactivity or protein needed for 2-D PAGE because the proteins are not spread out in two dimensions. Therefore, for H-2, Ia, and immunoglobulin molecules, samples consisting of immunoprecipitates from 1–2 $\times$ 10^6 radiolabeled lymphocytes are usually sufficient. If proteins are to be detected by Coomassie blue staining, there should be 0.5 μg or more of protein present.

2. *Sample preparation:* Given the recommendations for sample size

mentioned above, the following procedures are suggested for sample preparation. All samples for one-dimensional SDS slab gels must be heated in a boiling water bath to fully denature the proteins prior to electrophoresis.

a. *Concentrated samples:* Dilute proteins $\geq 1 : 10$ in $1\times$ SDS sample buffer, and heat for 90 seconds in a boiling water bath.

b. *Dilute samples:* Mix $1 : 1$ with $2\times$ SDS sample buffer, and heat.

c. *Samples in IEF sample buffer:* Samples previously prepared in IEF sample buffer can be adapted for SDS slab gel electrophoresis by adding a sufficient amount of SDS to remove the NP40 bound to the proteins. It is not necessary to add additional urea to the samples. Use the following proportions:

IEF sample	5 μl
10% SDS	10 μl
$2\times$ SDS sample buffer	15 μl

Heat in a boiling water bath.

3. *Sample storage:* Samples for SDS PAGE can be stored at $-20°C$ or $-70°C$.

19.5 TWO-DIMENSIONAL POLYACRYLAMIDE GEL ELECTROPHORESIS

The problem of separating complex mixtures of proteins into their component species was largely resolved when O'Farrell (1975) published a procedure for high-resolution two-dimensional electrophoresis of proteins in polyacrylamide gels. Proteins are first separated in cylindrical gels according to their charge; these gels are then laid across the top of an SDS slab gel and the proteins are separated according to their size. Individual proteins are resolved as discrete spots that can be visualized by protein stains or autoradiography. The high resolution and reproducibility of the separations in this system provide unique capabilities; for example, it is possible to resolve different biosynthetic forms of a single polypeptide chain and to recognize one mutant protein out of a thousand normal ones (Ivarie et al. 1977; Steinberg et al. 1977).

This chapter outlines the methodology for two-dimensional polyacrylamide gel electrophoresis (2-D PAGE) that has been described in a number of publications, with a few modifications. Two methods are presented for the first-dimension charge separation. The first, isoelectric focusing (IEF), is the procedure initially described by O'Farrell; it resolves proteins with isoelectric points between pH 4.5 and pH 7.

The second approach, nonequilibrium pH gradient electrophoresis (NEPHGE), was developed to allow the resolution of very basic as well as acidic proteins (O'Farrell et al. 1977). The version of NEPHGE outlined below resolves proteins ranging in pI from pH 4.5 to pH 9 and thus is the procedure of choice for analyzing immunoglobulins, which are basic proteins. For the second-dimension size separation, the modified Laemmli discontinuous SDS electrophoresis in slab gels described by O'Farrell (1975) is used.

The procedures described below can be varied as needed—for example, by running proteins in the nonreduced form, by altering the pH range of the ampholytes, or by varying the acrylamide concentration in the second-dimension gels. It is recommended that the original papers be read for additional details concerning the methodologies. Some of these procedures have also been outlined by O'Farrell and O'Farrell (1978).

The number of samples that can be included in individual 2-D PAGE experiments is limited primarily by the number of first-dimensional gels that can be handled satisfactorily at one time. Usually 24 gels is the limit, although experienced workers can run more by staggering the processing of the gels. It is not generally necessary to run duplicate gels. Most cylindrical gel tanks hold 12–18 gel tubes, so two tanks often are needed. Both tanks can be plugged into the same power supply, even if they contain different numbers of gels. Multiple second-dimension slab gels can be run simultaneously, as will be discussed later.

A. First Dimension (IEF and NEPHGE)

The choice of IEF or NEPHGE for the first-dimension charge separation of proteins depends on both the isoelectric points (pIs) of the proteins being studied and the nature of the sample. If the sample consists of a relatively small number of proteins, such as immunoprecipitated cell surface antigens, then the decision of which gel system to use can be based solely on the pIs of the proteins. IEF gels resolve protein with pIs from 4.5 to 7; the NEPHGE system described here can resolve proteins with pIs between 4.5 and ≥ 9. Therefore, if it is known that a protein has a pI below 7, IEF gels should be used; the proteins will be more spread out than they would be in NEPHGE gels. If the pI of a protein is unknown, it should be run first on NEPHGE gels.

Often it is desirable to electrophorese mixtures of large numbers of proteins, for example, whole cells or cell extracts. With such samples, which can produce more than 1000 spots, the wide pH range of NEPHGE gels tends to crowd the spots close together, making it difficult to pick out some of the spots of interest. Therefore, IEF gels should be used whenever possible for samples consisting of total cell proteins. However, if the pI of the protein is not known or if one wants to examine all of the cell proteins in one gel, the NEPHGE gels described below should be run. If the protein of interest is very basic, that NEPHGE system can be used, but a NEPHGE system designed to resolve *only* basic proteins might provide better separations. This type of NEPHGE, described by O'Farrell et al. (1977), is generated by altering the Ampholine composition and the voltage and/or time of electrophoresis.

The IEF and NEPHGE gels are very similar. The only difference in the gel composition itself is the Ampholines: IEF gels contain a 4 : 1 mixture of pH 5–7:pH 3.5–10 Ampholine, while the NEPHGE gels contain only pH 3.5–10 Ampholine. The more basic NEPHGE gel mixture requires slightly higher concentrations of ammonium persulfate and TEMED for polymerization. However, conditions of electrophoresis differ considerably between IEF and NEPHGE. In IEF gels a stable pH gradient is established by the Ampholines, and proteins are electrophoresed to equilibrium, that is, until the proteins reach a position in the gradient where they are uncharged. The proteins are loaded at the cathodal end; under these conditions the pH at this (the upper) end of the gel is 7, and more basic proteins do not focus within the gels. NEPHGE gels are run in the reverse direction, so that the cathodal (basic) end of the gel is at the bottom. NEPHGE is a *nonequilibrium* electrophoresis system; proteins are loaded at the anodal (acidic) end and electrophoresed just long enough to allow the most basic proteins to reach the bottom of the gel (determined empirically). See O'Farrell et al. (1977) for a more detailed discussion of the theory behind NEPHGE.

MATERIALS AND REAGENTS

Individual suppliers are named *only* if they are essential for the quality of the gels (supplier followed by an asterisk*) or if the item is not generally available.

Urea, ultrapure (Schwartz/Mann*)

Nonidet P40 (NP40; Particle Data Laboratories)

Acrylamide. Caution: Acrylamide is a neurotoxin; wear a mask when weighing and use gloves when handling solutions. Do not mouth pipet.

Bis-acrylamide

Ammonium persulfate

N,N,N',N'-tetramethylenediamine (TEMED)

Ampholines, pH 5–7 and pH 3.5–10 (LKB Instruments*); keep sterile

Phosphoric acid, 85% solution

Sodium hydroxide, $M_r = 40.0$
Potassium hydroxide, $M_r = 50.1$
Ethanol, 95%
Power supply ($\geq$ 800 V, 250 mA) to be used at constant voltage
Parafilm
Cylindrical gel electrophoresis tank (see Figure 19.1)
Cylindrical glass gel tubes (130 mm long, 2.5 mm inside diameter, see
  below)
Needle, 20 gauge, 8-inch length (BOLAB)

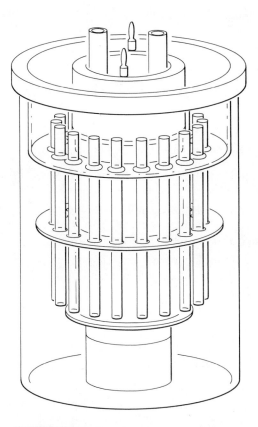

FIGURE 19.1
Cylindrical gel tank with gel tubes in place.
(Adapted from a Bio-Rad cylindrical gel tank,
with permission from Bio-Rad Laboratories.)

Syringe, 10 ml

Syringe, 5 ml with one inch of ⅜-inch diameter Tygon tubing attached

Rubber stoppers (Vacutainer stoppers for 14–16-mm diameter tubes) with ⅛-inch holes

Pipetman, 20 μl and 200 μl (Rainin Instrument)

Screw-cap glass tubes, 16 × 125 mm

Rocking platform or shaker

Solutions (recommended volumes for each solution are indicated)

1. Dichromate cleaning solution:

Sodium dichromate	60 g
Water	1000 ml
Sulfuric acid, concentrated	1600 ml

2. KOH-saturated ethanol (for cleaning gel tubes): Combine 188 g KOH with 500 ml 95% ethanol. Mix until dissolved (solution turns brown).

3. 30% acrylamide for IEF gels:

	Amount	Final concentration
Acrylamide	28.38 g	28.38 %
Bis-acrylamide	1.62 g	1.62 %
Add deionized water to	100.0 ml	

   Filter solution through Whatman #1 paper and store in refrigerator in opaque bottle.

4. 10% (w/v) NP40 stock solution: Dissolve 5.0 g of NP40 in deionized water to a total volume of 50 ml. The NP40 is a liquid and must be weighed. Store solution in refrigerator.

5. 10% ammonium persulfate: Dissolve 0.10 g ammonium persulfate in 1.0 ml deionized water. Make solution up fresh every two weeks. Store in refrigerator.

6. Anode electrode solution, 0.01 M phosphoric acid: Mix 1.0 ml 85% phosphoric acid in 1460 ml deionized water.

7. Cathode electrode solution, 0.02 M NaOH: Dissolve 0.80 g of NaOH pellets in 1000 ml deionized water.

For IEF gels:	Boil water 10 minutes; add NaOH dissolved in 5 ml water. Boil for additional 5 minutes. Evacuate and store under vacuum.
For NEPHGE gels:	Dissolve NaOH pellets. No boiling or evacuation necessary. Make fresh each time.

8. Sample overlay solution, 25 ml:

	Amount	Final concentration
Urea	13.52 g	9 M
pH 5–7 Ampholine	0.5 ml	0.8 %
pH 3.5–10 Ampholine	0.125 ml	0.2 %

Add deionized water to 25 ml. Store solution in 0.2-ml aliquots at $-70°C$.

9. IEF sample buffer: See Solutions in Section 19.4A.

10. SDS sample buffer: See Solutions in Section 19.4B.

Recipes for IEF and NEPHGE Gels: Both gels contain 9.2 M urea, 4% acrylamide, 2% NP40, and 2% Ampholines.

IEF gels

	Number of gels		
	8	16	24
Urea	2.75 g	5.5 g	8.25 g
30% acrylamide	0.665 ml	1.33 ml	2.0 ml
10% NP40	1.0 ml	2.0 ml	3.0 ml
Deionized water	0.98 ml	1.97 ml	2.95 ml
pH 5–7 Ampholines	200.0 μl	0.4 ml	0.6 ml
pH 3.5–10 Ampholines	50.0 μl	0.1 ml	0.15 ml
10% ammonium persulfate	5.0 μl	10.0 μl	15.0 μl
TEMED	3.5 μl	7.0 μl	10.5 μl
Final Volume	5.0 ml	10.0 ml	15.0 ml

NEPHGE gels

	Number of gels		
	8	16	24
Urea	2.75 g	5.5 g	8.25 g
30% acrylamide	0.665 ml	1.33 ml	2.0 ml
10% NP40	1.0 ml	2.0 ml	3.0 ml
Deionized water	0.98 ml	1.97 ml	2.95 ml
pH 3.5–10 Ampholine	0.25 ml	0.5 ml	0.75 ml
10% ammonium persulfate	7.0 μl	14.0 μl	21.0 μl
TEMED	4.0 μl	8.0 μl	12.0 μl
Final Volume	5.0 ml	10.0 ml	15.0 ml

PROCEDURE

Preparation of Cylindrical Glass Gel Tubes

1. Cut 130-mm long gel tubes from soft glass tubing of 2.5-mm inside diameter.

2. Before using the tubes for the first time, "season" them by polymerizing the acrylamide in them as described below (steps 3 and 4 under Procedure for Isoelectric Focusing).

3. Before using tubes for the first time and after *each* use, soak the tubes for 2–24 hours in dichromate cleaning solution, rinse in deionized water, soak for 2–24 hours in potassium hydroxide-saturated ethanol, rinse in deionized water, and dry. This treatment ensures that the gels will stick appropriately to the tubes, perhaps because it leaves the tubes slightly negatively charged. However, insufficient rinsing may lead to poor polymerization.

Isoelectric Focusing (IEF):

1. Prepare NaOH cathode electrode solution and evacuate several hours prior to use to allow the solution to cool.

2. Mark off 12.5 cm on glass gel tubes and cap bottom end of tubes with four layers of Parafilm.

3. Prepare the gel mixture. Dissolve all the urea by gently swirling before adding the ammonium persulfate. Then add the TEMED. This mixture will begin polymerizing after several minutes.

4. Using the 8-inch needle and 10-ml syringe, transfer the gel mixture to the glass gel tubes. Overlay gel mixture gently with deionized water.

5. After 1–2 hours, remove overlay and replace with 20 μl of IEF sample buffer. Overlay the sample buffer with deionized water. After an additional 1–2 hours, remove the overlay.

6. Load tubes into tube gel tank containing phosphoric acid anode solution in the lower reservoir by inserting tubes into the rubber stoppers. To make sure that there are no bubbles at the bottom end of tubes, jiggle the tubes.

7. Overlay gel with 20 μl IEF sample buffer and then with the NaOH cathode solution. Fill the upper reservoir with the NaOH solution.

8. To remove the ammonium persulfate from the gels, prerun the gels in the following sequence:

   a. 15 minutes at 200 V (constant voltage)

    b. 30 minutes at 300 V

    c. 30 minutes at 400 V

9. Turn power off and wait 1–2 minutes before opening tanks to allow the voltage to dissipate.

10. Remove the cathode solution and overlay. Apply samples (see Section 19.4 for sample preparation).

11. Overlay samples with 10 μl of sample overlay solution and then with NaOH cathode solution. Fill upper chamber with NaOH cathode solution.

12. Run at 300–400 V for a total of 4800 volt-hours (i.e., 12–16 hours).

13. Increase voltage to 800 V for 1 hour. This procedure tightens the protein bands and reduces streaking in the IEF dimension.

14. Shake out liquid at top and bottom of tubes. Using air pressure from the 5-ml syringe-Tygon tubing apparatus applied to the top end of the gels (the basic end), extrude each gel into 5-ml of SDS sample buffer in a screw cap tube.

15. Equilibrate gels with the SDS sample buffer by gentle rocking for a total of 2 hours. Gels can be frozen in the SDS sample buffer, using a dry ice-ethanol bath, any time after 30 minutes of equilibration. Store gels at $-70°C$ until ready for the second dimension. Just prior to running the second dimension, thaw the gels and continue equilibration until a total of 2 hours of equilibration is reached.

Nonequilibrium pH Gradient Electrophoresis (NEPHGE)

1. Using the NEPHGE gel mixture, pour gels and change overlays as described in steps 1 to 5 for IEF gels. (Gels can be poured the day before use and, after the overlay to the IEF sample buffer has been changed, the tops can be sealed with Parafilm to prevent evaporation. The next morning, replace the overlay with fresh IEF sample buffer.)

2. Place the NaOH cathode solution (made up fresh but not boiled) in the *lower chamber* of the tank. Load gels into tank. Avoid bubbles at bottom of tubes.

3. Remove overlay and load samples onto the gels. (No prerun is required.)

4. Overlay the sample with 10 μl of sample overlay solution and then with phosphoric acid anode solution. Fill the upper chamber with the phosphoric acid anode solution.

5. Using *reverse polarity,* run at 500 V for 6 hours.

6. Turn off power, wait 1–2 minutes, and remove tubes.

7. Shake liquid out from both ends of the gels and extrude gels in SDS sample buffer as described for IEF gels. However, apply pressure to the *bottom* end of the gels (i.e., always push from the basic end).

8. Equilibrate and store gels in SDS sample buffer as described for IEF gels.

COMMENTS

1. When extruding the gels from the glass tubes, always push from the basic end; for some reason it is easier than pushing from the acidic end. In some cases, especially for NEPHGE gels, putting a drop of SDS sample buffer in the gel tube at the basic end before extrusion is important to prevent the gel from tearing.

2. During the equilibration of the tube gels in SDS sample buffer, some of the proteins may diffuse out of the gel. This may be a problem especially for low molecular weight proteins. This problem can be avoided by a short-term equilibration in high-SDS sample buffer (see O'Farrell 1975). For most purposes, however, the protein loss due to diffusion does not present a problem.

B. Second Dimension (SDS Slab Gel Electrophoresis)

Each first-dimension tube gel is run on a single second-dimension SDS slab gel. With appropriate slab gel tanks and connections (described below), multiple tanks can be operated off a single power supply. Up to 12 slab gels can be processed at once after one has become familiar with the technique.

MATERIALS AND REAGENTS

Individual suppliers are named *only* if they are essential for the quality of the gels (supplier indicated by an asterisk*) or if the item is not generally available.

Acrylamide. Caution: Acrylamide is a neurotoxin; wear a mask when weighing it and use gloves when handling solutions. Do not pipet by mouth.
Bis-acrylamide
Ammonium persulfate

Sodium dodecyl sulfate (SDS; sodium lauryl sulfate,† BDH*)
Tris base (TRIZMA, Sigma Chemical)
Hydrochloric acid
Agarose, "SeaKem" (Marine Colloids Division)
Glycine
Bromphenol blue
Coomassie blue
Trichloroacetic acid (TCA)
Acetic acid
Ethanol (95%)
Power supply ($\geq$ 800 V, 250 mA), constant current
Parafilm
Slab gel electrophoresis tanks (see below under Procedure)
Slab gel plates (see below under Procedure)
Plastic strips, $6\frac{1}{4} \times \frac{1}{4}$ in., 0.030 in. thick (polyvinyl chloride, tabletop lamination plastic)
Silicon rubber tubing, 0.047 in. outer diameter, about 20 in. long (Silastic tubing, Dow Corning, #602-155)
Binder clips, No. 10 size (see Figure 19.4)
Epoxy glue (slow drying)
Teflon spacers, 0.030 in. $\times$ 1 in. $\times$ 5.125 in.
Staining dishes: 9 $\times$ 13-in. glass baking dishes
Whatman filter paper, #1 and #3MM
Gel dryer (Bio-Rad)
Alconox laboratory detergent
Boiling water bath
Test tube rack
Pipettes, disposable, 1 ml
10-ml syringe with 2-in., 23-gauge needle
30-ml syringe with 4-in., 20-gauge needle; bend the end of the needle to make a hook.

Solutions

1. 1$\times$ SDS sample buffer: See section 19.4B.

2. Lower gel buffer, pH 8.8, 1000 ml:

	Amount	Final concentration
Tris base	181.7 g	1.5 M
SDS	4.0 g	0.4%

---

† BDH refers to sodium dodecyl sulfate as sodium lauryl sulfate in their catalogue.

Add to 750 ml deionized water. Adjust to pH 8.8 with concentrated HCl and add deionized water to 1000 ml. Store solution in refrigerator.

3. Upper gel buffer, pH 6.8, 500 ml:

	Amount	Final concentration
Tris base	30.3 g	0.5 M
SDS	2.0 g	0.4%

Add to 350 ml deionized water. Adjust to pH 6.8 with concentrated HCl and add deionized water to 500 ml. Store solution in refrigerator.

4. 30% acrylamide for SDS gels, 1027 ml:

	Amount	Final concentration
Acrylamide	300.0 g	29.2%
Bis-acrylamide	8.2 g	0.8%

Add deionized water to 1027 ml. Filter solution through Whatman #1 paper. Store in a refrigerator in opaque bottles.

5. 1% agarose in SDS sample buffer: Two methods may be used to prepare this reagent.

   a. Dissolve 1.0 g agarose in 100 ml of SDS sample buffer by heating in a boiling water bath. Distribute hot solution into screw capped glass tubes and immediately store in refrigerator. Melt reagent in a boiling water bath prior to use.

   b. Place 100 mg of agarose in each of several screw-cap glass tubes. When needed, add 10 ml SDS sample buffer to the tubes and place tubes in a boiling water bath to dissolve the agarose. Use immediately.

6. SDS running buffer, 10 liters of 10× stock:

	Amount	Final concentration (1× buffer)
Tris base	303 g	0.025 M
Glycine	1440 g	0.192 M
SDS	100 g	0.1%

Add deionized water to 10 liters. The pH should be 8.3. Do not attempt to readjust pH. If the pH is off by more than 0.2 unit, discard. Buffer may be stored at room temperature. Dilute 1 : 10 with deionized water prior to use.

7. 0.1% bromophenol blue, 100 ml:

Bromophenol blue   0.1 g
Deionized water   100.0 ml

8. 0.1% Coomassie blue in 50% TCA, 2 liters:

Coomassie blue   2.0 g
50% TCA   2.0 liters

9. Destaining solution: 7% acetic acid

Recipes for SDS Gels

1. 10% acrylamide SDS gels, with a final concentration of 10% acrylamide, 0.1% SDS, and 0.375 M Tris-HCl, pH 8.8:

Number of gels

	1	2	3	4	6	8
Lower gel buffer	4.0 ml	8.0 ml	12.0 ml	16.0 ml	24.0 ml	32 ml
Deionized water	6.7 ml	13.4 ml	20.1 ml	26.8 ml	40.2 ml	53 ml
30% acrylamide	5.3 ml	10.6 ml	15.9 ml	21.2 ml	31.8 ml	42 ml
10% ammonium persulfate	25.0 μl	50.0 μl	75.0 μl	100.0 μl	150.0 μl	200 μl
TEMED	12.5 μl	25.0 μl	37.5 μl	50.0 μl	75.0 μl	100 μl

2. SDS stacking gel, with a final concentration of 4.75% acrylamide, 0.1% SDS, and 0.125 M Tris-HCl, pH 6.8:

Number of gels

	2	4	6	8	10
Upper gel buffer	2.5 ml	5.0 ml	7.5 ml	10.0 ml	12.5 ml
Deionized water	5.92 ml	11.83 ml	17.7 ml	23.66 ml	29.53 ml
30% acrylamide	1.58 ml	3.17 ml	4.76 ml	6.33 ml	7.93 ml
10% ammonium persulfate	30.0 μl	60.0 μl	90.0 μl	120.0 μl	150.0 μl
TEMED	10.0 μl	20.0 μl	30.0 μl	40.0 μl	50.0 μl

PROCEDURE

Slab gel electrophoresis tank

A slab gel tank suited for the second-dimension SDS slab gel electrophoresis can be constructed simply and inexpensively from acrylic plastic by a machine shop. Plans for such a tank are shown in Figures 19.2 (schematic) and 19.3 (detailed). This model is based on one

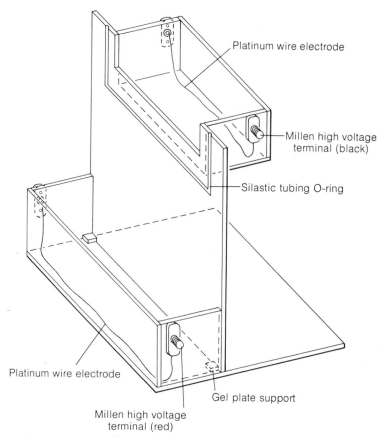

FIGURE 19.2
Slab gel tank: schematic drawing.

Labels in figure:
- Platinum wire electrode
- Millen high voltage terminal (black)
- Silastic tubing O-ring
- Platinum wire electrode
- Gel plate support
- Millen high voltage terminal (red)

designed by Dr. Patrick O'Farrell (Department of Biochemistry and Biophysics, University of California, San Francisco) and was modified by the author in conjunction with W. Harlow and M. Wise of the Department of Genetics, Stanford University School of Medicine. More complex chambers in which the gel plates are attached to the chamber prior to pouring the gel (such as Bio-Rad's models 220 and 221) are not satisfactory for this technique because they are not conducive to running a large number of gels. The Millen screw-type high voltage terminals shown in Figures 19.2 and 19.3 are recommended over the standard banana-plug terminals for safety; with the Millen screw-type terminals, no "live" surfaces are exposed. Having two terminals each for the upper and lower reservoirs facilitates connecting tanks to each other for running multiple gels simultaneously (as will be discussed later).

The slab gels are held in place on this apparatus by clamping the

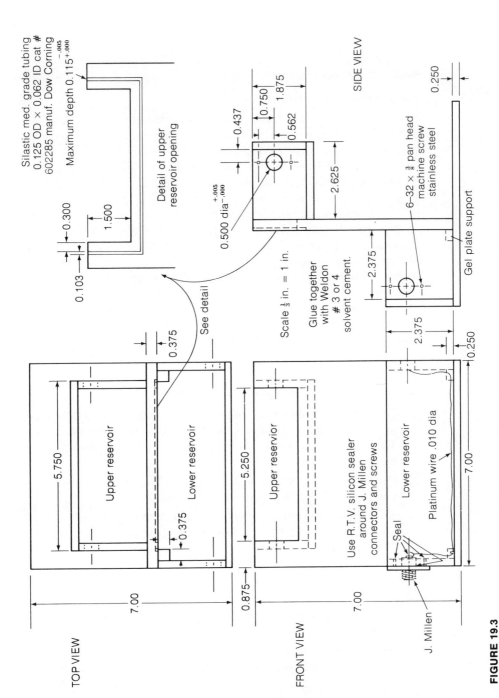

Silastic med. grade tubing 0.125 OD × 0.062 ID cat # 602285 manuf. Dow Corning

Maximum depth $0.115^{+.000}_{-.005}$

0.300

1.500

Detail of upper reservoir opening

0.103

0.500 dia$^{+.005}_{-.000}$

0.437

0.750

1.875

0.562

2.625

SIDE VIEW

2.375

$6\text{-}32 \times \frac{3}{8}$ pan head machine screw stainless steel

Gel plate support

0.250

0.375

See detail

Scale $\frac{1}{3}$ in. = 1 in.

Glue together with Weldon # 3 or 4 solvent cement.

5.750

Upper reservoir

Lower reservoir

0.375

7.00

TOP VIEW

5.250

Upper reservoir

Use R.T.V. silicon sealer around J. Millen connectors and screws

Seal

Lower reservoir

Platinum wire .010 dia

J. Millen

2.375

0.250

7.00

7.00

0.875

FRONT VIEW

FIGURE 19.3
Slab gel tank: precision drawing. (J. Millen high voltage terminal #37001 black or red: specify color.
Supplier: Zack Electronics.)

upper part of the sides of the gel plate to the sides of the tank with binder clip paper clamps.

Preparation of Slab Gel Plates

Slab gel plates are cut from ordinary $\frac{1}{8}$-in. window glass. The back plate is $6\frac{1}{2} \times 6\frac{1}{2}$ in. and the front plate has the same overall dimensions with a $\frac{3}{4} \times 5\frac{1}{4}$-in. notch in one side (Figure 19.4a); the bottom of the notch should be beveled as shown in Figure 19.4b. Several procedures can be used for assembling the gel plates before pouring the gels. We recommend gluing $6\frac{1}{4} \times \frac{1}{4}$-in. strips of polyvinyl chloride (PVC; tabletop lamination plastic, 0.030 in. thick) at the sides of the front plate with epoxy (Figure 19.4a). A piece of silicon rubber tubing (Silastic tubing, Dow Corning, #602-155, 0.047 in. outer diameter) placed around the edges forms a seal. The plates are clamped together with six large binder clips, and a small chip of polyvinyl chloride is inserted between the plates at the bottom to maintain the spacing at 0.8 mm (Figure 19.4c). After use, wash the plates with Alconox laboratory detergent (being careful not to dislodge the plastic strips) and rinse with tap water followed by deionized water. Just prior to use, clean the surfaces of the plates with 95% ethanol.

Second-Dimension Electrophoresis

1. Pour the gels 4–24 hours before needed. The 10% acrylamide gel mixture should be poured up to a line one inch from the notch. This mixture polymerizes rather slowly, so up to 5 minutes can be taken to pour the gels.

2. Overlay the gel mixture with 0.1% SDS. This is done most easily with a squirt bottle that produces a mist.

3. After 1.5–2 hours (twice the time it takes to see the polymerization line), remove the overlay (most easily done with a 2-in., 23-gauge blunt-end needle on a 10-ml syringe).

4. Replace overlay with 2–3 ml of a 1:4 dilution of lower gel buffer in deionized water containing ammonium persulfate and TEMED at the concentration present in the stacking gel (i.e., 3 μl of 10% ammonium persulfate and 1 μl of TEMED per ml of 1:4 diluted lower gel buffer).

5. To prepare gel for use, remove overlay and any material that may have settled onto the top of the gel.

6. Prepare stacking gel mixture and pour it up to the notch.

7. Insert Teflon spacer to a depth of 1–2 mm below the notch, being careful not to trap any bubbles.

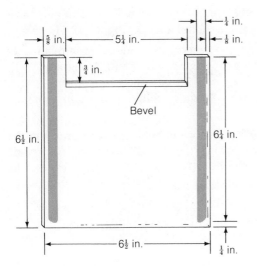

a. Notched front plate with PVC strips

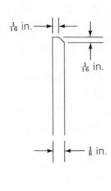

b. Cross section through bevel

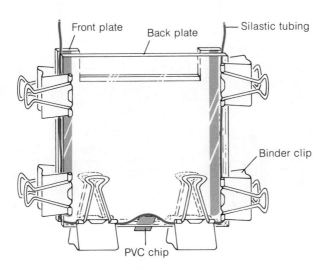

c. Assembled front and back plates

FIGURE 19.4
Dimensions and assembly of slab gel plates.

8. With a syringe and needle, remove any gel mixture that may have been trapped in front of the Teflon spacer (Figure 19.5).

9. Allow polymerization to proceed for 20 minutes. Meanwhile, set up the slab gel tanks (see Figure 19.6) and pour *used* SDS running buffer (see below, step 18) into the lower reservoir to a depth of $\frac{1}{2}$ to 1 inch. Also, prepare melted agarose in a boiling water bath.

10. After 20 minutes, remove the Teflon spacer and clean off upper surface of stacking gel with a tissue. Remove tubing or spacer used to seal the sides and bottom of the slab gel.

11. Number the gel with a marking pen.

12. Pour off the SDS sample buffer from the equilibrated tube gels (from the first-dimension runs). Place each tube gel on a piece of Parafilm and straighten the gel along the edge of the Parafilm (Figure 19.7a).

13. Place the slab gel slanted against a test tube rack (Figure 19.7b). Using a disposable 1-ml pipette, quickly pipette 1 ml of melted agarose onto the top of the stacking gel (Figure 19.7b) and immediately slide the tube gel into place using the Parafilm (Figure

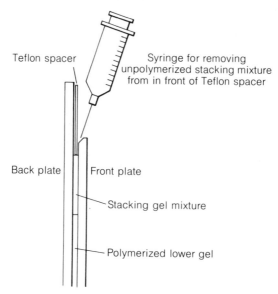

FIGURE 19.5
Removal of stacking gel mixture from in front of spacer.

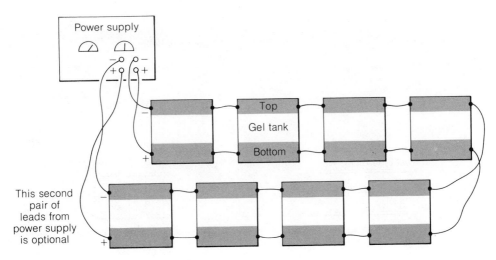

FIGURE 19.6
Connections of slab gel tanks for simultaneous
electrophoresis of multiple slab gels.

19.7c,d). Allow the gel to set for at least 30 seconds before moving it and several minutes before loading it into the tank.

14. Load gels into slab gel tanks with the notched front plate facing the upper reservoir.

15. Add 2 drops of 0.1% bromophenol blue to the upper chamber and pour in SDS running buffer (fresh, unused) until tube gel is covered.

16. Remove bubbles trapped between glass gel plates at bottom of gel by squirting running buffer into this space with a bent 4-in. needle on a 30-ml syringe.

17. Electrophorese at 20 mA/gel (constant current) until the bromophenol blue line reaches the bottom of the gel (3–4 hours).

18. After completing the run, turn off power, wait several seconds, then remove the gel. Separate the plates and discard the tube gel and stacking gel. (Save the SDS running buffer for use in the lower chamber during the next run.)

19. Place slab gels into stain (0.1% Coomassie blue in 50% TCA) in 9 × 13-in. glass pans for 20–30 minutes. Pour off the stain and save. Then destain with two changes of 7% acetic acid. The second change can be used as the first destaining solution for other gels.

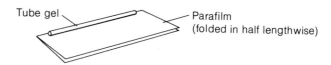

Tube gel ⎯⎯ ⎯⎯ Parafilm (folded in half lengthwise)

a. Placing tube gel on parafilm

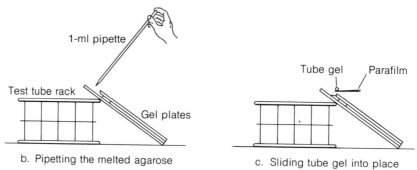

1-ml pipette

Test tube rack

Gel plates

b. Pipetting the melted agarose

Tube gel   Parafilm

c. Sliding tube gel into place

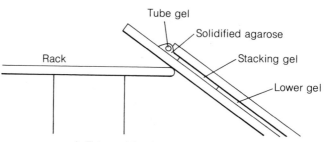

Tube gel

Solidified agarose

Rack

Stacking gel

Lower gel

d. Tube gel in place over slab gel

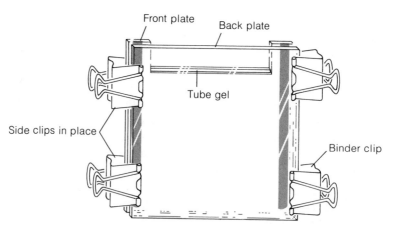

Front plate   Back plate

Tube gel

Side clips in place

Binder clip

e. Front view slab gel with tube gel in place
(bottom clips removed)

20. Place gels on a piece of Whatman #3MM paper and dry on a gel dryer.

21. See Section 19.7 for autoradiography procedure.

19.6 ONE-DIMENSIONAL SDS SLAB GEL ELECTROPHORESIS

This method for the size separation of proteins in one dimension is essentially the same system as the second dimension of the 2-D PAGE procedure (section 19.5B). SDS-PAGE in cylindrical gels has been used since the early 1970s for analyzing lymphocyte proteins; the slab gel system described here has several advantages over the cylindrical gels. First, autoradiography of the slab gels gives much greater resolution than does slicing the cylindrical gels and determining the radioactivity in the 1-mm slices. Second, the cost of scintillation vials and fluid is saved. Finally, it is much easier to analyze and accurately compare large numbers of samples with slab gels than with cylindrical gels.

MATERIALS AND REAGENTS

The materials, reagents, and solutions for the gels are all identical to those described for the second-dimension SDS gels (Section 19.5B). The only addition is a "comb" cut from 0.030 in. Teflon (1 × 5.125 in.) for forming 13 sample wells in the stacking gel (see Figure 19.8). The comb can also be cut to provide more than 13 wells.

PROCEDURE

1. Pour the slab gels and change the overlays as described for the second-dimension gels in Section 19.5B (steps 1 to 5).

2. Pour the stacking gel mixture to within approximately $\frac{1}{8}$ in. of the notch.

3. Slide in the Teflon comb to form sample wells in the stacking gel such that the teeth of the comb are completely below the notch.

4. With a syringe and needle, remove any gel mixture that may have been trapped in front of the comb (as described in Figure 19.5).

5. Allow gel mixture to polymerize for 15 minutes. Meanwhile, set

FIGURE 19.7
Placement of first-dimension tube gels on top of second-dimension slab gels. In b, c, and d, note that gel plates are still held together by binder clips at sides.

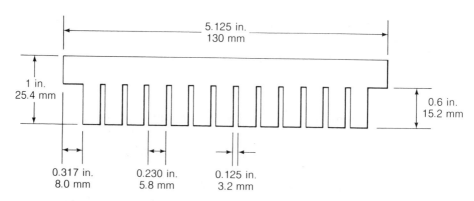

FIGURE 19.8
Dimensions of Teflon comb.

up gel tanks and pour used SDS running buffer into the lower
reservoir to a depth of ½ to 1 in.

6. If it has not been done previously, boil samples for 90 seconds.

7. Remove Teflon comb, rinse wells with deionized water, and then
   remove all liquid from the wells.

8. Place slab gels in tanks, and number the wells with a marking
   pen.

9. Remove any bubbles trapped between the glass plates at the
   bottom of the gel with a syringe and bent needle.

10. Load samples by touching the tip of the pipette to the back plate
    and letting the sample flow down into the well. Wells not being
    used should receive an equal volume of SDS sample buffer.

11. Wash each sample into the gel with a small amount of SDS
    sample buffer, equalizing the liquid levels in all wells (at ≤ ⅔ of
    well capacity).

12. Overlay with SDS running buffer, filling up the wells.

13. Add 2 drops of 0.1% bromophenol blue to the upper buffer
    chamber and fill with SDS running buffer until the wells are
    covered.

14. Continue as described in Section 19.5B, steps 17 to 20. These gels
    run slightly faster than the second dimension of the 2-D system
    (i.e., runs are complete in about 3 hours).

19.7 AUTORADIOGRAPHY

The autoradiographic procedure described below is appropriate for detecting ^{35}S and ^{125}I radioactivity. For ^{3}H and low levels of ^{14}C, which are less efficient at exposing film, fluorographic procedures in which a fluor is incorporated into the gel should be followed. These procedures are described by Bonner and Laskey (1974) and Laskey and Mills (1975).†

MATERIALS AND REAGENTS

Darkroom, with safety light (Kodak No. 6B)
Kodak No-Screen X-ray film (5 × 7 in.), Ready-Pak
Kodak X-ray Developer
Kodak Rapid Fixer
Tanks for developer, fixer, and rinse water
Film packs for holding gel and film during autoradiography; available from medical supply companies or homemade (see below)
Film rack for holding film during developing; available from medical supply companies or make from acrylic plastic

PROCEDURE

1. In a darkroom, place film up against dried gel and place in film pack. This can be done without commercial packs by using the Ready-Pak envelopes that the No-Screen film comes in. Insert the film into an envelope (Figure 19.9a), then cover the open side of envelope #1 with two additional envelopes that are opened on two adjacent sides (Figure 19.9b,c).

2. Place the pack between two boards and clamp together with binder clips (Figure 19.9d). For ^{35}S (and ^{3}H, and ^{14}C), multiple gels can be included together between one pair of boards since the radioactivity cannot penetrate paper. For ^{125}I, each gel must be wrapped individually to prevent cross-exposure of film.

3. After the desired period of time (see comment 1), develop the film in the darkroom using the following sequence:

   a. 4–5 minutes in developer (Kodak X-ray Developer)

   b. 1 minute rinse in water

   c. 9 minutes in fixer (Kodak Rapid Fixer)

---

† An alternative approach to the PPO-DMSO procedure of Bonner and Laskey is now available using the solution EN^{3}HANCE (New England Nuclear). It appears to work as well as PPO-DMSO but avoids the problem of skin penetration.

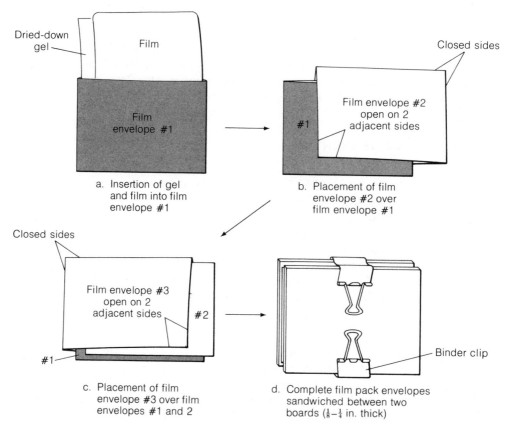

FIGURE 19.9
Wrapping gels and films for autoradiography.

    d. 30 minutes water rinse

    e. Air dry (hang from a "clothes line").

COMMENTS

1. The length of autoradiographic exposure depends on how much radioactivity is in the protein(s) of interest. Perhaps the best advice is to do a short exposure of 1–2 days, develop and examine the autoradiograph, and then put the gels back with new film for a longer exposure if necessary. Depending on the sample, exposure times can be varied from one day to several months.

2. The x-ray developer and fixer solutions can be used for several

months, depending on how much they are used. For fresh developer, use 4 minutes soaking time; extend this to 4.5 and 5 minutes as the developer gets older. The developer needs to be changed when major spots on the autoradiograms are grey instead of black.

3. For many purposes, No-Screen film is satisfactory for the autoradiography of ^{125}I-labeled proteins. However, when only small amounts of ^{125}I are present, intensifying screens can be used. These screens are placed on the opposite side of the film from the gel. Gamma rays from the gel pass through the film and strike the screen, resulting in the production of light. This light then hits the film, thereby increasing the effective film exposure. The most efficient combination of intensifying screen and x-ray film (according to a personal communication of Dr. James Goding, Stanford University School of Medicine) is as follows:

> Intensifying Screen: DuPont Cronex Lightning Plus (DuPont, Wilmington, Delaware).
> Film: Kodak X-OMAT-R (available from medical supply companies).

During exposure, the pack containing the gel, film, and screen should be kept at $-70°C$ for maximum efficiency. Under these conditions, the intensity of spots on the autoradiogram can be increased 10-fold over that obtained using No-Screen film.

REFERENCES

Ames, G. F-L., and K. Nikaido. 1976. Two-dimensional gel electrophoresis of membrane proteins. *Biochem. J.* **15**:616.

Baur, S., E. S. Vitetta, C. J. Sherr, I. Schenkein, and J. W. Uhr. 1971. Isolation of heavy and light chains of immunoglobulin from the surfaces of lymphoid cells. *J. Immunol.* **106**:1133.

Bonner, W. M., and R. A. Laskey. 1974. A film detection method for tritium labeled proteins and nucleic acids in polyacrylamide gels. *Eur. J. Biochem.* **46**:83.

Cone, R. E., and J. J. Marchalonis. 1974. Surface proteins of thymus-derived and bone-marrow-derived lymphocytes. Selective isolation of immunoglobulins and θ-antigen by non-ionic detergents. *Biochem. J.* **104**:435.

Cullen, S. E., and B. D. Schwartz. 1976. An improved method for isolation of H-2 and Ia alloantigens using immuoprecipitation induced by protein-A bearing staphylococci. *J. Immunol.* **117**:136.

Hayman, M. J., and M. J. Crumpton. 1972. Isolation of glycoproteins from pig lymphocyte plasma membrane using *Lens culinaris* phytohemagglutinin. *Biochem. Biophys. Res. Commun.* **47**:923.

Ivarie, R. D., D. H. Gelfand, P. P. Jones, P. Z. O'Farrell, B. A. Polisky, R. A. Steinberg, and P. H. O'Farrell. 1977. Biological applications of two-dimensional gel electrophoresis. In B. J. Radola and D. Graesslin (Eds.), *Electrofocusing and Isotachophoresis.* Walter de Gruyter, Berlin.

Kessler, S. W. 1975. Rapid isolation of antigens from cells with a staphylococcal protein-A antibody adsorbent: Parameters of the interaction of antigen-antibody complexes with protein A. *J. Immunol.* **115**:1617.

Jones, P. P. 1977. Analysis of H-2 and Ia molecules by two-dimensional polyacrylamide gel electrophoresis. *J. Exp. Med.* **146**:1261.

Laskey, R. A., and A. D. Mills. 1975. Quantitative film detection of ^{3}H and ^{14}C in polyacrylamide gels by fluorography. *Eur. J. Biochem.* **56**:335.

O'Farrell, P. H. 1975. High resolution two-dimensional electrophoresis of proteins. *J. Biol. Chem.* **250**:4007.

O'Farrell, P. H., and P. Z. O'Farrell. 1978. Two-dimensional polyacrylamide gel electrophoresis fractionation. *Meth. Cell Biol.* **16**:407.

O'Farrell, P. Z., H. M. Goodman, and P. H. O'Farrell. 1977. High resolution two-dimensional electrophoresis of basic as well as acidic proteins. *Cell* **12**:1133.

Oi, V. T., P. P. Jones, J. W. Goding, L. A. Herzenberg, and L. A. Herzenberg. 1978. Properties of monoclonal antibodies to mouse Ig allotypes, H-2 and Ia antigens. In M. Potter, N. Warner, and F. Melchers (Eds.), *Current Topics in Microbiology and Immunology.* Springer-Verlag, New York.

Schwartz, B. D., W. E. Paul, and E. M. Shevach. 1976. Guinea-pig Ia antigens: Functional significance and chemical characterization. *Transplant. Rev.* **30**:174.

Steinberg, R. A., P. H. O'Farrell, U. Friedrich, and P. Coffino. 1977. Mutation causing charge alterations in regulatory subunits of the cyclic AMP dependent protein kinase of cultured S49 lymphoma cells. *Cell* **10**:381.

APPENDIXES

A

Preparation and Testing of Reagents

A.1 FETAL CALF SERUM (FCS)

Fetal calf sera are essential reagents for primary immunization *in vitro* as well as for other cell culture work. They are, however, ill-defined complex mixtures of biologically active substances and there is considerable variability among different lots. Extensive testing of more than 300 lots of FCS indicates that a relatively small proportion (approximately 10%) are fully satisfactory for the generation of primary humoral immunity *in vitro* (Shiigi and Mishell 1975). These are termed "supportive" or "activating" because they support *in vitro* immunization and because they activate or induce accessory cells to secrete biological mediators (Mishell et al. 1978). Most of the remaining lots are "deficient" because they neither fully support primary immunity nor do they inhibit the responses of cultures supplemented with supportive FCS. Deficient FCS may be preferred for proliferative studies since they are adequate for these responses and generally cause less background incorporation of thymidine.

The ability of FCS to support primary immunization is affected by variations in individual spleen cell preparations. An occasional spleen cell preparation, presumably containing cells activated in the premorbid state, will respond in even a very deficient serum. Inclusion of activating substances such as 2-mercaptoethanol or bacterial lipopolysaccharide may also improve responses of cells cultured in otherwise deficient FCS. While much remains to be learned about the complex interactions of FCS and spleen cells, it is likely that the principal difference between supportive and deficient FCS is the presence of activating substances of bacterial origin in the former (Shiigi and Mishell 1975).

A testing protocol has been developed to characterize lots of FCS in order to identify those with strong supportive properties and those that are very deficient.

Testing of Sera

New samples of FCS are screened for the ability to support the induction of an *in vitro* primary humoral response against sheep red blood cells (SRBC) by the methods described by Mishell and Dutton (1967). The procedure is as described in Section 2.2, except that high cell concentrations (1.2×10^7 cells/ml) are used and 2-mercaptoethanol is omitted from the medium. Separate cultures are set up in medium containing control FCS and test FCS (5% or 10%) and fed daily with nutritive cocktail containing the appropriate serum. After 4 or 5 days incubation, the cultures are assayed for the number of plaque-forming cells per culture (PPC; Section 3.2).

The validity of individual screening tests is determined by employing two types of control sera: a control supportive FCS and a control deficient FCS. In a valid test, cultures supplemented with the control supportive FCS should generate 1000–5000 PPC on day 4 or 5, while cultures supplemented with the control deficient FCS should generate less than 20% of the PPC obtained with the positive control. Test sera that support responses equal to 80% or more of the positive controls are considered supportive. Very deficient sera that support <5% of control response are often lots that also provide exceptionally low background thymidine incorporation in proliferative assays. Occasionally, the deficient controls are too high (greater than 20% of the positive controls). Presumably, this occurs because of the presence in the spleen cell suspension of significant numbers of cells activated *in vivo*. Because of the complexity of the bioassay used, tests are repeated until three experiments with valid controls are obtained.

Occasionally, a lot of FCS that appears very deficient is in fact toxic. When deficient sera are to be used, they should be examined for toxicity by tests to determine whether they adversely affect the responses of cells cultured in control supportive sera. In performing toxicity tests, we add 0.2 ml of the test serum to 1-ml cultures containing 5% control supportive serum. At this concentration, inhibitory sera will reduce the response by 80% or more, while truly deficient sera will not reduce the response.

Storage of Sera

FCS may be stored for long periods (2–3 years) either frozen or at 4°C without loss of the ability to support primary immune responses *in vitro*. If the FCS is stored frozen, a precipitate may form when a sample is thawed. This precipitate seems to be of no consequence and may be removed by centrifugation or membrane filtration for esthetic reasons.

REFERENCES

Mishell, R. I., L. M. Bradley, Y. U. Chen, K. H. Grabstein, B. B. Mishell, J. M. Shiigi, and S. M. Shiigi. 1978. Inhibition of steroid-induced immune suppression by adjuvant stimulated accessory cells. *J. Reticuloendothel. Soc.* **23**:439.

Mishell, R. I., and R. W. Dutton. 1967. Immunization of dissociated spleen cell cultures from normal mice. *J. Exp. Med.* **126**:423.

Shiigi, S. M., and R. I. Mishell. 1975. Sera and the *in vitro* induction of immune responses. I. Bacterial contamination and the generation of good fetal bovine sera. *J. Immunol.* **115**:741.

A.2 COMPLEMENT: GUINEA PIG AND RABBIT SERA

Sera from guinea pigs and rabbits are commonly used as sources of complement, but must frequently be absorbed before use to eliminate either natural antibody or toxicity.

A. Absorption of Guinea Pig Sera for Use in Hemolytic Plaque Assays

To remove any antibodies naturally occurring in guinea pig serum to the red blood cells (RBC) being used in the hemolytic plaque assay, it is necessary to absorb the serum with whatever test red cells will be used; otherwise, general lysis may occur. The absorption can be done simultaneously with red cells from different species.

1. Remove directly from the supplier's bottle of RBC, a volume equal to $\frac{1}{3}$–$\frac{1}{2}$ the volume of complement to be absorbed.

2. Centrifuge these red cells at $400 \times g$ for 15 minutes (or 2 minutes in a Sero-Fuge). Remove and discard the supernate.

3. Wash the cells 3–4 times in large volumes of BSS (Appendix A.3).

4. After the last wash, draw off all BSS. Pour complement over packed RBC, resuspend cells, and transfer the suspension into a flask that is sufficiently large to enable the mixture to be buried in ice without having ice around the neck of the flask.

5. Incubate the mixture on ice 20 minutes, turning the flask occasionally to keep cells in suspension.

6. Pour into centrifuge tubes and centrifuge at $400 \times g$ for 15 minutes. The temperature of the centrifuge *must* be held at 4°C.

7. Remove complement to other tubes and repeat the centrifugation to remove all RBC.

8. Aliquot the absorbed complement keeping it cold. If necessary work in a cold room. Freeze the samples in an alcohol–dry ice mixture and store at −70°C.

9. In our experience, it is the rare lot of guinea pig serum that does not have satisfactory activity when diluted 10-fold. However, some lots are quite satisfactory at significantly greater dilutions (30–40-fold); we therefore titrate all lots of complement. Since complement can lose activity despite storage at −70°C, the titration should be repeated periodically prior to use.

B. Absorption of Guinea Pig or Rabbit Sera for Use in Mass Killing with Alloantisera

Guinea pig and rabbit sera tend to be cytotoxic for mouse cells and must be absorbed with agarose and/or mouse cells prior to use. Sera from rabbits 2–3 weeks old tend to be less cytotoxic than sera from adult rabbits. Agarose absorption is frequently effective in reducing the cytotoxicity. The complement must be checked for toxicity after absorption. Lots that are still cytotoxic after absorption may be used for other purposes, such as hemolytic plaque assays.

1. Mix agarose (Bio-Rad) and serum (80 mg of agarose per ml of serum) in a flask that is sufficiently large to enable the mixture to be buried in ice without having ice around the neck of the flask. Incubate on ice for 1 hour, turning the flask occasionally to keep the agarose in suspension.

2. Add a volume of cold BSS equal to the volume of serum and incubate an additional 30 minutes.

3. Centrifuge the mixture ($250 \times g$, 15 min).

4. Remove the serum from the packed agarose and sterilize the serum by membrane filtration (Appendix C.2). Aliquot and quick freeze the serum in an alcohol-dry ice mixture. Store samples at $-70°C$.

5. Before use, test for toxicity and titrate.

COMMENT

Agarose-absorbed rabbit and guinea pig sera, selected for high complement activity and low toxicity to mouse lymphocytes, are commercially available from Cedarlane Laboratories. The company also carries guinea pig sera absorbed with SRBC.

REFERENCE

Cohen, A., and M. Schlesinger. 1970. Absorption of guinea pig serum with agar. A method for elimination of its cytotoxicity for murine thymus cells. *Transplantation* **10**:130.

A.3   BALANCED SALT SOLUTION (BSS)

This balanced salt solution (Mishell and Dutton 1967) can be used during the manipulation of mouse cells prior to culture and for hemolytic plaque assays. A $2\times$ BSS is used with the hypotonic shock method of removing red blood cells (Section 1.16).

MATERIALS AND REAGENTS

Dextrose, $M_r = 180.1$
KH_2PO_4, $M_r = 136.1$
$Na_2HPO_4·7H_2O$, $M_r = 268.1$
Phenol red, 0.5% solution
$CaCl_2·2H_2O$, $M_r = 147.0$
KCl, $M_r = 74.6$
NaCl, $M_r = 58.4$
$MgCl_2$, anhydrous, $M_r = 95.2$ or $MgCl_2·6H_2O$, $M_r = 203.3$
$MgSO_4·7H_2O$, $M_r = 246.5$
Volumetric flask, 1000 ml
Membrane filtration equipment
Reagent bottles, sterile, 100 ml or 500 ml

PROCEDURE

1. The 10× BSS is made up as two stock solutions.

   Stock #1:

Dextrose	10.0 g
KH_2PO_4	0.6 g
$Na_2HPO_4 \cdot 7H_2O$	3.58 g
0.5% phenol red solution	20.0 ml

   Dissolve and bring up to 1000 ml with double-distilled water.

   Stock #2:

$CaCl_2 \cdot 2 H_2O$	1.86 g
KCl	4.0 g
NaCl	80.0 g
$MgCl_2$, anhydrous	1.04 g
(or 2.0 g $MgCl_2 \cdot 6H_2O$)	
$MgSO_4 \cdot 7H_2O$	2.0 g

   Dissolve and bring up to 1000 ml with double-distilled water.

2. Test the 10× stocks by making a sample of 1× BSS. Mix 10 ml of stock #1 and 10 ml of stock #2 and bring up to 100 ml with double-distilled water. The 1× BSS should be at pH 7.2–7.4 and have a conductivity of 14–16 mS.

3. 2× and 1× BSS are obtained by appropriate dilutions of the 10× stocks with double-distilled water. The 2× and 1× BSS can be sterilized by passage through a 0.22-μm filter (Appendix C.2).

COMMENTS

1. Store the 10× stocks at 4°C.

2. Make nonsterile 1× BSS for the hemolytic assays just prior to use. Discard 1× BSS after use.

3. Prepare sterile 2× and 1× BSS immediately after the 10× stocks are made. Then incubate the filtered BSS at 37°C for one week prior to use to detect bacterial contamination. The sterile BSS is stored at room temperature and appears to have an indefinite shelf life.

REFERENCE

Mishell, R. I., and R. W. Dutton. 1967. Immunization of dissociated spleen cell cultures from normal mice. *J. Exp. Med.* **126**:423.

A.4 HEPES-BUFFERED BALANCED SALT SOLUTION

The following recipe yields a balanced salt solution (Shortman et al. 1972) that is isotonic for mouse cells (osmolarity = 308 mOsm). It is useful for strong buffering that maintains the same pH in both air and 10% CO_2.

MATERIALS AND REAGENTS

KH_2PO_4, M_r = 136.1
K_2HPO_4, M_r = 174.1
HEPES (4-[2-hydroxyethyl]-1-piperazine-ethanesulfonic acid), M_r = 238.3
HCl, concentrated
KOH, M_r = 56.1
NaOH, M_r = 40.0
NaCl, M_r = 58.4
KCl, M_r = 74.6
$CaCl_2$, M_r = 111.0
$MgSO_4 \cdot 7H_2O$, M_r = 246.5

PROCEDURE

1. Make up the following solutions:
   a. Phosphate buffer: Dissolve 22.9 g KH_2PO_4 and 19.5 g K_2HPO_4 in 900 ml double-distilled water. Adjust to pH 7.2 with KOH or HCl. Make up to 1000 ml.
   b. HEPES buffer: Dissolve 80 g HEPES and 13.4 g NaOH in 900 ml double-distilled water. Adjust to pH 7.2 with NaOH or HCl. Make up to 1000 ml.
   c. 0.168 M NaCl: 9.83 g/liter.
   d. 0.168 M KCl: 12.5 g/liter.
   e. 0.112 M $CaCl_2$: 12.45 g/liter.
   f. 0.168 M $MgSO_4 \cdot 7H_2O$: 41.3 g/liter.
2. Mix the stock solutions in the following proportion:

Phosphate buffer	10 ml
HEPES buffer	30 ml
0.168 M NaCl	605 ml
0.168 M KCl	20 ml
0.112 M $CaCl_2$	15 ml
0.168 M $MgSO_4 \cdot 7H_2O$	5 ml
	685 ml

3. Sterilize the solution by membrane filtration (Appendix C.2) and store at room temperature or 4°C (do not freeze).

REFERENCE

Shortman, K., N. Williams, and P. Adams. 1972. The separation of different cell classes from lymphoid organs. V. Simple procedures for the removal of cell debris, damaged cells and erythroid cells from lymphoid cell suspensions. *J. Immunol. Meth.* **1:**273.

A.5 NUTRITIVE COCKTAIL

This recipe was developed by Mishell and Dutton (1967) and is used as a feeding supplement for many types of immunologic culture systems.

MATERIALS AND REAGENTS

Eagle's minimum medium, essential amino acids, 100× solution
Eagle's minimum medium, nonessential amino acids, 100× solution
L-glutamine, 200 mM solution
Dextrose
1 M NaOH (40 g/liter)
$NaHCO_3$: 7.5% (w/v) solution
Balanced salt solution (BSS; Appendix A.3)

PROCEDURE

1. Mix the following:

Essential amino acids	150 ml
Nonessential amino acids	75 ml
L-glutamine	75 ml
Dextrose	15 g
BSS	1050 ml

2. Adjust to pH 7.2 with 1M NaOH. Then add 225 ml of 7.5% $NaHCO_3$ solution.

3. Sterilize solution by membrane filtration (Appendix C.2). Aliquot into sterile tubes (Falcon, #2074 or similar) and store at −20°C. Each new lot of cocktail should be pretested in the primary humoral response system (as described in Section 2.2) prior to general use.

REFERENCE

Mishell, R. I., and R. W. Dutton. 1967. Immunization of dissociated spleen cell cultures from normal mice. *J. Exp. Med.* **126**:423.

A.6 2-MERCAPTOETHANOL (2-ME)

REAGENT

2-mercaptoethanol, 2-ME, M_r = 78.1 (Sigma Chemical); density = 1.114 g/ml, molarity = 14.3 M. Note: Concentrated 2-ME is extremely toxic and malodorous.

PROCEDURE

Preparation of 2-ME Stock: 5×10^{-2} M

Make a 1.0 M solution of 2-ME by diluting 0.5 ml 2-ME into 6.6 ml sterile double-distilled water. *Use a chemical hood and a Propipette.* Dilute 5 ml of the 1.0 M stock into 95 ml of sterile water to give a concentration of 5×10^{-2} M. Store at 4°C.

Addition of 2-ME to Culture Medium

Stocks of 5×10^{-3} M and 5×10^{-4} M 2-ME are obtained by making 1 : 10 and 1 : 100 dilutions of the 5×10^{-2} M stock in sterile balanced salt solution (Appendix A.3). 2-ME is usually used in culture at a final concentration of 5×10^{-5} M.

A.7 UNBUFFERED BALANCED SALT SOLUTION

This unbuffered balanced salt solution is isotonic with mouse cells and is used in the linear density gradient procedure described in Section 8.2.

MATERIALS AND REAGENTS

As described in Appendix A.4 with the omission of K_2HPO_4, HEPES, HCl, KOH, and NaOH.

PROCEDURE

1. Prepare the following stock solutions and combine them in the proportions indicated:

0.168 M NaCl	9.83 g/liter	121 ml
0.168 M KCl	12.5 g/liter	4 ml
0.112 M CaCl$_2$	12.45 g/liter	3 ml
0.168 M MgSO$_4$·7H$_2$O	41.3 g/liter	1 ml
0.168 M KH$_2$PO$_4$	22.9 g/liter	1 ml

2. Sterilize the solution by membrane filtration (Appendix C.2).

REFERENCE

Shortman, K., N. Williams, and P. Adams. 1972. The separation of different cell classes from lymphoid organs. V. Simple procedures for the removal of cell debris, damaged cells and erythroid cells from lymphoid cell suspensions. *J. Immunol. Meth.* **1**:273.

A.8 PHOSPHATE-BUFFERED SALINE (PBS), pH 7.2–7.4, 10X STOCK

Dissolve 20.5 g NaH$_2$PO$_4$·H$_2$O and 179.9 g Na$_2$HPO$_4$·7H$_2$O (or 95.5 g Na$_2$HPO$_4$) in about 4 liters of double-distilled water. Adjust to the required pH (7.2–7.4). Add 701.3 g NaCl and make up to a total volume of 8 liters. Dilute stock 1 : 10 prior to use, resulting in a final buffer of 0.01 M phosphate and 0.15 M NaCl.

A.9 BORATE-BUFFERED SALINE (BBS), 0.17 M BORATE, 0.12 M NaCl, pH 8.0

Dissolve 61.9 g H$_3$BO$_3$ and 43.9 g NaCl in 5 liters distilled water. Adjust to pH 8.0 with 0.15 M NaOH. Make up to a total volume of 6 liters.

A.10 1.0 M PHOSPHATE BUFFER, pH 7.6

1. Prepare the following stock solutions:
   a. 1.0 M KH$_2$PO$_4$: 136.1 g/liter.
   b. 1.0 M Na$_2$HPO$_4$·7H$_2$O: 268.1 g/liter. This solution may crystallize at room temperature. Warm to 45°C to dissolve.

2. Combine 910 ml of 1.0 M $Na_2HPO_4\cdot7H_2O$ and 90 ml of 1.0 M KH_2PO_4. If necessary, adjust to pH 7.6 with more 1.0 M $Na_2HPO_4\cdot7H_2O$.

A.11 GLUCOSE-PHOSPHATE-BUFFERED SALINE (G-PBS), pH 7.6

Combine the following and adjust to pH 7.6 if necessary:

1.0 M phosphate buffer, pH 7.6 (Appendix A.10)	10 ml
0.14 M NaCl: 8.2 g/liter	1000 ml
Dextrose	10 g

A.12 0.15 M PHOSPHATE BUFFER, pH 7.2–7.4

1. Combine the following solutions:

0.15 M $NaH_2PO_4\cdot H_2O$	20.7 g/liter	270 ml
0.15 M $Na_2HPO_4\cdot7H_2O$	40.2 g/liter	930 ml

2. Adjust to the required pH by addition of the appropriate 0.15 M phosphate solution.

A.13 0.28 M CACODYLATE BUFFER, pH 6.9

Dissolve 38.6 g cacodylic acid in 900 ml water. Adjust to pH 6.9 with 10 M NaOH (40 g/100 ml), using about 22 ml. Bring volume to 1000 ml with water.

Note: Cacodylic acid is poisonous; avoid skin contact and do not pipet by mouth. Synonyms: Hydroxydimethylarsine oxide and dimethylarsinic acid.

A.14 ALSEVER'S SOLUTION

Dissolve 20.5 g dextrose, 4.2 g NaCl, and 8.0 g sodium citrate in 1000 ml of water. Sterilize by membrane filtration (Appendix C.2) and store at room temperature.

A.15 MODIFIED CLICK'S MEDIUM

Prepare the incomplete and complete media by the following recipe, which is a modification of that described by Click et al. (1972).

Incomplete medium

Stocks for incomplete medium	Volume
1. Hanks' BSS, 10×†	100 ml
2. Essential amino acids, 50×†	40 ml
3. Nonessential amino acids, 100×†	50 ml
4. Nucleic acid precursors*	25 ml
5. Vitamins, 100×†	20 ml
6. HEPES, 0.5 M	30 ml
7. Double-distilled H_2O	650 ml
8. $NaHCO_3$, 7.5%	11.5 ml
9. NaOH, 2 M	~10 ml (pH to 7.0)
Total	~936 ml

Complete medium

Stocks for complete medium	Volume
1. Incomplete medium	93.5 ml
2. Penicillin/streptomycin, 5000 units/ml-5000 µg/ml†	2 ml
3. Glutamine, 100× (200 mM)†	2 ml
4. Sodium pyruvate, 100× (200 mM)†	2.5 ml
5. Gentamycin, 10 mg/ml	0.1 ml
6. Normal mouse serum	0.5 ml
7. 2-mercaptoethanol, 0.1 M	0.05 ml
Total	100.65 ml

* 100× precursors = 1 g/liter of adenosine, guanosine, uridine, and cytosine. This mixture can be sterilized by autoclaving (Appendix C.1). The solution must be heated to 56°C to dissolve.
† Grand Island Biological.

COMMENT

Incomplete medium can be filtered (Appendix C.2), aliquoted into small sterile bottles (fill to top and seal cap with tape to reduce CO_2 loss), and stored at 4°C.

REFERENCE

Click, R. E., L. Benck, and B. J. Alter. 1972. Immune response *in vitro*. I. Culture conditions for antibody synthesis. *Cell. Immunol.* **3**:264.

A.16   PARLODION-GENTIAN VIOLET SOLUTION

MATERIALS AND REAGENTS

Gentian violet

Amyl acetate

Parlodion strips, nitrocellulose, reagent grade (Tousimis Research Corp., #5051). Note: Parlodion degrades rapidly while in a solid state. However, when dissolved in amyl acetate, its shelf life is indefinite.

Glass beaker

Glass stirring rod

Aluminum foil

PROCEDURE

1. Add 4 g of Parlodion strips to 100 ml of amyl acetate. Stir the mixture periodically with a glass rod; complete dissolution takes 3–4 days at room temperature. (Cover the beaker with aluminum foil to prevent evaporation of the amyl acetate.)

2. After the Parlodion is completely dissolved, add 1.0 g of crystal violet to the solution. Stir the mixture periodically; complete dissolution takes 2–3 days at room temperature.

3. Store the solution in a tightly capped bottle.

A.17   ACIDIFIED WATER

Many investigators maintain their mouse colonies on acidified water. The weight at weaning is slightly lower than with animals given ordinary tap water, probably because of the sour taste of the acidified water; but the mice seem unaffected otherwise and soon reach normal size. Acidified water is particularly advantageous if the animals are to be x-irradiated: They should receive it for at least a week or two prior to irradiation; otherwise many of them will die from infections that result from bacteria not usually considered pathogenic, particularly those from the genus

Pseudomonas. Treatment of the drinking water with hydrochloric acid effectively reduces the incidence of *Pseudomonas* and other potentially pathogenic organisms. It used to be common practice to include chlorine in the water as well. However, there have been reports that chlorine has adverse effects and its use has been discontinued by many investigators.

1. *Stock HCl Solution:* Add 100 ml concentrated HCl to 8300 ml tap water (1 : 84 dilution).

2. *Drinking Water:* Add 5 ml of the stock HCl solution to 500 ml of drinking water (1 : 8400 final dilution). The pH is approximately 2.8 (useful range = 2.5–3.5). If the pH is below 2.5, the mice may consume an inadequate quantity of water.

Washing and Sterilization of
Laboratory Glassware

There are two essential requirements for tissue culture work: The laboratory ware that is used to prepare reagents and that comes into contact with cell suspensions must be scrupulously clean; in most instances, it must also be sterile.

B.1 WASHING OF GLASSWARE FOR TISSUE CULTURE WORK

MATERIALS

7X detergent (Linbro)
Distilled water
Double-distilled or glass-distilled water
Various sizes of bottle brushes
Pipette washing jars with racks

PROCEDURE

1. Immediately after use, rinse the glassware with tap water to remove medium, cells, etc. Fill containers (such as beakers, flasks,

reagent bottles) with tap water and completely submerge tubes and pipettes in tap water.

2. Using a brush, scrub the glassware (excluding the pipettes) with 7X detergent and warm tap water. Thoroughly rinse all traces of detergent from the glassware with warm tap water (a minimum of 5 times). Then, rinse a minimum of 3 times with distilled water and double-distilled water respectively.

3. Wash the pipettes by dipping them repeatedly into a washing jar filled with diluted 7X detergent. Transfer the pipettes to another washing jar filled with flowing warm tap water and rinse the pipettes until all traces of detergent have been removed. Finally, rinse the pipettes a minimum of 3 times each with distilled water and double-distilled water. Alternatively, automatic pipette washers may be used.

B.2 STERILIZATION OF LABORATORY GLASSWARE

MATERIALS

Autoclave
Sterile indicators
Cotton
Cheese cloth
Aluminum foil
Tape
Autoclaving bags
Pipette canisters with stainless steel caps

PROCEDURE

1. Prepare items to be autoclaved as follows:
   a. Tighten caps on reagent bottles, then loosen a turn. (Reagent bottles should have caps with intact sealers.)
   b. Plug flasks, graduated cylinders, etc., with cotton-filled cheese cloth plugs and cover the plugs securely with aluminum foil.
   c. Plug pipettes with cotton and burn off excess cotton with a Bunsen burner. Place pipettes, tips first, in the canisters (place a gauze padding on the bottom of the canisters to cushion the pipette tips) and place the caps on the canisters.

   d. Place items such as tissue homogenizers, membrane filter units, cotton swabs, etc., in autoclaving bags, label (with indelible ink), and seal.

2. Tape a sterile indicator to the glassware and canisters, and autoclave at 121°C for 20 minutes. We usually use a fast exhaust and a drying cycle.

C

Sterilization of Liquid Reagents

Reagents such as water, normal saline, and phosphate-buffered saline can be sterilized by autoclaving. Many other reagents, however, must be sterilized by membrane filtration since they contain heat-sensitive components.

C.1 STERILIZATION BY AUTOCLAVING

MATERIALS

Autoclavable reagent bottles with caps
Autoclave

PROCEDURE (For water, normal saline, and phosphate-buffered saline)

1. Fill reagent bottles two-thirds full of liquid. Cap tightly, then loosen cap one turn. Tape sterile indicator on bottles.
2. Place bottles in a steel tray with sufficiently high sides to catch liquid if bottles should break in the autoclave (especially important for autoclaving saline and PBS).

3. Autoclave at 121°C for 20 minutes, slow exhaust.

4. After autoclaving, let bottles cool and tighten caps. (If the reagents are to be used for chromatographic work, tighten the caps while the reagents are hot. This procedure will maintain the reagents in a degassed state.)

C.2 STERILIZATION BY MEMBRANE FILTRATION

MATERIALS AND REAGENTS

Cool normal saline
Sterile membrane filtration units, 0.22 μm or 0.45 μm (Millipore)
Disposable syringes and needles
Boiling double-distilled water

PROCEDURE

1. Carefully remove sterilized filter units from autoclaving bag and put needle (its cap still in place) onto unit.

2. Fill syringe with boiling water, attach filter unit, remove needle cap, and push a large volume of water through the filter. Recap needle, remove filter unit, fill syringe with cool normal saline, and pass the saline through the filter unit. (This procedure removes toxic wetting agents that are in the filters.)

3. Fill syringe with the reagent (media, buffers, antiserum, etc.) and pass through the filter unit into a sterile tube.

4. Finally, disassemble the filter unit to check whether the filter is intact. Occasionally, small cracks appear in the filters. If this occurs, refilter the reagent through another filter unit. Do not pull back on the syringe barrel while the filter unit is attached or the filter will tear.

COMMENTS

1. "Disposable" filter units can be recycled. Immediately after use, rinse the units thoroughly with tap water; then rinse 3 times with distilled water and 3 times with double-distilled water. Reassemble dry units with a new membrane filter, seal in a labeled autoclaving bag, and autoclave (121°C, 20 min.).

2. We usually use a 0.22-μm filter for sterilizing reagents not contain-

ing serum and either a 0.22-μm or 0.45-μm filter for sterilizing serum or reagents containing serum.

3. Growth media obtained from cultured cells usually need to be prefiltered to remove debris that can clog the 0.22-μm and 0.45-μm filters. Pass the media through nonsterile filters of decreasing pore size and finally through a sterile 0.22-μm or 0.45-μm filter. Alternatively, centrifuge the media at 12 000 × g for 20 minutes prior to filtering. Wash all filters with boiling water as previously described.

4. Nalgene filter units are satisfactory for larger volumes. Pretreat as described above.

5. When membrane filters are used to sterilize solutions containing low concentrations of macromolecules (such as serum-free medium containing immunoregulatory factors or chromatographically purified substances), considerable losses may occur due to adherence of the macromolecules to the filters. Treatment of the filters by flushing with small amounts of serum or protein (1% BSA) prior to passage of the biologically active solution reduces the likelihood of such losses.

D

Preparation of Dialysis Tubing

Dialysis tubing must be washed thoroughly before use to remove the chemicals that are used to make the tubing and that keep the tubing flexible during storage.

1. For Solutions Not Coming into Contact with Cells

Cut off sufficient lengths of tubing and soak them in a beaker of distilled water. Rinse the tubing thoroughly with several changes of distilled water. Bring tubing to a low boil in distilled water and immediately rinse with distilled water and soak in 0.01 M EDTA for 10 minutes (the EDTA helps to leach out metallic ions). Then rinse thoroughly (5–10 times) in distilled water and use tubing immediately.

2. For Solutions Coming in Contact with Cells

There seems to be no sure way of detoxifying dialysis tubing for use with solutions that will be used in culture. Each batch of prepared tubing must be tested for toxicity before use.

Follow the steps described above through the EDTA wash and rinse. Then complete a cycle of boiling and rinsing in double-distilled water 10 times. For the last cycle, cover the beaker with aluminum foil and bring to a full boil to sterilize the tubing; alternatively, autoclave the tubing in water as described in Appendix C.1. Store beaker at 4°C while maintaining sterility.

3. Toxicity Test

The toxicity of the tubing may be tested by incubating 0.5–1.0-cm pieces of autoclaved tubing in 10 ml of complete medium for several hours, sterilizing the medium by membrane filtration (Appendix C.2), and using the medium to culture normal spleen cells as described in Section 2.2. Toxic tubing inhibits the supportive properties of the preincubated medium.

E

Preparation of Allogeneic-Conditioned Medium

Allogeneic-conditioned medium is the supernatant fluid of cultured spleen cells from two strains of mice bearing different H-2 haplotypes. It contains factors that obviate the requirement for T cells in generating primary *in vitro* immune responses to red blood cell antigens. Allogeneic stimulation also generates suppressor factors. Synthesis of suppressor factors is, however, much reduced by treating the spleen cells with mitomycin C or irradiation.

MATERIALS AND REAGENTS

Spleen Cell Suspensions

As described in Section 1.2
Two strains of mice with different H-2 haplotypes
Mitomycin C (Section 10.3)

Cell Culture

As described in Section 2.2, with the following addition:

Tissue culture flask, 75 cm², 250-ml volume (Costar, #02139 or similar)

Cell Harvest

Centrifuge tubes, 50 ml
Equipment for membrane filtration (Appendix C.2)

PROCEDURE

1. Remove spleens from equal numbers of mice with differing H-2 haplotypes.

2. Treat both sets of cells with mitomycin C as described in Section 10.3 to reduce suppressor function.

3. Resuspend each set of spleens to $1-1.2 \times 10^7$ cells/ml in the medium described in Section 2.2. The FCS need not be particularly supportive of *in vitro* primary immunization (but should not be inhibitory).

4. Mix equal volumes of the spleen cell suspensions and distribute in 20-ml volumes to the tissue culture flasks. Cap flasks loosely and place in culture chamber. Exchange the air in the chamber with the gas mixture described in Section 2.2. When the pH of the medium has been adjusted, remove the flasks from the chamber and tighten the lids immediately. Incubate at 37°C without rocking or feeding (flat, not upright).

5. Harvest supernate on day 3. Pour the culture contents into 50-ml centrifuge tubes and pellet the cells ($400 \times g$, 10 min). Sterilize the culture supernate (allogeneic-conditioned medium) by membrane filtration and store at 4°C.

6. Titrate the conditioned medium prior to experimental use. Determine the capacity of the conditioned medium to restore the response of T cell depleted populations to SRBC (Sections 2.2, 9.2, and 11.2). We find that medium prepared as described above will replace T cell function in primary humoral responses when the conditioned medium constitutes 20% of the culture medium.

Freund's Adjuvant

Freund's adjuvant is frequently used to enhance the production of antibody. Equal portions of a diluent such as saline, in which the antigen is dissolved or suspended, and an emulsifier-mineral oil mixture (which may or may not contain mycobacteria) are mixed until a stable water-in-oil emulsion forms. It is important that the emulsion be complete if the antigen is a soluble protein. It is easier to obtain an adequate emulsion if the antigen is added in small increments to the mineral oil mixture and emulsified completely between each addition. After adding all the antigen, continue emulsifying the mixture until a drop of the emulsion placed on water remains intact and does not spread.

As noted throughout this book, Freund's adjuvant is potentially hazardous. Accidental injection into humans has been reported to cause severe, chronic inflammatory reactions. Luer-lock syringes should be used for injections. The spattering of Freund's adjuvant when a needle becomes disconnected from the syringe occurs quite frequently with disposable syringes. If Luer-lock syringes are unavailable, protective glasses should be worn. The spattering of Freund's adjuvant into the eyes can cause eye damage.

MATERIALS AND REAGENTS

Antigen, dissolved or suspended in saline (0.85% w/v NaCl) or in
balanced salt solution (BSS; Appendix A.3)
Freund's adjuvant, incomplete (without mycobacteria) or complete
(with mycobacteria) (Difco Laboratories)
Small beaker containing cold water
Equipment for preparing the emulsion:

1. Syringe (size depends on volume of materials)
   Needle, 13 gauge, blunt tip
   Beaker, small

   or

2. Luer-lock syringes, 2 each
   Needle, double hubbed

   or

3. Electric homogenizer (Virtis or similar)

PROCEDURE

1. If using complete Freund's adjuvant, resuspend the mycobacteria.
   Remove a volume equal to the volume of antigen and either place
   it in the small beaker or homogenizer or leave it in the syringe,
   depending on which method will be used for preparing the
   emulsion.

2. If using the syringe and blunt-tip needle, add a small amount of
   antigen to the adjuvant. Emulsify the mixture by repeatedly drawing the contents of the beaker into the syringe and expelling them.
   Continue, with repeated additions of antigen, until the emulsion is
   complete. The mixture will become white and very thick toward
   the end of the process.

3. If using the double-hubbed needle and Luer-lock syringes, place
   the antigen in one syringe and the adjuvant in the other; connect
   the two syringes by the double-hubbed needle. Prepare the emulsion by repeatedly expelling the contents of one syringe into the
   other. Air should be eliminated from the syringes and needle
   beforehand.

4. If using the electric homogenizer, follow the same principles; that
   is, add the antigen in small increments to the adjuvant during the
   preparation of the emulsion. In this instance, the mixture should
   be kept chilled in an ice bath during the process.

Manufacturers and Distributors

Accurate Chemical & Scientific Corp.
28 Tec Street
Hicksville, New York 11801
516-433-4900
800-645-7248

Aldrich Chemical Co., Inc.
940 W. St. Paul Avenue
Milwaukee, Wisconsin 53233
414-273-3850

Amersham Corporation
2636 S. Clearbrook Drive
Arlington Heights, Illinois 60005
312-593-6300
800-323-9750

Amicon Corporation
Scientific Systems Division
21 Hartwell Avenue
Lexington, Massachusetts 02173
617-862-7050

Arthur H. Thomas Co.
Vine Street at 3rd
P.O. Box 779
Philadelphia, Pennsylvania 19015
215-574-4500
215-574-4555

Arzol Chemical Co.
66 South Franklin Street
Nyack, New York 10960
914-358-2169

Astra Pharmaceutical Products, Inc.
Pleasant Street Connector
P.O. Box 1089
Framingham, Massachusetts 01701
617-620-0600

Atomergic Chemetals Corp.
100 Fairchild Avenue
Plainview, New York 11803
516-822-8800

J. T. Baker Chemical Co.
    222 Red School Lane
    Phillipsburg, New Jersey 08865
    201-859-2151

BBL
    Division of Becton, Dickinson and Co.
    P.O. Box 243
    Cockeysville, Maryland 21030
    301-666-0100

BDH Chemicals, Ltd.
    Dorset, England
    distributed by Gallard Schlesinger
    Chemical Mfg. Corp.

Beckman Instruments, Inc.
    Clinical Instruments Division
    2500 Harbor Boulevard
    Fullerton, California 92634
    714-817-4848

    Electronic Instruments Division
    3900 North River Road
    Schiller Park, Illinois 60176
    312-671-3300

    Scientific Instruments Division
    Campus Drive and Jamboree Boulevard
    Irvine, California 92713
    714-833-0751

Becton Dickinson FACS Systems
    500 Clyde Avenue
    Mountain View, California 94043
    415-969-6633

Becton-Dickinson Immunodiagnostics
(formerly Schwartz/Mann)
    Mountain View Avenue
    Orangeburg, New York 10962
    914-359-2700
    800-431-1237

Bellco Glass, Inc.
    340 Edrudo Road, P.O. Box B
    Vineland, New Jersey 08360
    609-691-1075

Bio-Rad Laboratories
    2200 Wright Avenue
    Richmond, California 94804
    415-234-4130

    220 Maple Avenue
    Rockville Center,
    New York 11570
    516-764-2575

BIOTEC Aktiengesellschaft
    CH-4124 Schöenenbuch/Basel
    Baselstrasse 59
    Basel, Switzerland

BOLAB, Inc.
    6 Tinkham Avenue
    Derry, New Hampshire
    603-434-4941

Calbiochem-Behring
    P.O. Box 12087
    San Diego, CA 92112
    800-542-6052
    800-854-2171

Cataphote Division, Ferro Corporation
    P.O. Box 2369
    Jackson, Mississippi 39205
    601-939-4631

Cedarlane Laboratories Ltd.
    5516 8th, Line R.R. 2
    Hornby, Ontario
    Canada LOP 1EO
    416-878-7800
    distributed by Accurate Chemical &
    Scientific Corp.

Cell Distribution Center
    Salk Institute
    P.O. Box 1809
    San Diego, California 92112
    714-453-4100, ext. 355

Clay Adams, Inc.
    Division of Becton, Dickinson and Co.
    299 Webro Road
    Parsippany, New Jersey 07054
    201-887-4800

Codman and Shurtleff, Inc.
    Pacella Drive
    Randolph, Massachusetts 02368
    617-961-2300

Colorado Serum Co.
    4950 York Street
    Denver, Colorado 80216
    303-623-5373

Commonwealth of Massachusetts
    Department of Public Health
    State Laboratory Institute
    305 South Street
    Boston, Massachusetts 02130
    617-522-3700

Cooke Laboratory Products
    see Dynatech Laboratories, Inc.

Corning Glass Works
    Customer Service
    Science Products Division
    Corning, NY 14830
    607-974-9000

Costar Division, Data Packaging Corp.
    205 Broadway
    Cambridge, Massachusetts 02139
    617-492-1110

Curtin Matheson Scientific Co.
    4220 Jefferson Street
    Houston, Texas 77001
    713-923-1661

Damon/IEC Division
    Damon Corp.
    300 Second Avenue
    Needham Heights, Massachusetts 02194
    617-449-0800
    800-225-8856

Davis and Geck Division
    American Cyanamide Co.
    Middletown Road
    Pearl River, New York 10965
    914-735-4879

Difco Laboratories, Inc.
    P.O. Box 1058A
    Detroit, Michigan 48232
    313-961-0800

Dow Corning Corp.
    P.O. Box 1592
    Midland, Michigan 48640
    517-496-4000

DuPont Co.
    Quillen Building, Concord Plaza
    Wilmington, Delaware 19898
    302-774-1000

E. I. DuPont de Nemours and Co.
    5215 Kennedy Avenue
    East Chicago, Indiana 46312
    219-398-2040

Dynatech Instruments, Inc.
    1718 21st Street
    Santa Monica, California 90404
    213-829-1902

Dynatech Laboratories, Inc.
(formerly Cooke Laboratory Products)
    900 Slaters Lane
    Alexandria, Virginia 22314
    703-548-3889

E & K Scientific Products, Inc.
    P.O. Box 822
    Saratoga, California 95070
    408-867-1157

Eastman Kodak Company
    343 State Street
    Rochester, New York 14650
    716-724-4000

Enzyme Center, Inc.
    33 Harrison Avenue
    Boston, Massachusetts 02111
    617-482-7123

Eppendorf Division
    Brinkmann Instruments, Inc.
    Cantiague Road
    Westbury, New York 11509
    516-334-7500
    800-645-3050

Falcon Products, Becton Dickinson Labware
    1950 Williams Drive
    Oxnard, California 93030
    805-485-8711
    800-235-5953

Fenwall Laboratories
    Division of Baxter-Travenol
    1 Baxter Parkway
    Deerfield, Illinois 60015
    312-948-4888

Fisher Scientific Co.
    711 Forbes Avenue
    Pittsburgh, Pennsylvania 15219
    412-562-8300

Flow Laboratories, Inc.
    Division of Flow General, Inc.
    936 West Hyde Park Boulevard
    Inglewood, California 90302
    213-674-2700

    7655 Old Springhouse Road
    McLean, Virginia 22101
    800-336-0424

Gallard Schlesinger Chemical Mfg. Corp.
    584 Mineola Avenue
    Carle Place, New York 11514
    516-333-5600

Gelman Sciences, Inc.
    600 S. Wagner Road
    Ann Arbor, Michigan 48106
    313-665-0651
    800-521-1520

General Electric Co.
    Plastic Business Division
    1 Plastics Avenue
    Pittsfield, Massachusetts 01201
    413-494-1110

GIBCO Diagnostics Laboratories
    2801 Industrial Drive
    Madison, Wisconsin 53713
    608-221-2218 or 221-2221

Goodfellow Metals
    Science Park, Milton Road
    Cambridge, England

Grand Island Biological Company
    3175 Staley Road
    Grand Island, New York 14072
    716-773-7616

    519 Aldo Avenue
    Santa Clara, California 95050
    408-988-7611

Hamilton Company
    4970 Energy Way
    P.O. Box 10030
    Reno, Nevada 89510
    702-786-7077

ICN Chemical and Radioisotope Division
    2727 Campus Drive
    Irvine, California 92715
    714-833-2500
    800-854-0530

ICN K&K Labs
    121 Express Street
    Plainview, New York 11803
    516-433-6262

ICN Nutritional Biochemicals
    Division of ICN Pharmaceuticals, Inc.
    26201 Miles Road
    Cleveland, Ohio 44128
    216-831-3000
    800-321-6842

Indubois, l'Industrie Biologique Francaise
   Gennevilliers, France
   distributed by Accurate Chemical &
   Scientific Corp.

Irvine Scientific
   2511 Daimler Street
   Santa Ana, California 92705
   714-957-8900

Johns Scientific
   219 Broadview Avenue
   Toronto, Ontario M4M 2G4
   416-469-5511

Kimble Products Division
   Owens-Illinois, Inc.
   P.O. Box 1035
   Toledo, Ohio 43666
   419-247-5000

D. Lee, Inc.
   932 Kintyre Way
   Sunnyvale, California 94087

Linbro Scientific, Inc.
   Subsidiary of Flow Laboratories, Inc.
   143 Leeder Hill Drive
   P.O. Box 6187
   Hamden, Connecticut 06517
   203-281-6371

Litton Bionetics, Inc.
   5516 Nicholson Lane
   Kensington, Maryland 20795
   301-881-5600

LKB Instruments, Inc.
   12221 Parklawn Drive
   Rockville, Maryland
   301-881-2510

Lux Scientific Corporation
   1157 Tourmaline Drive
   Newbury Park, California 91320
   805-498-3191

Marine Colloids Division
   Bio-Products Department
   FMC Corp.
   P.O. Box 308, Crockett Point
   Rockland, Maine 04841
   207-594-4436
   800-341-1574

MC/B Manufacturing Chemists
   Division of E. Merck
   2909 Highland Avenue
   Norwood, Ohio 45212
   513-631-0445

Microbiological Associates
   Building 100, Biggs Ford Road
   Walkersville, Maryland 21793
   301-898-7025
   800-638-8174

   11841 Mississippi Avenue
   Los Angeles, California 90025
   213-820-6851

Miles Research Products
   Miles Laboratories, Inc.
   1121 Myrtle, Box 2000
   Elkhart, Indiana 46515
   219-264-8804

Millipore Corporation
   Ashby Road
   Bedford, Massachusetts 01730
   617-275-9200
   800-225-1380

   448 Grandview Drive
   South San Francisco, California 94080
   415-952-9200
   800-632-2708 (California)
   800-227-0234 (western states)

Nalge Company
   Nalgene Labware Department
   75 Panorama Creek Drive, Box 365
   Rochester, New York 14602
   716-586-8800

New England Nuclear
   549 Albany Street
   Boston, Massachusetts 02118
   617-482-9595
   800-225-1572

Nuclepore Corporation
   7035 Commerce Circle
   Pleasanton, California 94566
   415-462-2230

Nunc Products
   Roskilde, Denmark
   distributed by Irvine Scientific and
   Vangard International

Nyegaard and Co.
   Oslo, Norway
   distributed by Accurate Chemical &
   Scientific Corp.

Otto Hiller Co.
   P.O. Box 1294
   Madison, Wisconsin 37013
   608-271-4747

Particle Data Laboratories, Ltd.
   115 Hahn Street
   Elmhurst, Illinois 60126
   312-832-5653

Pharmacia Fine Chemicals
   Division of Pharmacia Inc.
   800 Centennial Avenue
   Piscataway, New Jersey 08854
   201-469-1222
   800-526-3575

Pharmaseal Laboratories Division
   American Hospital Supply Corporation
   1015 Grandview Avenue
   Glendale, California 91201
   213-240-8900

Pierce Chemical Co.
   P.O. Box 117
   Rockford, Illinois 61105
   815-968-0747
   800-435-2960

Precision System, Inc.
   60 Union Avenue
   Sudbury, Massachusetts 01776
   617-443-8912

Rainin Instrument Co., Inc.
   94 Lincoln Street
   Brighton, Massachusetts 02135
   617-787-5050

Reheis Chemical Co.
   Division of Armour Pharmaceutical Co.
   235 Snyder Avenue
   Berkeley Heights, New Jersey 07922
   201-464-1500

Sargent-Welch Scientific Company
   7300 North Linder Avenue
   Skokie, Illinois 60076
   312-677-0600

Schwarz/Mann
   see Becton-Dickinson
   Immunodiagnostics

Scientific Products
   Division of American Hospital Supply
     Corporation
   1430 Waukegan Road
   McGaw Park, Illinois 60085
   312-689-8410

Sigma Chemical Company
   P.O. Box 14508
   St. Louis, Missouri 63178
   314-771-5765
   800-325-3010

Sigma Instruments, Inc.
   170 Pearl Street
   Braintree, Massachusetts 02184
   617-843-5000

Spectrum Medical Industries, Inc.
60916 Terminal Annex
Los Angeles, California 90054
213-323-1120

48 Middle Village Station
Queens, New York 11379
212-894-2200

TETKO Incorporated
525 Monterey Pass Road
Monterey Park, California 91754
213-289-9153

Tousimis Research Corp.
2211 Lewis Avenue
P.O. Box 2189
Rockville, Maryland 20852
301-881-2450

Tridom Chemical Inc.
255 Oser Avenue
Hauppauge, New York 11787
516-273-0110

Vangard International
1111 Greengrove Road
Neptune, New Jersey 07753
201-922-4900

Vector Laboratories
1479 Rollins Road
Burlingame, California 94010
415-344-6161

VWR Scientific, Inc.
Division of Univar Corp.
P.O. Box 3200 Rincon Annex
San Francisco, California 94119
415-469-0100
800-792-8030
800-792-8031
800-792-8032

200 Centere Square Road
Bridgeport, New Jersey 08014
609-467-2600
609-467-3333

Walter Sarstedt, Inc.
Route 1, P.O. Box 4090
Princeton, New Jersey 08540
609-452-1155

Wellcome Reagents Division
Burroughs Wellcome Co.
(radioactive products)
3030 Cornwallis Road
Research Triangle Park, North Carolina
27709
919-549-8371, ext. 417

Order Department (nonradioactive
products)
P.O. Box 1887
Greenville, North Carolina 27834
919-758-3436, ext. 215

West Coast Scientific, Inc.
Box 2947
Oakland, California 94618
415-654-2665

1627 Pontius Avenue
Los Angeles, California 90025
213-478-4396

7030 15th Avenue, NW
Seattle, Washington 98107
206-782-3727

Whatman, Inc.
9 Bridewell Place
Clifton, New Jersey 07014
201-777-4825

Winthrop Laboratories
Division of Sterling Drug Inc.
90 Park Avenue
New York, New York 10016
212-972-4141

Worthington Diagnostics (formerly
Worthington Biochemical Corp.)
    Division of Millipore
    Halls Mills Road
    Freehold, New Jersey 07728
    201-462-3838
    800-631-2142

Zack Electronics
    1444 Market Street
    San Francisco, California 94102
    415-626-1444

ADDENDUM

Linscott's Catalog of Immunological and Biological Reagents: This catalog is a guide to the major sources of biological reagents and standards used in immunological research. Updated periodically, the catalog gives the name, address, telephone and telex numbers of each source of reagents. For further information, write to:

Linscott's Catalog of Immunological and Biological Reagents
40 Glen Drive
Mill Valley, California 94941

Index